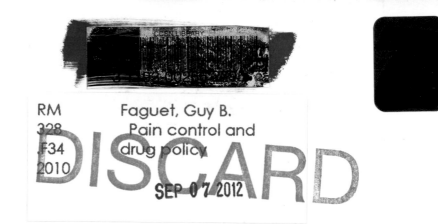

DISCARD

SEP 0 7 2012

D0428852

Pain Control
and Drug Policy

Pain Control and Drug Policy

A Time for Change

GUY B. FAGUET, MD

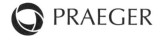 PRAEGER

AN IMPRINT OF ABC-CLIO, LLC
Santa Barbara, California • Denver, Colorado • Oxford, England

Library of Congress Cataloging-in-Publication Data

Faguet, Guy B.
   Pain control and drug policy : a time for change / Guy B. Faguet.
      p. ; cm.
   Includes bibliographical references and index.
   ISBN 978-0-313-38280-2 (alk. paper)
ISBN 978-0-313-38281-9 (ebook)   1. Narcotics—United States.   2. Drug
control—United States.   I. Title.
   [DNLM: 1. Analgesics, Opioid—therapeutic use—United States.   2. Drug
and Narcotic Control—United States.   3. Health Policy—United States.   4. Law
Enforcement—United States.   5. Pain—drug therapy—United States.
QV 33 AA1 F156p 2010]
   RM328.F34   2010
   615'.783—dc22   2009052223

ISBN: 978-0-313-38280-2
EISBN: 978-0-313-38281-9

14   13   12   11   10   1   2   3   4   5

This book is also available on the World Wide Web as an eBook.
Visit www.abc-clio.com for details.

Praeger
An Imprint of ABC-CLIO, LLC

ABC-CLIO, LLC
130 Cremona Drive, P.O. Box 1911
Santa Barbara, California 93116-1911

This book is printed on acid-free paper ∞

Manufactured in the United States of America

This book is dedicated to the blameless victims of the War on Drugs policy—especially to the millions of pain sufferers in the United States and their intimidated physicians, and to the millions of displaced foreign peasants whose property is stolen and whose human rights are trampled by exploiters of the illegal drug trade.

Contents

Preface

During my long career as a hematologist-oncologist, I witnessed the growing divergence between the enormous contribution of narcotics to pain management in the clinical setting and the entrenched perception of their lurking dangers. At issue is the belief that narcotics are extremely dangerous drugs that can easily and quickly turn an innocent and unsuspected victim into a drug abuser, at best, and into a crime-prone, self-destroying addict, at worst, whereas reality indicates otherwise. Indeed, the risk of addiction in populations taking narcotics as analgesics is extremely low in the absence of a prior history of drug abuse. As emphasized by the National Cancer Institute (NCI), "Extensive worldwide experience in the long-term management of cancer pain with opioid drugs has demonstrated that opioid administration in cancer patients with no history of substance abuse is only rarely associated with the development of significant abuse or addiction."[1] This strong endorsement of narcotics as nonaddictive painkillers concludes, "although the lay public and inexperienced clinicians still fear the development of addiction when opioids are used to treat cancer pain, specialists in cancer pain and palliative care widely believe that the major problem . . . is the persistent under treatment of pain driven by inappropriate fear of addiction." My own professional experience over more than 30 years of clinical practice confirms this. Similarly, patients taking opioids for noncancer pain have an extremely low risk of addiction. In three large studies involving 11,882, 10,000, and 2,369 hospitalized patients with no prior history of drug abuse who were administered opioids for chronic noncancer pain, only 7 patients, or 0.03%, showed signs of abuse or addiction.[2-4] On the other hand, the vast majority of addicts are not criminals to be incarcerated or victims of drugs or of their genes who threatened their communities but undisciplined individuals who *chose* to use drugs for pleasure and lost control over their level of consumption.[5] Hence, the popular dread of narcotics is not based on evidence but an example of *consent engineering* that creates "fear of just about anything after many years of intense propaganda designed to tame 'the great beast' by introducing panic."[6] The perception of drugs as the great beast of our time is reinforced by an obliging press, which confers legitimacy to detractors' even most extravagant claims. Relentless promulgation of this view, a replay of Prohibition, provided a fertile ground for the emergence of unsound drug control policies, first in the United States and then worldwide, that failed to achieve any of their goals. Indeed, neither drug production by producer countries nor drug supply, numbers of users, crime rates, or costs to society in consumer countries has decreased as a result.[7,8]

Yet, drug criminalization has had enormous unintended consequences. It has fomented repression, crime, and corruption at home reminiscent of Prohibition, where gangs of foreign and homegrown hard-core criminals build empires while 1.85 million Americans were arrested for drug violations in 2005 alone, including 696,074 for marijuana possession.[9] To these grim home-based statistics must be added massive human rights violations, large-scale population displacements, and social decay linked to the lucrative illegal drug trade pervasive in producer countries. In fact, perhaps drug policy's most tangible return on the $500 billion *investment* through 2005[10] has been to shift production from one region or country to another and to re-direct traffic routes, justifying the view "If you want to see money thrown at a problem to no good effect, you need look no further than America's 'war on drugs'."[11] This is because, as long as consumer demand for illegal drugs remains unabated and users risk public ostracism and incarceration to get their *fix*, traffickers and suppliers will defy, often violently, drug law enforcers and each other to preserve their livelihood, and farmers in producer countries with no realistic alternate sources of income will continue to rely on illicit crops to support their families. Hence, unless current drug policy that created and sustains the black market of illegal drugs is abolished, the core of the problem, perpetuation of the status quo is assured.

Another unintended but devastating consequence of narcotics control laws in the United States is on patients with chronic or terminal illnesses associated with intractable, daily pain who benefit the most from the use of narcotics, especially because they are the most potent and the safest painkillers on the market. Indeed, millions of American pain sufferers are victims of physicians' reluctance to prescribe narcotics in appropriate doses for as long as necessary,[12,13] in part to diminish their patients' highly improbable risk of addiction but mainly to steer clear of possible entanglements with the Drug Enforcement Administration (DEA). Indeed, the DEA aggressively persecutes narcotics-prescribing physicians for the flimsiest of reasons, ignoring what 30 state attorneys general pointed out in their protest of its misguided policy: that drug diversion prevention should not hinder physicians' ability, indeed duty, to provide "the best pain relief available to alleviate suffering" that only narcotics can offer.[14] Likewise, many patients take less than the prescribed dose of narcotics or increase the dosing intervals enduring daily pain, often severe, for fear of addiction but also to avoid the prospects of having to justify a daily narcotics dose or a total supply deemed excessive according to unwritten and shifting criteria conceived by medically untrained and naïve DEA agents. The consequence of insufficient prescribing and inadequate medicating is an unprecedented pain management crisis of national scope where most pain patients are undertreated and optimal pain control is seldom achieved. This is as unacceptable as it is unconscionable especially for terminally ill patients who, after months or years of a devastating and painful illness, die in pain.

President Richard Nixon launched the War on Drugs as a means to promote his political career, claiming drugs are inherently addictive and foster a life of crime. Nixon's drug war has been continued with renewed vigor by his successors despite the falsehood of the claims that set it in motion, its failure to achieve its goals, and its devastating if unintended consequences at home and abroad. Is so much suffering inflicted on so many by the War on Drugs justified by the harm drugs and drug offenders inflict on society? The answer to these questions is suggested by the portrayal of the average incarcerated American drug offender by a disaffected senior member of the drug enforcement establishment. "Imagine yourself as a 20-year-old man in a mid-sized American city. Not only are you a high school dropout, you are, for all intents and purposes, illiterate. You are addicted to crack cocaine. Your only source of income is small-time thievery and drug pushing. Poverty, substance abuse, and failure have followed your family for three generations. You have no concept of a work ethic or of contributing to society. Your plans for the future go as far as this afternoon's score. However, instead of scoring crack, you are arrested for stealing a car phone and are carted off to jail—not an unusual circumstance for you. As a repeat offender, the judge sentences you to 18 months in state prison. What I have described is the average prison inmate. Not a grisly murderer. Not a predatory rapist. Just a young man with absolutely nothing going for him. This is the typical inmate received in Ohio's prison system over and over again, day after day, month after month, year after year."[15]

This book focuses on the DEA interference with American medical practice that caused the pain management crisis, examined within broader historical, socioeconomic, and geopolitical perspectives. It shows that, in addition to penalizing millions of blameless American pain sufferers and hundreds of thousands of nonviolent American drug offenders, and devastating societies in producer countries, drug policy has not, cannot, and will not reduce the supply of drugs on American streets or elsewhere as long as the illegal drug trade remains in place. Frontline Drug Wars documentary's headline said it best, "from both sides of the battlefield, a 30-year history of America's war on drugs—a war with no rules, no boundaries, no end."[16]

Nevertheless, an end to the status quo is achievable albeit politically unpalatable. It requires overturning policies that created and sustain the black market for illicit drugs and handling drug use as a health issue rather than as a criminal matter. Hence, I call for the repeal of all drug laws, the relegalization of all illicit drugs, and the dismantlement of all drug enforcement agencies and of their infrastructures. Such a thoroughly revisionist strategy, the only approach capable of solving the American pain management crisis and worldwide crime, corruption, and human rights violations associated with the illicit drug trade, is based on six compelling arguments drawn from empirical evidence. First, the War on Drugs was launched and is sustained by false claims (drugs are addictive and induce crime). Second, human behavior cannot be successfully legislated, especially in democratic countries. Third, the criminalization of drugs gave rise to a highly lucrative black market that entices criminals and fuels crime and corruption in consumer countries and massive societal disruptions in producer countries. Fourth, drug policy implementation penalizes large segments of the population who use opioids for medical purposes or illicit drugs for recreation, most often in moderation, briefly, reversibly, and without ill effects to themselves or to society. Fifth, the socially acceptable and legally permissible alcohol and tobacco each impose a much greater burden on society, in terms of economic and human costs, than all illicit drugs combined. Sixth, illicit drug users are not enemies to be confronted by their own governments but imperfect human beings in need of society's indulgence and assistance.

This book argues that current political environment, popular sentiment, and advocates' self-interest complicate enormously the implementation of such a radical change in direction. In large measure this is because "drug war supporters have so demonized drugs, drug users, and drug war opponents that most public figures dare not raise questions."[17] In fact, "Trying to stem the tide of fatuous laws that emanate from our incontinent legislatures . . . is a luckless and thankless task."[18] However, the reform I propose is an approach worthy of enlightened societies ruled by laws that punish criminal activity rather than repress harmless behavior. Undoubtedly, to achieve such a paradigm shift in drug policy requires the emergence of a new breed of judicious and bold political leaders who, emulating policy makers of the 1930s, will acknowledge past legislative errors and repeal the far more egregious and socially pernicious War on Drugs. Only then, will both the United States enjoy a drug policy worthy of its Constitutional principles to "promote the general welfare," including pain control for all Americans, and world governments be at peace with their drug using citizens.

PART I

History and Politics of Mind-Altering Drugs

CHAPTER 1

Prohibition:
An Historical Precedent

Prohibition . . . goes beyond the bounds of reason in that it attempts to control a man's appetite by legislation and makes a crime out of things that are not crimes.

> —Abraham Lincoln, speech to the
> Illinois House of Representatives, December 18, 1840

I'd rather that England should be free than that England should be compulsorily sober. With freedom, we might in the end attain sobriety but in the other alternative, we should eventually lose both freedom and sobriety.
> —W. C. Magee, Archbishop of York, sermon at Peterborough, 1868

Today's attempt by the U.S. government to control mind-altering drugs is a replay of Prohibition, albeit with international scope and colossal human and financial resources at its disposal, but without Prohibition's constitutional anchor. Hence, by reviewing the failures and consequences of Prohibition it will become clear that the current drug policy and implementation strategies, drawn on similarly fallacious principles and unachievable goals, are destined to fail and, if left standing, will continue to cause harm to our nation and foster crime, corruption, and human rights violations abroad. Prohibition, ironically called *the noble experiment*, refers to the period in American history when the manufacture, transportation, import, export, purchase, and sale of alcoholic beverages was prohibited, and also to the temperance movement that sponsored such a policy. Prohibition began on January 17, 1920, when the 18th amendment of the constitution went into effect, and was abolished by Congressional passage of the Blaine Act on February 17, 1933; it became the first and only amendment ever repealed later that year with ratification of the 21st amendment. National Prohibition was the culmination of much earlier regulatory efforts at state level. Indeed, as early as 1905 Kansas, Oklahoma, and Mississippi had enacted *dry* laws, and over the ensuing 10 years, another 23 American states had joined in. Hence, between 1915 and 1920 over 60% of the U.S. population was already under some sort of prohibition. Likewise, because the 21st amendment explicitly gives states the right to enact their own laws on the purchase, sale, and consumption of alcohol, Prohibition remained the law of the land in several states for years after its repeal, with Mississippi being the last state to finally repeal Prohibition in 1967. Today, the last remnants of Prohibition are dry county and city ordinances and widespread Sunday bans that compel consumers to stock up on weekdays or to pay a Sunday visit to wet establishments located just outside dry jurisdictions.

However, the history of alcohol control in the United States reaches much farther in time. Its evolution and outcome are of interest to us as a study of a complex issue with personal, societal, financial, political, and religious overtones often difficult to reconcile that led to conflicting measures with unintended consequences. It must be observed that, contrary to popular belief, alcohol consumption was not frowned upon by Puritans, as suggested by the 42 tons of beer and 10,000 gallons of wine they carried on their voyage to Massachusetts compared to 14 tons of water.[1] Likewise, production, sale, or consumption of alcoholic beverages was not forbidden in early colonial times, though drunken behavior and sales to Indians were unlawful. As intemperance and rowdy behavior by drunks upset the moral sensitivities of abstemious neighbors, colonial legislators passed laws attempting to curb excessive drinking. For example, in 1629, the Virginia Colonial Assembly ruled that "Ministers shall not give themselves to excess in drinkinge, or riott, or spending their tyme idellye day or night."[2] Four years later, the Plymouth Colony prohibited the sale of *more than 2 pence worth of spirits to anyone but strangers just arrived,* and in 1637, Massachusetts ordered that no one should stay in a tavern *longer than necessary.*[2] Nevertheless, it became clear that while liquor consumption and human behavior were not easy to regulate, they could become sources of revenue and were easy to enforce.[3] Hence, license fees, taxes, and fines multiplied. Soon, production of most types of alcoholic beverages was taxed at the source; a sales license fee was imposed; and selling to drunks or Indians, selling without a license, and drunkenness were subject to fines. However, attempts at prohibition did not appear until the following century, when notable politicians, physicians, and church leaders voiced concerns about real or perceived effects of alcohol. For example, in 1760, John Adams wrote that taverns were "becoming the eternal haunt of loose, disorderly people . . . the nurseries of our legislators . . . [who] by gaining a little sway among the rabble of the town . . . secure the votes of taverner and retailer and of all."[4] In 1785, Dr. Benjamin Rush, the Surgeon General of Washington's Continental Army, added health arguments to the claims of the temperance movement, listing "unusual garrulity, unusual silence, captiousness . . . an insipid simpering . . . profane swearing . . . certain immodest actions . . . and extravagant acts which indicate a temporary fit of madness."[5] He also circulated thousands of copies of an *Intemperance Thermometer* designed to gauge one's alcohol consumption restraint or lack thereof.[6] Likewise, most evangelical churches saw alcohol as the devil's tool and had their members sign a pledge of temperance. However, because a voluntary pledge left many uncommitted souls exposed to eternal damnation, churches became a driving force in the prohibition movement. Indeed, it is said that without the religious influence "the temperance revolution of the past century would yet remain to be accomplished."[2] As early as 1773, John Wesley was preaching for the prohibition of manufacturing and sale of alcoholic beverages; a demand echoed by the Presbyterian, Methodist, Universalist, and Baptist churches.[2]

Nonreligious groups also sprang up to discourage the use of spirits, such as the Free African Society, the Organization of Brethren, and the Connecticut Association of *"the most respectable farmers,"* which culminated in the well-organized American Temperance Society in 1826, the Congressional Temperance Society in 1833, and the Sons of Temperance in 1842.[2] Their membership was mostly middle-class, self-righteous, rural WASPs (White Anglo-Saxon Protestant) who believed their stock to be *"the most improved, hardiest, and fittest."* With their combined evangelic zeal and Messianic vision they felt destined to bring the Kingdom of God to the United States, and alcohol had no place in it. Under Alexander Hamilton, a federal tax was included in the Revenue Act, and the Second Congress of the United States enacted license fees, taxes, and fines for lawbreakers. However, Pennsylvania farmers mobbed tax collectors, and a 15,000-man militia was called in to suppress what became known as the *Whiskey Rebellion*.[7] Liquor taxes were later repealed, and the liquor industry enjoyed a tax-free period between 1818 and 1862, only to be taxed again in 1863 at a rate of 20 cents per gallon initially, which rose to $2.00 per gallon by 1868.[8] Predictably, while tax rates went up, total collections did not, due to massive tax evasion. Another consequence of high liquor taxes was the birth of the first industry lobby, the United States Brewers Association.[2] After intense lobbying by the Association, Congress reduced the tax to 50 cents in early 1869, resulting in a dramatic rise in tax collections, from $13.5 million in 1868 to $45 million in 1969.[8] During this period, a wave of state prohibition laws were passed by several state legislatures, only to be vetoed by governors, declared unconstitutional by state supreme courts, or repealed by the same legislatures that had enacted them in the first place, suggesting that the majority of the people did not support prohibition laws. The U.S. Army had adopted a dry stance in 1830, at least officially. But soldiers, who put their lives on the line, could not be asked to remain abstinent and were granted a daily alcohol allowance by their commanders. Drinking was generally condoned except while on guard duty or during battle. Additionally, during the Civil War, alcohol was a surgeon's trusted friend that, since times immemorial, was used to clean battlefield wounds and to numb the senses of wounded soldiers undergoing surgery. Once released from duty, most soldiers were more interested in resuming their lives than in becoming temperance advocates.

Nevertheless, the late 1890s saw another wave of prohibition laws, statues, or constitutional amendments at state level, or local options that emerged from broad-based activism over a variety of social issues. A common denominator was the evils of saloons, which were denounced as hotbeds of corruption and vice. By 1895, this movement had evolved into the Anti-Saloon League (The league born of God).[2] Most of the League's claims were unsupported. Common denunciations included, "liquor is responsible for 19% of the divorces, 25% of the poverty, 25% of the insanity, 37% of the pauperism, 45% of child desertion, and 50% of the crime in this country."[9] With massive disinformation campaigns, the League was able to "force closure of saloons, influence the election of dry candidates, and published its own periodicals,"[10] including *The American Issue* and *The New Republic, The National Daily,* and *The Scientific Temperance Journal.* The continuous barrage of propaganda began to sway public opinion against saloons and against alcohol in general. While most religious denominations espoused the League's views, the Episcopal, Lutheran, Catholic, and Jewish churches did not. As the issue of drinking and its effects on society and on the country moved further into the limelight, workers' unions and business interests weighted in the debate, mostly based on self-interest. Businesses viewed drinking as an impediment to productivity and wanted to *keep God* on their side. Henry Ford later declared, "The country could not run without Prohibition; that is the industrial fact." On the other hand, workers generally resented temperance laws they thought were directed at them. Yet, workers' unions and the Socialist Party, both claiming to look after laborers' interests, endorsed temperance laws as a means to advance their agenda. The latter declared, in 1908, "any excessive indulgence in intoxicating liquors by members of the working class is a serious obstacle to the triumph of our cause since it impairs the vigor of the fighters in political and economic struggle."[11] The temperance movement was aided by widespread prejudice against immigrant populations, especially Catholics who arrived with their *drinking intemperance* to our Protestant shores at the turn of the 20th century and by a wave of anti-German sentiment that swept the country before and during World War I. The latter was fueled by chauvinistic newspaper stories that Germany was attempting to addict the entire American population by spiking cosmetics with powder heroin, a powerful and mysterious opium derivative developed in 1898 by the German company AG Bayer. The fact that the U.S. Brewers Association, with members named Pabst, Schlitz, and Blatz, associated itself with the German-American Alliance to oppose the temperance movement added fuel to the anti-German fire prevailing at the time that led to the Wartime Prohibition Act, passed in 1918. Self-serving politicians also embraced alcohol prohibition as a banner to seek notoriety and advance their careers and fortunes.

Perhaps the most prominent such profiteering figure was captain Richmond Hobson (1870–1937), an unlikely Spanish–American war hero.[12] After escaping court martial for failing his mission, Hobson was decorated by President McKinley and began touring the country on behalf of the U.S. Navy. Portraying himself as the champion of the forces of good that would save Western civilization from the scourge of Japanese military power, which he called the *Yellow Peril*, he argued for American naval supremacy, as being *the Will of God*. At first, he was a very popular speaker attracting public and media attention, but he soon realized that a new, more immediate and public-arousing *enemy* was needed for his self-serving rhetoric to succeed. He identified alcohol, which he called *the Great Destroyer*, as the target for his new crusade that would make him the best-paid speaker in America and win him a seat in the U.S. Congress. His apocalyptic depiction of alcohol was just as reckless as the Anti-Saloon League's and that of many other prohibitionists. Based on statistics concocted for the occasion, he made claims such as: "alcohol is killing our people at the rate of nearly two thousand men a day, every day of the year . . . ninety-five percent of all acts and crimes of violence are committed by drunkards . . . a hundred and twenty-five million white men today are wounded by alcohol."[12] The latter claim was especially absurd because the total U.S. population in 1930 was 122,775,046.[13] He argued that alcohol cost *16 billion dollars*, a figure picked out of thin air that at the time represented 25% of the national budget. Ironically, passage of the 18th amendment put an end to congressman Hobson's antialcohol crusade, but he soon found a new cause: heroin, a German product. The new *greatest evil*, as he called it, had the advantage over home-produced alcohol of being a foreign import that could rally the public anti-German xenophobia around the emerging antidrug sentiment. He published several books denouncing drugs, including *Drug Addiction: A Malignant Racial Cancer*, in 1933. Half a century later, a similar approach would be espoused and refined by several unscrupulous politicians to launch the War on Drugs. For instance, Harry J. Anslinger, Commissioner of the U.S. Bureau of Narcotics from 1930 to 1962, waged a press campaign during World War II to convince the American public that Japan had mounted an *Opium Offensive* to addict the entire American population. During the Korean War, it was the turn of Communist China to be smuggling massive amounts of heroin into the United States to *weaken American resistance*, according to Anslinger. Indeed, the politics of narcotics legislation in the United States that resulted in the War on Drugs is no less fascinating and tragic than Prohibition's, as briefly summarized in chapter 3, section 1.

The final drive that brought about the 18th constitutional amendment was spearheaded by the Anti-Saloon League and coordinated by the National Temperance Council. The League's petition was formally presented to Congress in 1913. The first congressional resolution failed to secure the

two-thirds majority necessary to submit the amendment for state ratification. A second resolution didn't make it past the Judiciary Committees of
both houses. Eventually, a resolution was passed by Congress and sent to
the states for ratification in 1917.[2] It stated, "After one year from the ratification of this article the manufacture, sale, or transportation of intoxicating liquors within, the importation thereof into, or the exportation thereof
from the United States and all territory subject to the jurisdiction thereof
for beverage purposes is hereby prohibited." Mississippi was the first state
to ratify, on January 16, 1918. One year and eight days later, the ratification
process was completed when Nebraska became the 36th state to ratify.[1]
Ratification took place in a national atmosphere of religious zeal when
preachers, capitalizing on the 1918 influenza epidemics that killed over
half a million Americans, blamed sin and the wickedness of an intemperate nation as the causes. On October 28, 1919, Congress enacted the *National
Prohibition Act*, also known as the *Volstead Act*, that made alcohol prohibition the law of the land beginning on January 17, 1920. Andrew Volstead,
an ultradry congressman from Minnesota, successfully included wine and
beer under the rubric *intoxicating liquors,* intended by the drafters of the
amendment to target *eighty proof* liquors rather than beverages of lower
alcoholic content, and his Act passed, overriding President Wilson's veto.
A highly puritanical, albeit unrealistic, impact of Prohibition on society
was expressed by Billy Sunday, a noted evangelist. He stated: "The reign
of tears is over. The slums will soon be only a memory. We will turn our
prisons into factories and our jails into storehouses and corncribs. Men will
walk upright now, women will smile, and the children will laugh. Hell will
be forever for rent."[14] While the Anti-Saloon League and other promoters
of the temperance movement were jubilant about their impressive victory,
they probably could not have predicted the mayhem that would follow.
Indeed, as the amendment went into effect, half a million dollars worth of
liquor was stolen from Government warehouses. Within a couple of years, 20
Prohibition enforcement agents had been murdered, and there was more
to come, much more. Herbert Asbury, a Prohibition historian, describes the
new national scene as follows: "The American people had expected to be
greeted, when the great day came, by a covey of angels bearing gifts of peace,
happiness, prosperity and salvation, which they had been assured would
be theirs when the rum demon had been scotched. Instead they were met
by a horde of bootleggers, moon shiners, rum-runners, hijackers, gangsters,
racketeers, triggermen, venal judges, corrupt police, crooked politicians,
and speakeasy operators, all bearing the twin symbols of the eighteenth
amendment; the Tommy gun and the poisoned cup."[15]

Prohibition ended for a variety of real or imaginary reasons. However,
shared interests by Washington and the alcohol industry, both eager to protect their respective revenues, became a decisive anti-Prohibition coalition.
In fact, Prohibition was an economic disaster for the federal government,
for while excise taxes on alcohol amounted to 27% of the total tax revenues

in 1917, they dropped to 1.7% four years later and remained at that level throughout the 1920s.[8] Additionally, while the temperance movement's strategy of voting only for *dry* candidates ensured the loyalty of elected representatives at a local level, national politicians were eager to reclaim generous campaign funds contributed by the alcohol industry, which also provided employment in their districts; both powerful arguments in favor of repeal. However, a major catalyst for the Prohibition repeal camp was Franklin D. Roosevelt's acceptance speech before the National Convention of the Democratic Party held in Chicago in 1932. He stated: "I congratulate this convention for having had the courage, fearlessly to write into its declaration of principles what an overwhelming majority here assembled really thinks about the 18th Amendment. This convention wants repeal. Your candidate wants repeal. And I am confident that the United States of America wants repeal."[4] Roosevelt went on to win the Presidency; the repeal amendment was introduced February 14, 1933, approved by the Senate (63 to 23) and by the House (289 to 121) within a week and ratified by the states later that year.

ALCOHOL MANUFACTURE AND CONSUMPTION

Given the intended purpose of the 18th amendment, law enforcement and compliance should have brought down the manufacture and consumption of alcohol drastically. However, records show a very different picture; one that clearly indicates that the law was ignored or circumvented, and liquor production and consumption continued almost unabated, albeit illicitly. In fact, the 1931 report by the Wickersham Commission, appointed by President Herbert Hoover, established to investigate conditions under Prohibition, concluded that the country had "prohibition in law but not in fact." It also noted, "the drys had their prohibition law and the wets had their liquor."[16] For example, because wine was forbidden, wine makers switched to produce and sell grape juice that after a few simple steps could be converted to wine. Demand for the juice was such that the 97,000 acres planted with vines in 1919 grew to 681,000 acres by 1926.[17] The number of seized illicit distilleries exploded from only a few prior to Prohibition, to 95,933 in 1921, jumping to 282,122 in 1930. These seizures resulted in 34,175 arrests in 1921, jumping to 75,307 in 1928, with most being convicted.[14] In addition to bootlegged domestic production, liquor was smuggled across the Canadian border, from Belgium and Holland,[18] and many vessels stayed anchored outside U.S. territorial waters, easily accessed by entrepreneurial mongers. Saloons went underground as *Speakeasies* (illicit taverns or stores selling liquor illegally), where the *wets* gathered to consume alcohol and indulge in other, often illegal, activities. It is estimated that up to 500,000 such establishments were in existence throughout the United States at the end of Prohibition,[14] double the number of pre-Prohibition saloons. During Prohibition, alcohol consumption rose by 11.64%[19] and that of hard liquor increased from 1.46 gallons per capita during the 1910–1914 period to 1.63 gallons in the late 1920s, according to the U.S. Department of Commerce and Statistics.[19,20] Two prominent economists contested these estimates and contended that alcohol consumption actually dropped at the beginning of Prohibition.[14,21] However, the downward trend in question had begun in 1910, was greater in the first year post-Prohibition, and subsequently reversed course despite rapidly rising resources devoted to enforcement.[14] Hence, claims that Prohibition was successful in reducing alcohol consumption are based on the interpretation of partial data, at best, or a deliberate distortion of the facts, at worst. On the other hand, spending on alcohol was higher after than before Prohibition as expected for an outlawed product. Additionally, the tenets of *The iron law of Prohibition*[22] were fully at work during Prohibition: First, sales shifted from beer to more potent, profitable, and easier to conceal liquors,[23] and the price of the bulkier beer increased by 700%, whereas spirits rose only rose by 270%.[21] Hence, most alcohol production and consumption was of liquors, distilled spirits, and fortified wines instead of equivalent amounts of beer and unfortified wine;[21] a reversal from pre-Prohibition habits. Secondly, the potency of all alcoholic beverages rose by 150% according to some estimates. A notable example is the legendary *White Mule Whiskey*, a whiskey with a particularly strong *kick*.[21] Thirdly, the lack of production standards led to home-distilled moonshine by amateurs and to often adulterated and unsafe beverages produced by unlawful enterprises. Health consequences were not far behind.

HEALTH EFFECTS

Adverse health effects observed during Prohibition resulted from increased alcohol consumption and from drinking more potent or adulterated liquors. Increased alcohol consumption during Prohibition occurred within three groups of patrons:[24] the young, attracted by the lure of an illegal product; previous nondrinkers recruited by savvy marketers seeking to expand their base; and individuals resentful to be told by government not to drink. In addition, there were those who drank permissible, high-content alcohol products, known as *Nostrum* or *Patent medicines* because they enjoyed royal endorsement; or medicinal alcohol (95% pure), the sale of which rose by 400% between 1923 and 1931; or sacramental wine. In 1925, the Federal Council of the Churches of Christ observed, "the withdrawal of wine on permit from bonded warehouses for sacramental purposes amounted in round figures to 2,139,000 gallons in the fiscal year 1922; 2,503,500 gallons in 1923; and 2,944,700 gallons in 1924. There is no way of knowing what the legitimate consumption of fermented sacramental wine is but it is clear that the legitimate demand does not increase 800,000 gallons in two years."[4] Young men and young women took up to drinking alcohol at an earlier age (20.6 and 25.8 years, respectively) after passage of the 18th amendment than before (21.4 and 27.9) or after its repeal (23.9 and

31.7).[25] One particularly serious adverse health effect of Prohibition was the progressive rise of alcoholic psychoses cases, as indicated by the following statement, "these facts appear to indicate that since 1920, Prohibition [was] increasingly impotent as a means of preventing excessive use of alcohol to an extent productive of serious mental disorders and untimely death. 1920 marks the end of the decline and the beginning of the rise in the trends of alcoholic mental diseases and of deaths from alcoholism in the general population."[26] This is confirmed by hospital admissions for alcoholic psychoses, which in 25 states and the city of New York rose from 485 in 1920 to 1,380 in 1929.[26,27] Likewise, death rates from alcoholism, which had decreased steadily from 5.8 cases per 100,000 people in 1916 to 1.0 per 100,000 in 1920, rose year after year subsequently, reaching 4.0 per 100,000 in 1928.[26,28,29] Yet, these statistics actually understate the facts, as reported by New York's Chief Medical Examiner, "in making out death certificates (which are basic to Census Reports) private or family physicians commonly avoid entry of alcoholism as a cause of death whenever possible. This practice was more prevalent under the National Dry Law than it was in pre-prohibition time."[19] Finally, the ban and high price of liquor enticed a consumer segment to switch to tobacco, hashish, marijuana, and narcotics, bringing users into contact with another set of criminals.[30] Some might argue that statistics in the 1920s and 1930s were unreliable by today's standards and that some of the diagnoses of alcoholic psychoses and death from alcoholism at that time might have been mislabeled or mistaken. However, statistics were not less reliable during than before or after Prohibition. Moreover, what is unarguable and undeniable is the fact that no health benefits accrued from Prohibition and that the inverse is the most accurate and rational interpretation of available data.

CRIME AND CORRUPTION

The expectation of temperance enthusiasts that Prohibition would usher in a world without crime and solve untold social ills, including poverty, was not to be. In fact, America had experienced a declining rate in serious crime over much of the 19th and early 20th centuries.[30] However, "a major wave of crime appears to have begun as early as the mid-1920s . . . increased continually until 1933 . . . when it mysteriously reversed itself."[31] For example, the incidence of homicides increased from 5.6 per 100,000 persons in the 1900–1910 period, to 10 per 100,000 in the decade of the 1920s. Arrests for violating Prohibition laws increased across the board: 81% for DUI (driving under the influence), 41% for drunkenness and disorderly conduct. Likewise, arrests for thefts and burglaries rose by 9% and by 13% for assault, battery, and homicides,[31] despite rising law enforcement budgets. As a result, local, state, and federal prisons became overcrowded. For example, the number of federal convicts increased 561%, from 3,000 in 1914 to 26,589 in 1932, most of them for violations of Prohibition laws.[24] In response to the exploding prison population, the federal budget for penal institutions grew by tenfold between 1915 and 1932.[24] More ominously, given the high margin profits associated with the underground alcohol industry, much of production and distribution was taken over by organized criminal groups, often combined with gambling and prostitution. These groups resorted to violent crimes in order to protect their turfs and income, giving birth to infamous crime syndicates and to street gangs, "a criminal element that first surfaced during Prohibition."[30] By 1927, Al Capone controlled not only all illicit commerce in Illinois, from alcohol to gambling to prostitution, but also the majority of the politicians, most police commissioners, the mayor of Chicago, and the governor. But Illinois was not an aberration. It was an open secret that "everyone from major politicians to the cop on the beat took bribes from bootleggers, moonshiners, crime bosses, and owners of speakeasies,"[30] leading the Commissioner of Prohibition to conclude in 1931: "The fruitless efforts at enforcement are creating public disregard not only for this law but for all laws. Public corruption through the purchase of official protection for this illegal traffic is widespread and notorious. The courts are cluttered with prohibition cases to an extent, which seriously affects the entire administration of justice."[16] The Bureau of Prohibition had to be reorganized, without much success, to combat corruption in its midst. Finally, Prohibition presided over an enormous increase in the size and reach of the Bureau of Prohibition. Other federal agencies, with expanded roles to backup the Bureau of Prohibition, also experienced a phenomenal growth. For instance, "between 1920 and 1930 employment at the Customs Service increased 45 percent, and the service's annual budget increased 123 percent. Personnel of the Coast Guard increased 188 percent during the 1920s, and its budget increased more than 500 percent between 1915 and 1932."[30] Thus at the strike of a pen, the 18th amendment turned drunkenness and petty offenses by a few into a nation where crime and corruption were rampant at all levels of society, the government, and the judicial system.

In conclusion, Prohibition was an unmitigated disaster as it failed to achieve its main goal of reducing alcohol consumption, had adverse health consequences for the public, and promoted, albeit unintentionally, an unprecedented rise in crime and corruption on a grand scale.[11,30,32,33] Organized crime grew into regional empires, and corruption permeated the government, law enforcement, and the judicial system and lasted throughout the Prohibition years, which in turn fostered general disrespect for the law. Tens of thousands of citizens were prosecuted and incarcerated for activities that were legal both before the enactment of the 18th amendment and after its repeal. Prohibition stimulated an exponential growth and reach of a repressive federal government that failed to retrench after its repeal. *The noble experiment* clearly demonstrates that proscription of mutually agreeable exchanges is doomed to failure primarily because arbitrary laws cannot regulate human behavior.[26] Moreover, laws designed to protect people from themselves are an assault on individual and collective freedoms of the governed and on the prestige of government, as observed by Albert Einstein upon reaching U.S. shores. He declared, "The prestige of government has undoubtedly been lowered considerably by the prohibition law."[34] With such credentials, future federal undertakings, based on equally fallacious principles that parallel those that gave rise to Prohibition, would seem unlikely to emerge. Yet, the blueprint for the War on Drugs is a *déjà vu* copy of Prohibition's, though the social disruptions and economic costs caused by the former are much greater at home and, given its unprecedented internationally reach, abroad.

CHAPTER 2

The Lure of Mind-Altering Substances

The first recorded drug phenomenon was traced to the late tenth century. It appeared in the holy city of Mecca with opium brought from Persia, Egypt, and neighbouring countries. Persia, in the late eleventh century, was the centre of the Assassins, who used opium, hashish, and other spices and potent drugs to induce mental and physical euphoric feeling and excitement.
    —Dr. Sami K. Hamarneh, scholar on the history
                of medicine under Muslim rule

The purpose of this chapter is to illustrate the impact of drugs on ancient and modern societies, especially on their health, social fabric, and historical course, and how the drug trade was exploited by some colonial powers eager to enhance their geopolitical agenda of domination and to profit from the process. Our focus is on poppy (*Papaver somniferum*), the source of the mind-altering substance with the longest recorded history and the most enduring and because, as the precursor of narcotics, it is central to this book's core themes: *pain control* and *drug policy*. Examples of early societal involvement with drugs, reviewed in the first part of this chapter, were selected based on the reliability of available records and as a prelude to today's drug scene that confirms the enduring relevance of the old adage "plus ça change plus ça reste la même chose" (the more it changes the more it stays the same). They also demonstrate that the often-repeated quote, "those who ignore the lessons of history are bound to repeat its mistakes" should be restated for the benefit of policy makers to: History repeats itself endlessly because its lessons are seldom learned. However, in modern times drug abuse involves not only poppy but countless licit and illicit drugs and extends to ordinary substances, dietary products, and even intemperate behaviors, which is addressed in the second part of this chapter and in chapter 4.

POPPY AND OPIUM THROUGH THE AGES

Antiquity

Poppy was known to man circa 5500 B.C.E., as shown by poppy-adorned religious artifacts unearthed in southern Spain. Archaeological evidence suggests that a precursor poppy plant might have originated in northwestern Africa, Spain, and southern France, but the plant seems indigenous to Asia Minor and northern Mesopotamia, Persia, and India, where it is still cultivated.[1] The wild strain of poppy growing in the Mediterranean basin is thought to be the forerunner, by centuries of breeding and cultivation, of *Papaverum somniferum*, the only species used to produce opium today. Fossil remains of poppy seed cake and poppy-pods have been found in Neolithic Swiss lake dwellings, circa 2000 B.C.E. The historical trail of poppy begins around 3400 B.C.E. with a Sumerian tablet unearthed at Nippur (south of modern Baghdad). In cuneiform script it describes, "early in the morning old women, boys and girls collect the juice, scraping it off the notches [of the poppy-capsule] with a small iron [questionable for the iron age began around 1200–1300 B.C.E.] blade, and place it within a clay receptacle."[2] Moreover, they referred to poppy as the *Joy plant* for its euphoric effects, suggesting that poppy had gained certain popularity in Sumerian culture. Sumerians passed their knowledge on the cultivation of the plant and the extraction and use of opium to the Assyrians. Opium, the latex extracted from poppy, was likely the most powerful substance of the time as it had distinct sedative and calming effects in small doses, hypnotic properties in moderate doses, and rendered the user insensitive to pain in higher doses.[3,4] Hence, it is not surprising that the Babylonians adopted opium and in turn passed it to the Egyptians. The earliest record of poppy use in Egypt is found in the Eber papyrus (circa 3500 B.C.E.) where it is advised that the use of sap from the unripe poppy seedpod "prevents the excessive crying of children." Two millennia later, in the 1300s B.C.E., the Thebes (modern Luxor) area of Upper Egypt became a major center of poppy growing, especially during the 18th-dynasty Pharaohs, from Tuthmosis IV (1419–1386 B.C.E.) through Tutankhamen ("King Tut," 1333–1324 B.C.E.). *Poppy rhoeas* (red poppy), a variety imported from Asia Minor and the Palestine region that is closely related to *Papaver somniferum*, was grown in the gardens of pharaoh Tuthmosis III and in the temple of Amum at Karnak; it was regularly depicted in vases, paintings, and ornaments of the time.[1,5,6] Traders, mostly Phoenicians and Minoans, took this lucrative crop they called *opium thebaicum* across the Mediterranean Sea into Greece, North Africa, and Southern Europe.[7] These ancient people used poppy and hemp mainly for medicinal purposes and religious rituals, and there is no credible evidence of drug abuse among them. In fact, their languages did not include a term indicating abuse, dependence, or addiction. The Persians, who conquered much of Assyria and Babylonia, also inherited part of those civilizations' customs, though the first mention of opium (*malidéh or afiuum*) only occurs in circa 600 B.C.E. Likewise, the Hebrews, living in an area where poppy and its extracts were known since antiquity, must have known and used poppy and opium. In fact, it has been suggested that a mixture of vinegar and poppy juice (*rosh* in Hebrew) was the drink given to Christ on the cross in order to alleviate His suffering.[8]

The Ancient Greeks

The poppy culture became pervasive among the ancient Greeks. They portrayed their divinities Hypnos (sleep), Nyx (night), and Thanatos (death) covered with poppy capsules or carrying poppies on their heads, and they similarly decorated the statues of Apollo, Pluto, Aphrodite, Isis, Demeter, and many other gods.[2] According to legend, Demeter, in despair over the seizure of her daughter Persephone by Pluto, ate poppies in order to fall asleep and forget her grief. Archaeological findings also unearthed poppy capsules depicted on Greek pottery, ornamental figures, vases, coins, and jewelry; a symbolic association with love, healing, fertility, and immortality. Their classical texts also bear testimony of poppy use. In fact, the first written mention of poppy in ancient Greece is found in Homer's *Iliad* (circa 800 B.C.E.), "and as a poppy which in the garden is weighed down by fruit and vernal showers, droops its head on one side." In his other epic work, *Odyssey*, Homer mentions *Nepenthes*, a substance assumed to derive from poppy, which Helen gave to Telemachus and his comrade to "lull all pain and anger, and bring forgetfulness of every sorrow." However, others have cast doubt on the nature of Nepenthes, claiming to refer to Helen's charms instead. Hesiod (circa 700 B.C.E.) wrote about a Corinthian town named *Mekonê* (poppy-town) for the extensive cultivation of poppy in the area, "when the gods and mortal men were divided at Mekonê, even then Prometheus was forward to cut up a great ox and set portions before them, trying to beguile the mind of Zeus."[9]

Ancient Greeks also recognized the medicinal and healing properties of poppy. It is to be noted that while the ancient Greek language included the word *pharmakon*, signifying drugs, the term had a positive (healing) and a negative (poison) connotation. In its positive connotation, pharmakon also applied to herbs of all kinds, especially exotic ones brought from the orient, whether used for healing by physician-herbalists, for household cooking, or for their fragrance. Additionally, in pre-Hippocratic times, when medicine was magical and the province of the gods and of physician-magicians, *pharmakon* referred to an incantation or a spell as often as it meant a physical substance. Like that of other ancient civilizations, the ancient Greek language lacked terms for drug abuse or addiction, suggesting that such concepts and behavior were alien to them. Hippocrates (460–377 B.C.E.), the *father of medicine*, repeatedly referred to the hypnotic, narcotic, and styptic properties (capable of stopping wound bleeding) of opium and recommended its use for the treatment of various ailments.[10,11] He distinguished between the white, fire-red, and black poppy and mentioned the nutritive properties of poppy seeds. Of interest is the use of poppy for euthanasia purposes among a segment of the Ancient Greek population, as described by Herakleides of Pontus (circa 340 B.C.E.) in his work *On Government*.[11] He described the *Keian custom* practiced in the island of Keos of the South Aegean Sea: "Since the island is healthy and the population lives to a ripe old age, especially the women, they do not wait until they are very old for death to take them, but before they grow weak or disabled in any way, take themselves out of life, some by means of the poppy, others with hemlock."[2]

Centuries later, poppy and opium were still prominent in Hellenic culture. Pliny the Elder (23–79 C.E.) is credited to having been the first to use the word *opium* to describe the juice of the poppy.[2] Dioscorides of Anazarba (circa 100 C.E.) and especially Galen of Pergamon (Claudia Galena, 129–210 C.E.), two of the most renowned Greek medical practitioners, described, prescribed, and recommended the use of poppy extracts and opium juice. Either could be taken internally or applied externally, for their therapeutic benefits extended to a variety of illnesses and ailments. Galen, the second most famous physician of the ancient world after Hippocrates and the physician to three Roman emperors, was a brilliant anatomist, philosopher, and poet and a most prolific writer with a corpus of 500 works. He bridged the Greek and Roman medical worlds and enshrined Hippocratic principles as the foundation of all medical knowledge that, with the collapse of Greco-Roman civilization after the fall of Rome in 476 C.E., was preserved by Muslim translators until the Middle Ages. According to Galen, opium had numerous medical properties. It "resists poison and venomous bites, cures chronic headache, vertigo, deafness, epilepsy, apoplexy, dimness of sight, loss of voice, asthma, coughs of all kinds, spitting of blood, tightness of breath, colic, the lilac poison, jaundice, hardness of the spleen stone, urinary complaints, fever, dropsy, leprosy, the trouble to which women are subject, melancholy and all pestilences."[12]

The Muslims

Poppy was unknown in pre-Islamic Arab lands. It made its entrance into Arabia's drug armamentarium around 800 C.E. when Hjunayn ibn Ishaq and others[1] translated Greek works or their Syriac versions into Arabic. In his seven-volume treatise *Firdous al-Hikmat*, the first medical encyclopedia published in Arabic, Ali Ibn Rabban Al-Tabari (838–870), teacher of the distinguished physician Zakariya al-Razi (a.k.a. Razes), recommended opium as ointment for external application and in tablet form for migraine and colds. The latter was administered in increasing daily doses until the desired effect was achieved. He also prescribed poppy seeds, along with psyllium, dandelion, and other seeds, for childhood coughs and consumption.[13] Jabir ibn Hayyan, the most famous Arabic alchemist, and other Muslim alchemists of the ninth century considered opium as a poison to be used as a remedy with extreme caution.[14] The *Medical Compendium,* written by Sabtur Ibn Sahl (?–869) and utilized in the prestigious Adudi hospital in Baghdad, listed opium and poppy in tablet, powder, decoction, electuary (a medicine sweetened with honey), enema, and other preparations for the treatment of various ailments, and as an antidote. In his *al-Qanun fi al-Tibb* (Canons of Medicine), Ibn Sînā (a.k.a. Avicenna, 981–1037), philosopher, mathematician, astronomer, and the most famous physician of his time described how to extract opium from poppy. He warned, it "dulls the intellect, impairs consciousness, thwarts good counseling, weakens digestion, and causes death by freezing the natural faculties."[1,15] Likewise, Al-Birûnî (973–1048), one of Avicenna's contemporaries and a famous astronomer, mathematician, physicist, physician, geographer, geologist, and historian, cautioned that opium could cause death. He wrote, "I have seen a case where a person died from the use of an opium suppository. Therefore it should be used with extra care."[1] More importantly, he keenly observed and correctly interpreted the psychological implications of a new social phenomenon developing in the Muslim world. It is in all likelihood the first report of recreational use and abuse of a mind-altering drug. He wrote, "People who live in the tropics or hot climates, especially those in Mecca, get into the habit of taking opium daily to eliminate distress, to relieve the body from the effects of scorching heat, to secure longer and deeper sleep, and to purge superfluities and excesses of humors. They start with smaller doses which are increased gradually up to lethal dosages."[cited in 16] According to a current Muslim scholar, "examination of historical evidences in Islam shows that abusers, seeking flight from reality, brought dangerous consequences upon the whole Muslim community and its cultural, religious, and economic life."[1] He further points out that this drug-permissiveness was possible because "neither hemp nor opium was then known [in pre-Islamic Arabia] . . . no specific prohibition was made against their use in the Qur'an."

The drug abuse phenomenon occurred at a time when Islam was expanding exponentially on the physical, political, and religious fronts, reaching India and even China to the East, controlling North Africa as far as Morocco, and ruling most of the Iberian Peninsula in Europe. The conquerors brought with them and propagated to the conquered peoples, especially converts to Islam, the good and the bad of their culture, including addiction to opium. Political unrest arising from religious sectarianism of all shades and colors that sprung up in the Muslim world compounded the social landscape and threatened the stability of the central government: the

Caliphate. *Ikhwãn al-Safã* (Brethren of Purity) and *Qaramitites* were two of the best know ideological societies that attracted large following and considerable political influence. Many of their adepts used drugs, presumably to withstand long hours of praying, meditation, and fasting, leading to addiction in some. It has been observed that this and other practices represented a "dreadful prostitution of religion [that] was often a cover for the pernicious influences of secret societies and the horrors of unbridled political ambitions."[1] Perhaps the most radical sect of Ismaili Muslims known for its extreme political dissidence and drug abuse was *Al-da'wa al-jadĩda* (the new doctrine) founded by Hasan-I-Sabbâh (1090–1124 c.e.), also known as *Hashshashin,* or *Assassins* as they were known in the West. The name of the sect is said to mean Hashish-eaters or hashish-smokers, either because they "would take hashish before missions in order to calm themselves . . . to turn themselves into madmen in battle . . . [or] to show the neophyte the sensual pleasures awaiting him in the afterlife."[17] However, whether this is myth or fact has never been determined. Indeed, there are many stories connected with the Assassins, especially because their contacts with the Crusaders and the writings of Marco Polo awakened the imagination of European storytellers inclined to believe reports of wickedness among distant people of another race or religion, becoming part of Western folklore. They called themselves *Fedayeen,* "one who is ready to sacrifice their life for a cause," and were known for their blind obedience to their spiritual leader and for their use of murder to eliminate foes, especially of the *Abbasid* and *Seljuq* dynasties. Under the pretense of religious zeal, they engaged in conspiracy, murder, and terrorism, undermining the moral values of Islam.[1] In a well-documented article, one Muslim scholar attributes the decline of the Muslim world after the 13th century in part to "the addiction problem in a nation which subscribed very actively to the use and misuse of drugs since the 900s."[17] However, this self-inflicted curse pales in comparison with the plight of the Chinese, eight centuries later, whose drug problem was imposed by a foreign power.

India and China

It is believed that opium was introduced to India by the armies of Alexander the Great (356–323 b.c.e.) and to China by Arab traders (circa 400 c.e.). In the 15th century, poppy was cultivated along the coast of India, mainly for medicinal purposes. At the time of the Mogul Empire, poppy was extensively cultivated and, as a state monopoly, became a profitable crop for trading with China and other eastern countries. During the reign of Mogul Jalaluddin Muhammad Akbar (1556–1605), the British and the Dutch conducted a lucrative opium trade between India and China. After the fall of the Mogul Empire, the monopoly over opium production and sale shifted to a group of merchants in Patna. However, a few years after the British conquered the province of Bengal in 1757, and on the order of Lord Warren

Hastings, the Bengal's British Governor-General, the Indian opium production was transferred to the *British East Indian Company* (1773–1833). As a tool of British colonial policy, the Company established a monopoly on the cultivation and sale of opium that was to oppress Indian peasants, turn millions of Chinese into addicts, and promote two wars. Faced with the social impact of opium on his people, the Chinese emperor imposed a ban on opium smoking and trading in 1729. In order to circumvent the Chinese ban on opium importation, the British East Indian Company purchased tea from Guangzhou (Canton) on credit and paid in Calcutta with Indian opium, leaving opium smuggling to third parties.[18] In 1799, the Chinese reiterated the ban on the importation of opium and in 1810 decreed, "Opium has a very violent effect. When an addict smokes it, it rapidly makes him extremely excited and capable of doing anything he pleases . . . but before long, it kills him . . . we should also order the general commandant of the police and police-censors at the five gates to prohibit opium and to search for it at all gates. If they capture any violators, they should immediately punish them and should destroy the opium at once."[19] The decree had little effect given the Chinese central government's lack of control over opium smuggling through southern ports thousands of miles away from Beijing, the strong demand by increasing numbers of Chinese users, and the greed of the British East Indian Company and of its surrogate smugglers. As a result, the amount of opium brought to China skyrocketed from 15 tons per year in 1730, to over 900 tons in the early 1820s, to 4,000 tons in 1836. By that year, an estimated 8 million Chinese had become opium addicts. Alarmed about the health and social problems caused by opium, the Emperor of China, Tao-kuang, appointed Commissioner Lin Tse-hsü to completely rid China of opium and opium addiction. Lin, an incorruptible official, established rehabilitation centers for addicts; banned all trading with Western merchants, demanding they turned over to him their opium stockpile; and had opium dealers arrested and publicly executed. He also blockaded the city of Guangzhou and surrounding towns where most of the opium trade took place. Although Charles Elliot, the British Chief Superintendent of Trade and British Minister to China, and other merchants complied by surrendering to Lin all remaining stockpiles of opium, many traders and British ships moved their illegal activities further south along the coast. Lin also wrote to Queen Victoria asking, "I have heard that your country very strictly forbids the smoking of Opium . . . why do you let it be passed on to the harm of other countries?" to no avail. And, although Charles Elliot, the British chief superintendent of trade and British minister to China, and other merchants complied by surrendering to Lin all remaining stockpiles of opium, many traders and British ships moved their illegal activities further south along the coast.

On July 12, 1839, a group of drunken British sailors rampaged through the village of Kowloon, near Hong Kong, destroying a temple and killing Lin Weixi, one of the villagers. When the British rejected the Quing government's legal jurisdiction over their seamen and refused to sign a bond pledging not to smuggle opium, an infuriated Lin ordered all exports to Britain be halted immediately. He also ordered the freshwater streams used by the British to be poisoned. This temporarily drove the British out of China only to come back in late August of that year with 28 war ships that seized Hong Kong and easily defeated a second-rate Chinese navy. The first Opium War (1839–1842) had begun. Emperor Tao-kuang blamed Lin for the war and exiled him. In August 1842, China signed the vanquished nation-style treaty of Nanjing that committed the Quing government to cede Hong Kong *in perpetuity* and grant *extraterritoriality* to Britain (British subjects accused of crimes committed in China to be tried by British law), to open major Chinese ports to all traders, and to pay the British government a considerable indemnity. It included, "6,000,000 of dollars as the value of the opium which was delivered up at Canton in the month of March, 1839 and as a ransom for the lives of Her Britannic Majesty's Superintendent and subjects, who had been imprisoned and threatened with death by the Chinese High Officers . . . 3,000,000 of dollars, on account of debts due to British subjects . . . 12,000,000 of dollars, on account of the expenses incurred."[20] The treaty of Nanjing paved the way for resuming and expanding the lucrative drug trade and opening up Chinese society to Western missionaries. A smuggler's chant of the time illustrates the treaty's outcome: "Those were days to be remembered, when our good ship sailed away. From the old home port behind us, to Calcutta or Bombay; When we sold the Heathen nations runt and opium in rolls, And the Missionaries went along to save their sinful souls."[21] However, there was more to come, much more.

In the 1850s, the British, eager to expand their hold on the China trade, petitioned the Quing government to renegotiate the treaty of Nanjing. The most notable British demands included opening all of China to British merchants, the exemption of foreign imports from internal transit duties, and, its ultimate goal, the legalization of the opium trade. The Imperial court rejected the new demands. In the same timeframe (October 8, 1856), Quing officials arrested 12 Chinese sailors after boarding the *Arrow*, a Chinese-owned, Hong Kong–registered ship suspected of piracy and smuggling for the British. The British authorities in Guangzhou demanded the seamen's immediate release on the grounds that the ship had been previously British-registered and that the British flag, which they claimed was flown that day, had been desecrated. Concurrently, the British attacked Guangzhou, finding no Chinese resistance. Moreover, based on the *Arrow Incident* report prepared by Harry Parkes, British Consul to Guangzhou, the British Parliament voted to assault China and asked France, the United States, and Russia to join in, marking the beginning of the second Opium War (1858–1860). France accepted, using as a pretext the execution of Father August Chapdelaine by Chinese authorities in Guangxi province. James

Bruce, 8th Earl of Elgin (whose father stole "whole boatloads of ancient sculpture from Greece's capital city, [including] a large amount of fifth-century B.C.E. sculpture taken from the Parthenon,"[22] and brought them to the British Museum where they now stand) and Baron Jean Baptiste Louis Gros commanded the British and French armies, respectively. The United States and Russia chose to send no armies but dispatched envoys to Hong Kong to assist with planning the assault on China. Guangzhou soon fell into the hands of the aggressors and was plundered. Ye Mingshen, governor of Guangdong and Gyangxi provinces, was captured, and a puppet government was installed that would last four years. The defeat of China led to the lopsided treaties of Aigun and Tientsin. The former, signed with Russia on May 28, 1858, revised the 1689 Nerchinsky Treaty granting Russia additional territory bordering the Aigun River and the Pacific Coast, establishing the modern borders of the Russian Far East. The latter, signed in June 1858, gave Britain, France, the United States, and Russia certain navigation and travel rights, allowed them to establish diplomatic missions, and forced China to pay an indemnity. The latter amounted to 2 million *taels* (a former Chinese monetary unit worth 1 1/3 Oz of silver) to each Britain and France, plus 2 million *taels* to Britain as compensation for destruction of property. However, Chinese refusal to allow Western embassies in Beijing the following year, the capture and torture of Harry Parkes, and the murder of several members of his entourage were used as a pretext for a new Anglo-French military offensive. The allied forces captured and looted Beijing on October 6, 1860, and Lord Elgin ordered the Imperial Summer Palace be razed to the ground. Through the *Convention of Peking*, the Chinese granted freedom of religion and consented to allow Western diplomatic missions in Beijing once again. They were also forced to legalize opium trade and to pay a new indemnity to Britain and France, this time of 8 million *taels* each. Inexplicably, two weeks later, Russian envoy General Nicholas Ignatiev convinced the Chinese government to sign the *Sino-Russian Supplementary Treaty of Peking*, which ceded to Russia an additional 300,000 squares miles of its territory.

DRUGS IN THE 21ST CENTURY

Worldwide Drug Consumption

Today, the choice of illicit and licit drugs and other substances available for abuse is considerable. In addition to the everlasting marijuana, cocaine, and heroin, choices include alcohol (beer, wine, and distilled spirits), central nervous system stimulants (tobacco, caffeine, and ritalin), hallucinogens (GHB [or Gamma hydroxybutyrate], LSD [or Lysergic acid diethylamide], PCP [or Phencyclidine], ecstasy, ketamine, methamphetamine, rohypnol, mescaline, and psilocybin), inhalants (glue, solvents, aerosols), and prescription drugs ranging from anabolic steroids to opioids. However, in modern societies addictive behavior has transcended drugs to embrace many activities that, to most people, are ordinary and routine such as eating chocolate or having sex. This fact must be taken into account when exploring the nature and the possible causes of addiction (see chapter 4). According to the United Nations Office on Drugs and Crime (UNODC) World Drug Report 2006, "The total number of drug users in the world is now estimated at some 200 million people, equivalent to about 5 percent of the global population age 15–64. Cannabis remains by far the most widely used drug (some 162 million people), followed by amphetamine-type stimulants (amphetamines, 25 million people and ecstasy, 10 million people). The number of opiate abusers is estimated at some 16 million people, of which 11 million are heroin abusers. Some 13 million people are cocaine users."[23]

Drug prevalence varies throughout the world (Table 1). While cannabis and cocaine are the most abused drugs in North America (32% and 31% prevalence, respectively), opiates represent approximately 60%–65% of abused drugs in Asia, Oceania, and Europe; cannabis predominates in Africa (63%); and cannabis and opiates dominate the illicit drug market in Australia and New Zealand. Likewise, the prevalence of the five most common drugs varies widely by region and by country. Singapore has the lowest prevalence of drug abuse, ranging from a low of 2 cocaine users to a high of 5 amphetamine users per 100,000-population aged 15–64. In contrast, Canada, Iran, Philippines, the United States, and Australia report the highest drug abuse prevalence: an average of 16.8 users per 100 population aged 15–64 for cannabis, 6.0% for amphetamines, 4.0% for ecstasy, and 2.8% for each opiates and cocaine. However, these figures are not actual statistics but "estimates by drug experts from each country"[23] reporting to the UNODC. Yet, if these estimates on illicit drugs sound ominous and would appear to justify the War on Drugs at the national and international levels, they pale in comparison to the higher prevalence and greater economic and human impact of abused *licit* substances. Indeed, as emphasized in the UNODC World Drug Report 2006, "The picture is more bleak for licit psychoactive substances. Tobacco, a particularly addictive substance, is a case in point. About 28 per cent of the world's adult population is estimated to use tobacco, which exceeds, by far, the number of people using illicit drugs (4 per cent for cannabis and 1 per cent for amphetamine-type stimulants (ATS), cocaine and opiates combined)."[23] More ominously, "with its 3,000-plus chemical components, including at least 43 carcinogens, tobacco is the leading preventable cause of disability and deaths in the US and the world. As a major contributor to the four leading causes of premature death (heart disease, cancer, strokes, chronic lung disease), cigarettes kill as many Americans as the next 10 causes combined . . . In the US, illnesses attributable to smoking accounted for 430,000 premature deaths in 1990, of which 189,700 were from cancer."[24]

Table 1
Lowest and highest annual prevalence rates (%) of abuse in populations, aged 15–64[23]

Region	Cannabis	Amphetamines	Opiates	Cocaine	Ecstasy
Europe	0.80–11.3	0.01–1.5	0.05–1.2	0.02–2.7	0.10–2.5
North America	1.30–16.8	0.1–1.5	0.10–0.6	0.4–2.8	0.01–1.1
Central America	1.30–16.1	0.2–1.1	0.01–0.4	0.1–2.5	0.10–0.7
South America	0.50–5.6	0.1–0.7	0.01–0.6	0.3–1.9	0.10–0.3
Asia	0.004–6.4	0.005–6.0	0.004–2.8	0.002–0.03	0.004–0.8
Oceania	0.1–29.5	3.4–3.8	0.50–0.5	0.5–1.2	2.2–4.0
Africa	0.05–21.5	0.01–0.9	0.01–2.3	0.01–0.8	0.01–0.4

However, the most widely used and abused mind-altering substance worldwide is alcohol. According to the World Health Organization's (WHO) *Global Report: Alcohol Policy:*

[T]here are about 2 billion people worldwide [approximately 48% of the world's population aged 15–64 the year of the report] consuming alcoholic beverages and 76.3 million with diagnosed alcohol use disorders. From a public health perspective, the global burden related to alcohol consumption, both in terms of morbidity and mortality, is considerable in most parts of the world. Globally, alcohol consumption causes 3.2% of deaths (1.8 million) and 4.0% of the Disability-Adjusted Life Years lost (58.3 million). Overall, there are causal relationships between alcohol consumption and more than 60 types of disease and injury. Alcohol consumption is the leading risk factor for disease burden in low mortality developing countries and the third largest risk factor in developed countries . . . besides the numerous chronic and acute health effects, alcohol consumption is also associated with widespread social, mental and emotional consequences.[25]

Trends in Global Drug Consumption

According to the Executive Summary of the UNODC World Drug Report 2006, "There is evidence that, over the last hundred years, it [the multilateral drug control system] has reduced and contained the drug problem at the global level. While tracking a trend over a century is difficult because there are few facts, some baselines can be found. The best is for the opium problem, because it was investigated at the Shanghai Commission in

1909."[23] This statement is based on a "world opium production estimated to have been at least 30,000 metric tons . . . [which] nearly a hundred years later . . . is down to about 5,000 metric tons," despite a nearly six-fold rise in the world population. However, a greater scrutiny of worldwide estimated drug production (called *potential manufacture;* e.g., amounts of drug that *could* be manufactured from *estimates* of produced base product), seizure, and consumption for the most prevalent drugs reported in the same document reveals quite a different picture, as briefly outlined here.

Cannabis (162 million users estimated worldwide). Cultivation of cannabis herb (marijuana) is widespread worldwide, including in the homes of many consumers, especially Americans. The main sources of Cannabis resin (hashish) are Morocco, Afghanistan, and Pakistan. Data available from Morocco indicate that cultivation decreased from 120,500 hectares in 2004 to 72,500 hectares in 2005 to which a probable 30,000 hectares must be added for Afghanistan and an unknown cultivation area for Pakistan. Potential manufacture of cannabis resin in Morocco declined from 3,070 metric tons in 2003 to 2,760 metric tons in 2004 and 1,070 metric tons in 2005. Additionally, global seizures of cannabis herb and cannabis resin reached all-time highs of over 6,000 and 1,470 metric tons, respectively, in 2004. Yet, despite official claims of sharply declining cultivation and production and of increased seizures, the same report acknowledges, "cannabis use increased by more than 10 per cent at the global level" since the early 1990s.[23]

Amphetamine-Type Stimulants (35 million users estimated worldwide). Potential manufacture of amphetamine-type stimulants was estimated at 480 metric tons in 2004, a sharp fall from 2000 levels. However, seizures declined by 53% from 2000 levels, to 19.5 metric tons. As a result, worldwide use increased by nearly 5% from 1992 to 2004.

Opiates (16 million users estimated worldwide). Between 1990 and 1997, worldwide poppy cultivation dropped from approximately 250,000–280,000 hectares to an average of 151,500 hectares over the period. Despite this sharp reduction in poppy cultivation, official figures revealed that improved cultivation techniques and better land irrigation helped maintain 2005 potential manufacture of opium at 4,600 metric tons, of which 4,100 metric tons came from Afghanistan. These production figures are little changed since 1993 except for 1994 and 1999 when opium production surpassed 5,500 metric tons and for 2001 when a strict ban by the Taliban regime almost eliminated Afghanistan's poppy cultivation. Global seizures of opiates (opium, morphine, and heroin) increased from approximately 10 metric tons in 1992 to 120 metric tons in 2004. However, these gyrations in cultivation area, production yield, and seizures had no impact on the street price of opiates. Indeed, between 1990 and 2004 the per-gram price for opium fell steadily from an average of (inflation-adjusted) US$250 in the United States and US$420 in Western Europe to $78 and

$157, respectively. As a result, opium use increased globally by approximately 0.3% annually between 1992 and 2005.

Coca and Cocaine   (13 million users estimated worldwide). Today, most coca leaves (54%) are cultivated in Colombia, followed by Peru (30%) and Bolivia (16%). The total area under coca cultivation was 159,600 hectares in 2005, a level little changed since 2003 but much lower than a high of approximately 220,000 hectares reported for 1999 and 2000. Similarly, the potential manufacture of cocaine remained virtually unchanged over the last decade, at 910 metric tons. Seizures reached 588 metric tons in 2005, the highest figure ever. However, between 1990 and 2004 the street price per gram fell from an average of (inflation-adjusted) US$175 in the United States and US$275 in Western Europe to $87 and $104, respectively. The net result is little change in cocaine use since 2002, after rising 0.3% annually in the previous decade.

Trends in U.S. Drug Consumption

In 19th-century America, the importation of opium was unregulated and its consumption unrestricted. Hence, myriad elixirs, tonics, potions, concoctions, liniments, and other remedies containing alcohol and/or opium and all sorts of other undisclosed ingredients inundated the market. Opium was very popular for its presumed medicinal properties, including as an analgesic and hypnotic, to ward off fevers, to treat various ailments, and to soothe teething infants, among others. The recreational use of opium also rose alongside its medicinal use, from an annual per capita consumption of about 12 grains (equivalent to 0.78 grams) in 1840 to roughly 52 grains towards the end of the century. As a result, addiction to opium rose, reaching a peak of 250,000 at the turn of the century in a total population of approximately 76 million; the highest rate ever reported in the United States. Likewise, cocaine became very popular throughout the country in the first two decades of the 20th century. However, all figures and quotes on recreational drugs and addiction were mere estimates by individuals or groups with a moral or prohibitionist agenda rather than the product of painstaking surveys, as is the case today. At this writing (2007–2008), solid data are available in the United States on drug use and, to a lesser extent, abuse for different age groups albeit buried in a sea of unsubstantiated, exaggerated, or deceitful reports. Reliable data are gathered by federal agencies and by other independent research groups. Perhaps the most thorough and authoritative drug use data collection in the United States is generated from surveys conducted by the *Monitoring the Future* (MTF) project at the Institute for Social Research of the University of Michigan. These ongoing surveys, which began with the class of 1976 and cover use of illicit drugs plus alcohol and cigarettes by population cohorts ranging from 8th graders to adults age 45, are conducted biennially through age 30 and every five years for cohorts aged 35, 40, and 45. An analysis of their 2008 report[26] suggests the following conclusions.

The Highest Use Prevalence Rates: Teenagers and Young Adults (percentages of users within a specific timeframe) for any illicit drug use. In 2007, the annual and 30-day prevalence rates for *any* illicit drug use for the 18- to 26-year-old age groups ranged from 29% to 36% and from 17% to 22%, respectively, dropping to 18% and 10%, respectively, at age 45 (Figure 1).

The Single Most Widely Used Illicit Drug: Marijuana In 2007, the annual and 30-day prevalence rates for marijuana use by the 18- to 26-year-old age groups ranged from 25% to 33%, and 14% to 19%, respectively, dropping to 13% and 7%, respectively by age 45 (Figure 2).

Figure 1
Any illicit drug. Lifetime, annual, and 30-day prevalence rates by age group (Reproduced from reference 26, Figure 4-1)

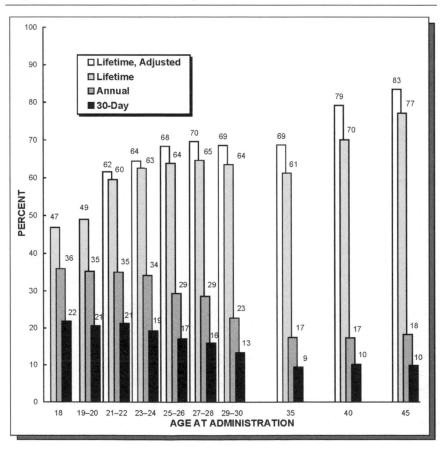

Figure 2
Marijuana. Lifetime, annual, and 30-day prevalence rates by age group
(Reproduced from reference 26, Figure 4-3)

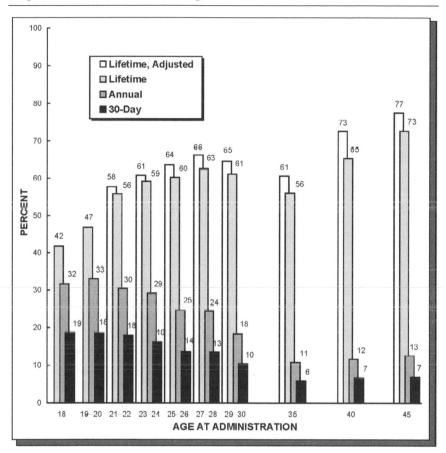

Drug Use Varies Widely From Year to Year   After peaking in 1980–1982, the annual prevalence rates of illicit drug use (marijuana excluded) among 8th, 10th, and 12th graders and young adults (18 to 22) declined through 1992, after which they rose for teenagers and young adults but stabilized to approximately 10% for the 35 to 45 age group (Figure 3). Annual prevalence rates for marijuana followed a comparable pattern, but for a much sharper rise in the decade of the 1990s (Figure 4). Indeed, as noted in the MTF report (2006), "during the 1990s, the annual prevalence of marijuana use tripled among 8th graders (from 6% in 1991 to 18% in 1996), more than doubled among 10th graders (from 15% in 1992 to 35% in 1997), and nearly doubled among 12th graders (from 22% in 1992 to 39% in 1997). Among college students, however, the increase in marijuana use . . . was much more gradual."[27] As a result, peak rates occurred in 1996 for 8th graders, 1997 for 10th and 12th graders, 2001 for college students, and 2004 for young adults. Interestingly, use patterns do not rise and fall in tandem. For example, the annual prevalence for cocaine peaked in 1985–1986 at 12% to 24% for the 18 to 26 age group before falling over the next decade to approximately 5%. Similarly, the annual prevalence rate for MDMA (commonly known as ecstasy) peaked in 2001 at 7% to 11% for the 18- to 24 year-old cohort before falling to less than 5% in 2005. In contrast, the annual prevalence rate for heroin remained stable at or below 1% for all cohorts since 1975, with only a slight rise between 1995 and 2001 for the 18 to 22 cohort. Remarkably, these variations in drug use patterns over three decades were independent of drug availability (increased) and street price (decreased).

The Lowest Use Prevalence Rates: Cohorts 35 and Older   In 2007, the annual prevalence rates for illicit drugs other than marijuana (Figure 1) and for marijuana (Figure 2) for the 35, 40, and 45 cohorts are the lowest of any surveyed age group and have been so since these age groups were included in the surveys (Figures 3 and 4). Comparable findings apply to the 30-day prevalence rates. Hence, high overall prevalence rates among teenagers and young adults do not predict drug addiction later in life. This is because annual and 30-day prevalence rates represent casual, mainly recreational, drug use rather than a compulsion associated with addiction. In contrast, the 30-day prevalence of daily use, a better indication of heavy drug use, drops sharply with age for all illicit drugs. For instance, while the 30-day prevalence of daily use of marijuana in 2007 ranged from 4.1% to 5.2% between ages 18 and 26, it fell to approximately 2.7% by age 45 (Figure 5). Similarly, while 44% of the surveyed 45 age group admitted lifetime use of cocaine, only 2% reported use within the 30-day period preceding the interview (Figure 6).

Use Prevalence Rates Are Higher for Licit than Illicit Drugs in All Ages As stated, among all prevalence criteria, the 30-day prevalence of daily use best describes the pattern likely to represent drug abuse that might lead to addiction. From available data, alcohol and tobacco abuse is generally defined as drinking five drinks of alcohol in a row within the two-week period preceding the survey, and smoking half a pack of cigarettes or more daily, respectively. Using these criteria of abuse reveals that alcohol and tobacco abuse are a much greater problem than abuse of any illicit drugs. Indeed, as shown in Table 2, tobacco and alcohol abuse by young adults far exceeded abuse of any illicit drugs in 2005, including marijuana, the most prevalent, by 2.5- and 7-fold, respectively. Moreover and in contrast to illicit drugs, the prevalence of tobacco (one-half pack per day) and of alcohol abuse (daily in the past 30 days) is age-independent (Figures 7 and 8, respectively). In fact, the prevalence of alcohol abuse (five or more drinks in a row within two weeks or daily use within 30 days) is highest for the

Figure 3
Illicit drugs other than marijuana. Trends in annual prevalence by age group (Reproduced from reference 26, Figure 5-2)

Age	'76	'77	'78	'79	'80	'81	'82	'83	'84	'85	'86	'87	'88	'89	'90	'91	'92	'93	'94	'95	'96	'97	'98	'99	'00	'01	'02	'03	'04	'05	'06	'07
18 Years	25.4	26.0	27.1	28.2	30.4	34.0	30.1	28.4	28.0	27.4	25.9	24.1	21.1	20.0	17.9	16.2	14.9	17.1	18.0	19.4	19.8	20.7	20.2	20.7	20.4	21.6	20.9	19.8	20.5	19.7	19.2	18.5
19–20 Years			28.6	30.2	33.3	34.2	32.4	29.8	27.5	26.9	24.7	22.2	21.3	17.6	16.5	13.8	13.4	13.5	14.6	18.6	17.6	17.6	17.4	18.7	19.6	18.0	19.6	19.9	20.2	20.2	18.1	17.8
21–22 Years					35.5	37.0	34.2	33.7	31.6	29.5	29.1	25.6	22.8	19.4	17.4	14.9	15.4	13.5	14.1	15.2	13.7	17.7	15.3	14.1	17.0	20.0	18.9	20.7	21.2	20.5	22.0	19.7
23–24 Years									29.4	33.4	29.3	22.6	21.0	18.8	17.5	14.6	14.8	12.9	12.9	11.5	13.1	12.1	12.5	14.8	15.0	14.1	17.2	20.1	21.2	18.0	19.4	19.1
25–26 Years									30.2	30.3	25.5	25.7	21.0	17.6	16.6	14.4	13.4	13.0	12.0	11.6	10.0	10.7	10.6	11.6	12.5	13.3	14.6	14.5	16.3	19.7	16.9	17.0
27–28 Years											26.5	23.3	20.4	18.2	15.2	13.6	13.2	11.5	11.1	10.9	10.7	8.4	8.8	8.6	9.9	11.4	11.4	15.1	14.6	14.2	15.1	16.9
29–30 Years													20.0	17.4	12.4	13.2	11.6	9.9	10.8	11.0	10.3	11.0	7.8	8.1	7.4	9.9	10.9	11.6	11.8	15.8	15.3	13.0
31–32 Years[a]															13.8	13.1	10.7	9.5	11.5	8.2	10.2	10.8	9.6	8.3	7.4	9.7	—					
35 Years																			11.2	10.4	11.4	10.0	8.2	9.3	9.3	8.8	9.6	9.5	11.0	10.5	10.8	11.0
40 Years																								7.9	7.7	7.3	9.7	6.7	8.3	9.4	9.8	11.3
45 Years																												8.9	9.3	8.4	10.3	10.7

YEAR OF ADMINISTRATION

Figure 4

Marijuana. Trends in annual prevalence by age group (Reproduced from reference 26, Figure 5-3a)

Chart: PERCENT (y-axis, 0–100) vs. YEAR OF ADMINISTRATION (x-axis, '76–'07)

Legend — Respondent Age: 18 Years; 19–20 Years; 21–22 Years; 23–24 Years; 25–26 Years; 27–28 Years; 29–30 Years; 31–32 Years; 35 Years; 40 Years; 45 Years

Age	'76	'77	'78	'79	'80	'81	'82	'83	'84	'85	'86	'87	'88	'89	'90	'91	'92	'93	'94	'95	'96	'97	'98	'99	'00	'01	'02	'03	'04	'05	'06	'07
18 Years	44.5	47.6	50.2	50.8	48.8	46.1	44.3	42.3	40.0	40.6	38.8	36.3	33.1	29.6	27.0	23.9	21.9	26.0	30.7	34.7	35.8	38.5	37.5	37.8	36.5	37.0	36.2	34.9	34.3	33.6	31.5	31.7
19–20 Years			52.8	51.0	49.7	49.0	44.9	43.0	41.4	40.3	39.1	35.8	36.2	32.2	28.4	25.4	26.9	27.9	31.8	34.8	34.2	37.9	37.2	37.0	37.0	37.9	36.4	35.9	34.5	34.9	33.2	33.1
21–22 Years					50.1	51.1	45.8	45.4	42.1	40.9	39.6	37.4	33.7	31.6	28.2	23.2	26.9	26.1	29.2	28.1	30.6	30.6	31.9	31.5	33.2	37.5	34.3	33.1	32.5	32.6	31.1	30.5
23–24 Years							46.0	43.8	38.6	42.0	36.6	33.7	32.0	27.3	26.6	21.8	26.6	26.5	24.6	25.8	25.8	25.1	25.5	27.4	26.9	28.3	31.8	30.0	27.7	26.8	28.5	29.3
25–26 Years									38.3	39.2	34.1	35.4	29.7	26.2	24.1	21.3	23.5	22.2	22.6	24.4	21.7	23.3	21.2	21.8	22.7	25.0	24.5	24.3	27.6	26.4	24.0	24.7
27–28 Years											32.5	31.4	26.8	26.8	22.6	20.9	21.2	21.3	20.1	20.4	20.6	18.0	19.9	18.2	18.8	19.4	19.4	21.2	22.4	19.7	20.9	24.7
29–30 Years													25.4	24.7	20.0	21.0	20.1	18.8	19.0	18.2	19.5	18.0	16.9	16.0	18.4	17.1	17.5	17.0	16.4	18.9	19.9	24.4
31–32 Years[a]															19.8	19.9	17.7	19.9	18.6	17.2	16.3	17.5	15.8	14.8	14.5	16.7	—	—	—	—	—	18.3
35 Years																			14.5	17.2	16.3	17.5	14.9	14.7	13.8	14.8	13.7	13.0	13.0	12.9	11.4	10.8
40 Years																							17.1	13.8	13.7	12.5	14.6	13.4	13.9	14.3	11.0	11.6
45 Years																												14.0	11.9	11.7	11.6	12.6

Figure 5
Marijuana. Trends in 30-day prevalence of daily use by age group (Reproduced from reference 26, Figure 5-3c)

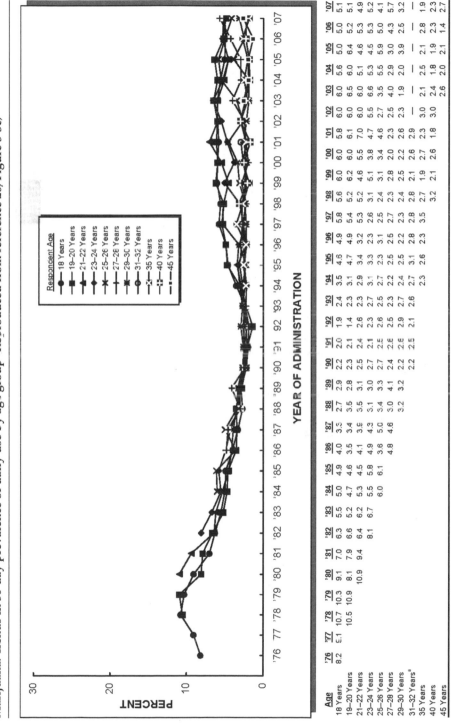

Age	'76	'77	'78	'79	'80	'81	'82	'83	'84	'85	'86	'87	'88	'89	'90	'91	'92	'93	'94	'95	'96	'97	'98	'99	'00	'01	'02	'03	'04	'05	'06	'07
18 Years	8.2	9.1	10.7	10.3	9.1	7.0	6.3	5.5	5.0	4.9	4.0	3.3	2.7	2.9	2.2	2.0	1.9	2.4	3.5	4.6	4.9	5.8	5.6	6.0	6.0	5.8	6.0	6.0	5.6	5.0	5.0	5.1
19–20 Years		10.5	10.9	8.1	7.9	6.6	5.2	4.7	4.6	3.5	3.4	3.5	2.8	2.3	2.1	1.4	2.3	3.1	4.7	4.9	5.4	5.2	6.2	6.0	6.1	6.0	6.5	6.0	6.4	5.2	5.1
21–22 Years				10.9	9.4	6.4	6.2	5.3	4.5	4.1	3.8	3.5	2.8	2.5	2.4	2.6	2.3	2.9	3.4	3.2	5.3	5.2	6.5	5.5	7.0	6.0	6.0	5.1	4.6	5.3	4.9
23–24 Years							8.1	6.7	5.5	5.8	4.9	3.8	3.1	3.0	2.7	2.4	2.3	2.7	3.1	3.3	2.3	5.3	3.1	5.1	3.8	4.7	5.5	6.6	5.3	4.5	5.3	5.2
25–26 Years									6.0	6.1	3.6	5.0	3.4	3.3	2.7	2.6	2.6	2.5	2.7	2.3	3.1	2.5	2.4	3.1	3.4	4.6	2.7	3.5	5.5	5.9	5.0	4.1
27–28 Years											4.8	4.6	3.0	4.1	2.4	2.6	2.5	2.3	2.2	2.5	2.5	2.7	2.3	2.8	2.0	2.3	2.5	4.0	2.9	3.0	4.3	5.7
29–30 Years													3.2	3.2	2.2	2.6	2.9	2.3	2.4	2.2	2.2	2.7	2.4	2.5	2.2	2.3	2.3	1.9	2.0	3.9	2.5	3.2
31–32 Years[a]															2.2	2.5	2.1	2.6	2.7	3.1	2.8	2.8	2.8	2.1	2.6	2.9	—	1.9	1.9	2.1	—	1.9
35 Years																			2.3	2.6	2.3	3.5	2.7	1.9	2.7	2.3	3.0	2.1	2.5	2.1	2.8	2.3
40 Years																								2.1	2.6	1.8	3.0	2.4	1.8	1.9	2.3	2.3
45 Years																							3.2					2.6	2.0	2.1	1.4	2.7

Figure 6
Cocaine. Lifetime, annual, and 30-day prevalence by age groups (Reproduced from reference 26, Figure 4-7)

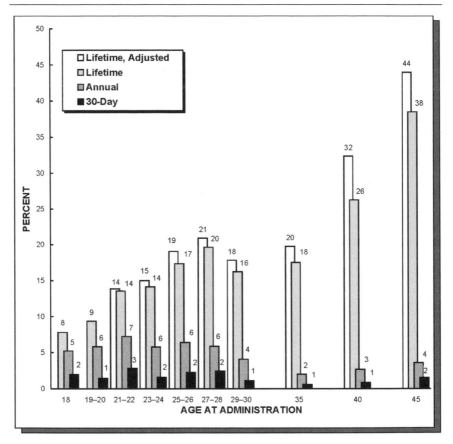

45-year old cohort (9%) than any previous age group (3% to 8%), as shown in Figure 8.

Costs of Illicit Drug Use. Social liabilities (crime, disease, drugs, risks, hazards, or natural events) can be assessed by their economic and human costs. Economic costs include direct (e.g., disease treatment cost) and indirect costs (e.g., lost productivity). Human costs are judged by the *morbidity* (e.g., asthma caused by pollutants) and *mortality* (e.g., death from drug overdose) they cause. Mortality caused by a disease, risk, or natural event is reported in terms of actual deaths per year or per population group, or are calculated to reflect *years of potential life lost* (a statistical measure of premature death). Although all such data are mere estimates rather than factual figures, they serve to quantify, rank, and compare their costs to other

Table 2
Thirty-day prevalence of daily use of various licit and illicit drugs: Ages 19–28

Licit and Illicit drugs	Percent
Marijuana	4.9
Cocaine	0.1
Amphetamines	0.1
Alcohol	
Daily	4.2
5 drinks in a row in past 2 weeks	37.0
Cigarettes	
Daily	19.6
Half-pack or more daily	12.5
Sample size (n)	5,400

social liabilities. The best annual cost estimates for all illicit drugs combined and for alcohol and tobacco individually are shown in Table 3. As shown, the number of deaths from all drugs (licit and illicit) in the United States was 19,102 in 1999.[28] In contrast, *alcohol-associated mortality* was estimated at over 75,000 annually between 1995 and 1999[28] and at over 440,000 for *cigarette smoking* in 2001.[29] The same reports estimated the concomitant annual years of potential life lost at over 2.2 million for alcohol and 5.6 million for cigarette smoking. Finally, a study prepared by the Lewin Group for the National Institute on Alcohol Abuse and Alcoholism reported, "The economic cost to society from alcohol and drug abuse was an estimated $246 billion in 1992. Alcohol abuse and alcoholism cost an estimated $148 billion, while drug abuse and dependence cost an estimated $98 billion."[30] The total economic cost for tobacco use in the United States has been estimated at $158 billion in 1999 or $3,391 for each of the 46.5 million smokers.[30] The overall cost to society of drug abuse has continued to rise, surpassing $143 billion in 1998.[31]

In conclusion, humans have sought and used mind-altering substances since the dawn of time. Archaeological findings and early recorded history seem to indicate that drug use was driven mainly by curiosity, as is the case today, but no records exist of untoward effects to users or their entourage, and their languages had no word for addiction. However, two later societies appear to have suffered greatly from drug abuse: the Muslim world at the turn of the first millennium and the 18th-century Chinese. To the former, it represented a self-gratification behavior that apparently

Figure 7
Cigarettes. Annual, 30-day, and half-pack-a-day prevalence rates (Reproduced from reference 26, Figure 4-21)

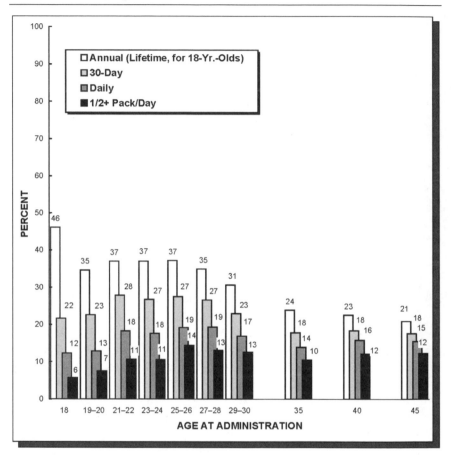

permeated large segments of the population and contributed to the decline of that prosperous and advanced culture. To the latter, it became a curse fomented by a foreign power eager to enhance its geopolitical agenda of domination and to profit from the process. In modern America, mind-altering drugs are used by nearly one in two teenagers. It denotes natural curiosity, self-discovery, rebellion against *grown-up* rules, the lure of the *forbidden fruit*, and the omnipresent albeit overrated *peer pressure*; an excuse claimed by the inattentive parents of every troubled youngster and the refuge of investigators at a loss to explain the causes of drug abuse. The natural history of drug abuse suggests that following peaks of problem behaviors in adolescence and early adulthood recovery is the norm for

Figure 8
Alcohol use. 2-week prevalence of 5 or more drinks in a row and 30-day prevalence of daily use (Reproduced from reference 26, Figure 4-20b)

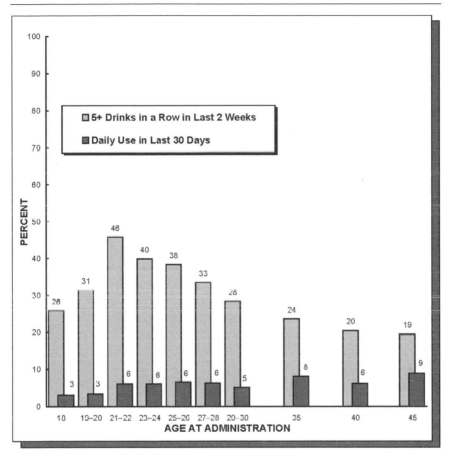

most users. Indeed, the high prevalence rates of drug use among teenagers decline progressively with age for all *illicit* drugs, whereas they increase slightly for *alcohol* and *tobacco*, the two drugs that, despite exhibiting the highest morbidity and mortality rates and the highest cost to society, are *licit*. As a result, while about 5% of the global population age 15–64 use drugs (cannabis in 80% of cases), about 28% use tobacco and approximately 48% consume alcohol on a regular basis. As shown in Table 3, the economic and human costs of each alcohol or tobacco in the United States far exceed the costs of all illicit drugs combined. Moreover, as stated in the Lewin Group's report, even the comparatively low mortality rates attributed to illicit drugs included deaths caused by "drugs, medicaments, and

Table 3
Economic and human costs (U.S., 1995–2001 data): Illicit drugs, alcohol, and tobacco

Costs	All Illicit Drugs	Alcohol	Tobacco
Human			
Deaths	19,102	75,000	440,000
YPLL*	NA	2.2[1]	5.6[1]
Economic	$97.7[2]	$148.0[2]	$157.7[2]

* Years of potential life lost.
[1] Million life-years.
[2] Billions.

biologicals." Likewise, the report explained, "more than half of the estimated costs of drug abuse were associated with drug-related crime";[30] an obvious consequence of the criminalization of drugs. In contrast, very little of the economic costs of alcohol or tobacco are related to crime because possession and use of both these substances are legal. Hence, on the bases of economic and human costs, it is difficult to justify a *War on* [illicit] *Drugs* while the use and abuse of alcohol and tobacco, the two most deadly and costly substances to society, are *licit*. Moreover, illicit drugs are not enemies to be vanquished, as in a *War*, but manageable problems to be ranked alongside other societal liabilities aiming at developing appropriate public prevention or interventional policies, and for allocating resources for their implementation.

CHAPTER 3

The Politics
of Drug Legislation

A CONVOLUTED AMERICAN POLITICAL SAGA

> There are 100,000 total marijuana smokers in the US, and most are Negroes, Hispanics, Filipinos, and entertainers. Their satanic music, jazz and swing, result from marijuana usage. This marijuana causes white women to seek sexual relations with Negroes, entertainers, and any others.
>
> —Harry J. Anslinger, former commissioner of the
> U.S. Bureau of Narcotics, in testimony to Congress
> in support of the Marijuana Tax Act, 1937

> Keep our Commission in line . . . [so] it [does] not appear that the Commission's frankly just a bunch of do-gooders . . . [but] if you're just a bunch of do-gooders that are going to come out with a "soft on marijuana" report, I'll destroy it right off the bat.
>
> —Richard M. Nixon to Raymond P. Shafer, head of his
> Presidential Commission on Marijuana and Drug
> Abuse, declassified Oval Office tapes, 1971–1972

A visitor from outerspace or an idealistic observer from earth could imagine drug policy to have emerged after a careful review of all available evidence by policy makers, advised by experts in the legal, social, medical, economic, and other relevant realms, aimed at developing a far-reaching program likely to impact millions of lives. Yet, both would be wrong, for political reality is far more cynical.

As previously mentioned, the annual per capita opium consumption in the United States rose steadily from about 12 grains in 1840 to approximately

52 grains toward the end of the century. Opium was popular as an analgesic and hypnotic, to ward off fevers and illnesses, and to soothe teething infants, among many popular uses. Addiction to opium is said to have risen alongside, reaching a peak at the turn of the century estimated at 250,000 addicts in a total population of approximately 76 million—the highest rate ever reached in the United States. It is said that there were tens of thousands of heroin addicts in New York City and that cocaine was massively consumed throughout the country in the first two decades of the 20th century. However, such statistics are inherently unreliable and should be viewed with suspicion as they were driven by motives often disconnected from reality, as is still the case today. What is known with certainty is that the 19th and early 20th centuries witnessed the unimpeded availability in America of myriad elixirs, tonics, potions, concoctions, liniments, and the like containing alcohol and/or opium and all sorts of undisclosed ingredients. Indeed, the importation of opium in 19th- and early 20th-century America was unregulated and its consumption unrestricted, and the status of medicine was chaotic. It has been characterized as follows: "The United States had no practical control over the health professions, no representative national health organizations to aid the government in drafting regulations, and no controls on the labeling, composition, or advertising of compounds that might contain opiates or cocaine. The United States not only proclaimed a free marketplace; it practiced this philosophy with regard to narcotics in a manner unrestrained at every level of preparation and consumption."[1] The main reason for this was the American form of government where mostly autonomous states were free to enact or not to enact regulatory drug laws. Because of this autonomy, state drug control initiatives with different goals precluded the emergence of uniform regulatory bodies and of nationwide health groups suitable to regulate the manufacture, content, and distribution of drugs and other health products. For instance, the American Medical Association and the American Pharmaceutical Association, founded in 1847 and 1851, respectively, remained parochial, unorganized, and unrepresentative until World War I, lacking any authority to license or regulate practitioners. Likewise, American medical schools were unregulated, and many were little more than diploma mills. Medical licensing, a state prerogative to this day, began in the late 19th century. However, efforts to raise health standards coupled with the federal government exercise of its right to regulate interstate commerce led to the Pure Food and Drug Act of 1906, which imposed modest labeling requirements for over-the-counter drugs and certain health products.

As the temperance movement led to the enactment of the National Prohibition Act on October 28, 1919, described in chapter 1, drug laws where not far behind, for drug addiction was being targeted in certain circles as a new cause for action. As a prelude to events of half a century later, physicians were finger-pointed and opium prescriptions were regulated, though the manufacture of opium-containing *patent medicines* remained unimpeded and their sale ubiquitous. However, the road to what would years later become the federally based, led, and funded War on Drugs began with the acquisition of the Philippines through the Spanish-American War. Unlike American states that were and remain semiautonomous, the Philippines came under the direct and sole control of the U.S. federal government. This was an opportunity for Congress to exercise its power and for its members to respond to public pressure and to the interests of influential constituents. At the time, Spanish authorities held a monopoly on the sale and distribution of opium in the Philippines, presumably destined to Chinese living in that country. William Taft, the newly appointed American Civil Governor of the Philippines, continued the monopoly and earmarked profits of the opium trade to educate Filipinos. When American missionaries in the Philippines and religious organizations in the United States learned of the project, they were outraged that *tainted* money from opium sales would be channeled to education and prevailed on President Theodore Roosevelt to order Governor Taft to kill the bill. The latter appointed the Philippine Opium Investigation Committee to explore how the *opium problem* was dealt with in Asian countries and to make recommendations. Departing from the Committee's recommendations, the U.S. Congress decreed to register adult non-Filipinos opium smokers, allowing them a three year opium supply that would be reduced gradually to zero over the final 6 months of the grace period. Nonmedicinal opium was banned for all other inhabitants of the Philippines.

As mentioned earlier, at the end of the 19th century, China had tried to free itself from British-imposed opium trade and was making vigorous efforts to address its opium addiction problem. In the meantime, Chinese laborers hired to build the western states' railroads were being mistreated, and unhappy Chinese government, industrialists, and merchants were planning retaliatory measures. In order to placate the Chinese government and in attempts to reduce the flow of opium to the Philippines but not necessarily to the United States, President Roosevelt convened in Shanghai the International Opium Commission, which led to the First International Opium Convention signed in The Hague, on January 23, 1912. The signatories of the latter were "determined to bring about the gradual suppression of the abuse of opium, morphine, and cocaine as also of the drugs prepared or derived from these substances, which give rise or might give rise to similar abuses."[2] The Convention was convened on behalf of heads of participating states. They included, the Presidents of the United States, France, and Portugal and the Majesties or Imperial Majesties of nine Kingdoms or Empires, raging from His Majesty King of Italy to His Majesty the King of the United Kingdom of Great Britain and Ireland and of the British Dominions Beyond the Seas, Emperor of India. In the meantime, the U.S. government had passed the 1909 anti-opium law designed to placate China's outrage for the mistreatment of Chinese workers in the United States. Dr. Hamilton Wright, newly appointed opium commissioner, proposed a federal law to curtail the dispensation of narcotics to addicts using the government's power of taxation as a pretext to circumvent the states' autonomy on drug regulation. In April 1910, Republican Congressman David Foster of Vermont introduced a bill to that effect that included cocaine, cannabis, and chloral hydrate (a hypnotic agent) in addition to opium. However, its passage had to await the Democratic majority of the 62nd Congress when it became the law of the land as the *Harrison Act*, after Congressman Francis Burton Harrison of New York.

The Harrison Act was less draconian than the Foster bill for it accommodated both demands from southern congressmen eager to preserve racial segregation laws and the lobbying pressure of the recently formed National Drug Trade Conference, which represented drug trade associations. As a result, cannabis and chloral hydrate were dropped, penalties were reduced, record keeping was relaxed, and *patent medicines* containing small amounts of narcotics were allowed. It provided "for the registration of, with collectors of internal revenue, and to impose a special tax on all persons who produce, import, manufacture, compound, deal in, dispense, sell, distribute, or give away opium or coca leaves, their salts, derivatives, or preparations, and for other purposes." The U.S. Senate passed the Harrison bill in August 1914, and President Wilson signed it into law in December of that year. In 1902, the AMA had labeled as *highly addictive* the new drug heroin (from the German *heroisch*—heroic) developed in 1898 by the German company AG Bayer that it marketed as a *nonaddictive painkiller*. Prior to enactment of the Harrison Act, heroin was being prescribed to treat morphine addiction. However, it became the recreational drug of choice in New York and other major cities and was blamed for an increasing incidence in violence and crime. More ominously, it was rumored that heroin, mixed with cosmetics, was being smuggled from Germany in attempts to addict the entire U.S. population. These were powerful arguments for prohibitionists and isolationists who rallied around Stephen G. Porter, then Republican chairman of the House Committee on Foreign Relations, to stop all heroin production in the United States beginning in 1924. However, while the U.S. government banned drugs at home, it was unable to convince the international community to do likewise at the Geneva's revised International Opium Convention of 1925, which dealt with cocaine as well as opium and was later monitored by the League of Nations' Permanent Opium Central Board. In fact, in a display of undiplomatic obstinacy over other nations' refusal to curb poppy and coca production, the American delegation walked out of the conference. In addition to losing to the League of Nations its leading position in the global antidrug movement it had gained in Shanghai and The Hague, the United States was unable to join the League due to Senate opposition led by Henry Cabot Lodge of Massachusetts and other influential Republican senators.

In addition to criminalizing opium and cocaine, the Harrison Act set in motion a witch-hunt that targeted physicians and pharmacists, especially those willing to prescribe maintenance narcotics to addicts; a practice the U.S. Supreme Court ruled constitutional in 1916.[3] The net result was that fewer of them were willing to risk their livelihood and a prison sentence for prescribing or dispensing narcotics. Addicts, no longer freely maintained by prescription narcotics, turned to crime in order to support their habit, or so it was claimed. In response to this narcotics prescription vacuum and a perceived need for registering and assisting addicts rid themselves of their habit, several states and cities sponsored *narcotics clinics*. Today's methadone maintenance clinics are but a rebirth of this approach to the treatment of drug addiction. However, some clinics became indiscriminate narcotics distribution centers, selling heroin and morphine to all visitors. More ominously, in March 1919, the U.S. Supreme Court reversed itself in a five to four ruling that a narcotics prescription intended to supply maintenance doses to a *mere* addict could not be considered a true prescription given in the proper conduct of medical practice. Armed with these two powerful arguments, the Treasury Department proceeded to close down *narcotics clinics* and to arrest narcotics-prescribing physicians and narcotics-dispensing druggists unless preapproved by a narcotics agent. As mentioned earlier, over 25,000 professionals were arrested and more than 3,000 were imprisoned. Whether because of the implementation of the Harrison Act or as a reflection of fluctuations in social mores, the number of addicts in the United States is said to have dropped dramatically, though from an unrealistic and unsubstantiated high of one million cases *estimated* by a U.S. Treasury Department committee in 1918.

In the interim, another *war* loomed on the horizon, and this time, the target was *marijuana*. As animosity toward Chinese laborers had galvanized public opinion against opium at the turn of the century, anti-Mexican prejudice of the early 1930s provided impetus that led to the Marijuana Tax Act of 1937. Mexicans had come to the United States during the prosperous years of the 1920s to work as laborers in the fields of southwestern and western states. Many Mexicans grew and smoked marijuana; a benign custom initially tolerated, as it caused no ill effects in their adopted communities. However, as the Great Depression took its toll on the U.S. job market Mexicans were finger-pointed as taking American jobs and engaging in drugs, violence, and crime. That was the classical and recurrent justification put forth by those who intuitively or on moral or religious grounds distrust minorities, especially if they exhibit physical, cultural, or behavioral traits that set *them* apart from *us*, the majority. The fact that they smoked marijuana was used as a confirmation of their deviant nature and of their danger to others. At first, the Federal Bureau of Narcotics and its head, Harry J. Anslinger, former Commissioner of the U.S. Bureau of Narcotics during Prohibition, were hesitant to get involved in banning a drug grown domestically as compared to opium and cocaine, which were *evil imports*. However, realizing he could expand the reach of his office and his personal power and driven by his racist zeal, Anslinger soon reversed course, becoming the most outspoken and tireless, if deceitful, antidrug campaigner. In speeches and articles, he described how *Orientals* used drugs to entice "women from good families" into brothels and how marijuana addiction was responsible for "over 50% of violent crimes among Mexicans, Turks, Filipinos, Greeks, Spaniards, Latino-Americans, and Negroes" and had brought about "an epidemic of crimes committed by young people."[4] While his racially inflammatory antidrug rhetoric found no boundaries, he was supplying morphine to the infamous Senator Joseph McCarthy "so that communists could not blackmail this great American senator for his drug dependency weakness."[5]

A fortuitous event took place that provided the U.S. Bureau of Narcotics an opportunity to take action: the Firearms Act of 1934 that made it illegal to transfer a machine gun without the payment of a transfer tax. As soon as the U.S. Supreme Court upheld the *Firearms Act,* the Treasury Department petitioned and obtained from Congress a marijuana tax law, which became known as the Marijuana Tax Act of 1937. Under the Act, marijuana could not be sold, bartered, or given away without the proper federal stamp. However, funds to implement the Marijuana Tax Act were not granted. It remained an irrelevant piece of legislation until the 1960s when it became "a law enforcement weapon directed against America's youth, the foreign-born, and non-conforming minorities."[5] Within the atmosphere of antidrug paranoia of the 1930s and 1940s, there was an occasional voice of sanity. Suspicious of the U.S. government claims on drugs, Fiorello La Guardia, mayor of New York City from 1934 to 1945, appointed a special committee to conduct a thorough sociological and scientific investigation into the effects of marijuana use in New York City. After six years of research, the commission concluded that marijuana use: created in the user a feeling of adequacy, relaxation, verbal disinhibition, self-confidence, and sometimes anxiety; was not widespread among school children; was not associated with juvenile delinquency or major crimes; did not lead to hard drug use; and was more prevalent among individuals of limited social adaptive capacity.[6] These findings echoed those of the British Indian Hemp Drug Commission of 1894 and of the Panama Canal Zone Report of 1925. Significantly, its findings were to be validated by four subsequent American and foreign studies on marijuana (the Advisory Committee on Drug Dependence and Cannabis of 1968, the Canadian LeDain Commission Report of 1970, the National Commission on Marijuana and Drug Abuse of 1973, and the National Academy of Science Report: Marijuana and Health of 1982). The La Guardia report was strongly opposed by the Narcotics Bureau and by Anslinger who, true to form, attacked the integrity of the scientists involved in the study. Undeterred by his lack of medical, biological, or psychiatric training, he prepared his own unfounded version of *The Psychiatric Effects of Marijuana Intoxication,* which inexplicably and inexcusably was published by the *Journal of the American Medical Association.*[7] Disregard for the facts was Anslinger's trademark during his 32 years at the helm of the U.S. Bureau of Narcotics, as is further documented in an interesting book on the politics of America's War on Drugs.[8] The book describes,

During World War II, Anslinger waged a press campaign to convince the American public that Japan was systematically attempting to addict its enemies, including the American people, to opium, in order to destroy their civilization. Although there was no other evidence of the putative "Japanese Opium Offensive," Coast Guard ships and Internal Revenue Service investigative units were directed to work with Anslinger's bureau. In 1950, during the Korean War, Anslinger again used the Hobsonian theme [from Richard Hobson's book *Drug Addiction—A Malignant Racial Cancer*], leaking a report to the press that "subversion through drug addiction is an established aim of Communist China," and that the Chinese were smuggling massive amounts of heroin into the United States to weaken American resistance.[8]

Such misrepresentation of the facts, widely adopted and kept alive by drug enforcement agencies and drug prohibitionists of the time, continues to this day.

Anslinger's disregard for the facts and his targeting drugs as a springboard to promote his own political agenda would have a legion of intellectual successors over the years, most notoriously President Richard M. Nixon, creator of the DEA and the Central Intelligence Agency (CIA), and Governor Nelson A. Rockefeller. *Big Bill* Rockefeller's great grandson, Nelson A. Rockefeller became a master manipulator of the media as the coordinator of inter-American affairs for President Franklin Delano Roosevelt, backed by a $150 million budget to run a propaganda agency in Latin America. His approach was to distribute daily articles, editorials, and photographs of anecdotic or dramatic stories with titillating titles with the appearance of *news* to journalists not inclined to check the sources, motives, or politics behind the stories. While Rockefeller's mission ostensibly was to promote a positive image of America in that part of the world, his experience in manipulating the South American media proved invaluable in his subsequent political career at home. After delegates at the 1964 Republican Convention rejected him, Rockefeller realized he needed to appeal to hard-line, law-and-order Republicans and to ordinary citizens concerned about their family and property *threatened by addicts,* according to polls he commissioned. Drawing on his South America experience, he launched a media blitz proposing the most draconian antidrug policies in America in order to win the Governorship of New York, which upon his election became known as the Rockefeller Drug Laws, which took effect in May 1973. Rockefeller had boldly claimed that heroin was like an infectious disease that would spread to unsuspecting victims, and he declared that the *epidemic of addiction* in New York state had reached plague proportions that threatened the lives of innocent children. He played loose with statistics and with the size of the addict population and their cost to New York state taxpayers, according to the needs of the moment. He portrayed his antidrug campaign as a "treatment and rehabilitation program for addicts" to appease his liberal supporters, while pushing for "an all-out war on drugs and addiction" to satisfy his right-wing patrons.

The Rockefeller Drug Laws established mandatory prison sentences for possession and sale of controlled substances based on the weight of the drug involved. The statues mandated that anyone convicted of selling two ounces or more of heroin, morphine, or marijuana, or of possessing four ounces or more of these drugs, receive a minimum of 15 years to a maximum of life. As a result, the state's prison population and the costs involved escalated year after year. Yet, the Rockefeller Drug Laws failed to reduce the number of addicts and drug-related crime despite incarcerating thousands of drug offenders, imposing mandatory sentences that are longer than those for rapists and murderers, choking prisons and the judicial system, and escalating incarceration and facility construction costs. In 1977, the Committee on New York Drug Law Evaluations, a partnership between the Association of the Bar of the City of New York and the Drug Abuse Council, Inc., issued a highly critical report on the Rockefeller Drug Laws.[9] The Committee found that heroin use and heroin-related crime, the main issues that inspired the Rockefeller Drug Laws, were as prevalent in 1976 as they had been prior to enactment of the laws. It described the experiment as a *dismal failure* despite its high cost and the appointment of scores of additional judges to handle thousands of cases prosecuted under the new laws. It can be objectively concluded that, as all prior and subsequent prohibition statutes, the Rockefeller Drug Laws did not serve the interests of justice nor did they reduce drug abuse or crime attributed to drugs in New York state.

Throughout the 1960s, marijuana use was widespread on college campuses and among liberal circles as an expression of dissent and as a symbol of rebellion against the Vietnam War and the *establishment*. During the Johnson and Kennedy administrations, public attitudes on drug control shifted from supporting punishment to one of laissez faire, a view ignored by the law enforcement community. Indeed, while there were only 169 marijuana felony convictions in 1960, marijuana arrests rose to 188,000 in 1970.[5] During that decade, treatment of addicts was authorized by the Narcotic Addict Rehabilitation Act of 1966, which provided voluntary, pretrial civil commitment, as well as forced treatment of convicted addicts. In 1968, the Alcoholic and Narcotic Addict Rehabilitation Amendments authorized funding of rehabilitation and treatment services by states and private organizations. Congress later enacted the Comprehensive Drug Abuse Prevention and Control Act of 1970, which consolidated all previous federal drug laws, acts, and statutes, including the Harrison Act, in order to regulate legitimate drug use and curtail importation and distribution of illicit drugs throughout the United States. Because it stratified mind-altering drugs into five *classes* according to their *accepted medical use* and *substantial potential for abuse*, it has become known as the Controlled Substances Act (CSA). It also included a relatively benign provision that lowered the maximum penalty for possession of an ounce of marijuana to one year in jail and a $5,000 fine, with the option of probation or a conditional discharge at the judge's discretion. After President Nixon signed the Act in October 1971, it soon became obvious that he planned an overall assault on the production, selling, and use of all illicit drugs. Under Nixon, drugs were catapulted to national prominence, and drug policy became the political centerpiece of his administration.

From a very humble background, Nixon attended Duke University Law School on a scholarship and graduated among the top of his class. However, when his attempts to join prestigious New York law firms were dashed, apparently for lack of connections, he returned to Whittier, CA, his hometown. He espoused the fear of the time, *the menace of international communism*, and ran as the Republican nominee for the congressional seat held by Jerry Voorhis, a liberal Democrat, which he won in 1946. His adept exploitation of the national fear of Communism won him reelection to the U.S. Congress (1948), a seat in the U.S. Senate (1950), and the U.S. vice presidency (1952). After loosing his bids first for the U.S. Presidency to John F. Kennedy and then for the California Governorship to Pat Brown, Nixon's political career seemed to be over. However, he resurfaced in 1968 as the Republican nominee for the Presidency of the United States, this time on a platform of law and order, inspired by the widely publicized success of Robert F. Kennedy, the attorney general for the Kennedy administration. However, once in office (1969 to 1974), the lack of jurisdiction and the powerlessness of federal institutions to effectively curtail street crime became apparent to the Nixon administration. In fact, national statistics for crime, arrests, prosecutions, and convictions rose nationwide during 1969 and 1970, a fact that was not lost to a critical press. Hence, a new approach was needed for Nixon to fulfill his tough law and order campaign rhetoric. Some of his campaign trail slogans had included, "In New York City more people between the ages of fifteen and thirty-five years die as a result of narcotics than from any other single cause,"[10] and "Doubling the conviction rate in this country would do more to cure crime in America than quadrupling fund for Humphrey's war on poverty."[5] Additionally, there was a perceived need to divert popular attention from the highly unpopular Vietnam War and to steer attention to domestic issues with popular appeal; drugs seemed the obvious choice, especially because of the high incidence of addicts among soldiers servicing in Vietnam. Besides, Governor Rockefeller was scoring major political points by waging a highly publicized war on the *drug menace* and on addicts few cared about.

Once again, the Hobsonian thesis that addicts cause most street crime, up to 75% according to one claim, provided the political cover and an easy way to reduce crime statistics, or so they thought. At first, the Domestic Council, a White House group created and used by John Ehrlichman to further his own political ambitions, advocated to shift "the burden for responsibility in controlling crime to the state and local governments, which have jurisdiction over local law enforcement."[8] However, this obvious abdication of Nixon's campaign pledges was rejected by the White House, which opted for a triple antidrug strategy instead. The strategy called for the Bureau of Narcotics to crack down on drug dealers and peddlers; for the Department of Health, Education and Welfare to expand treatment programs for addicts; and for the State Department to coax producer countries to curtail the production of drugs entering the United States. In his Special Message to the Congress on Drug Abuse Prevention and Control, June 17, 1971, Nixon stated "America does not grow opium—of which heroin is a derivative—nor does it manufacture heroin, which is a laboratory process carried out abroad. This deadly poison . . . is, in other words, a foreign import . . . No serious attack on our national drug problem can ignore the international implications of such an effort, nor can the domestic effort succeed without attacking the problem on an international plane. I intend to do that . . . It is clear that the only effective way to end heroin production is to end opium production and the growing of poppies."[10] In what would become a highly controversial international drug cultivation eradication program endorsed by each subsequent administration, he added, "I am asking the Congress to provide $2 million to the Department of Agriculture for research and development of herbicides which can be used to destroy growths of narcotics-producing plants without adverse ecological effects." *Time Magazine* reported, "The Administration's strategy has been to try to pinch off the drug routes before they reach New York, Miami or the Mexican border, the main U.S. entry points. The effort involves long, Le Carré-style work by dozens of globe-ranging narcotics agents, as well as diplomatic pressure on 57 countries that are concerned with the trade in one way or another. But the effort has been frustrating."[11]

According to plan, Mexico was identified as the first target of *Operation Intercept,* as it presumably produced 85% of the heroin entering the United States, and most of the marijuana, the claimed *stepping-stone* to heroin addiction. That fictitious claim is now called a *gateway drug* by the drug enforcement establishment and prohibitionists for lack of objective evidence that marijuana is harmful to users or fosters crime. Soon, 2,000 customs and border-patrol agents were deployed along the Mexican border for what was touted as the country's largest peacetime search and seizure operation by civil authorities. At first, the White House was pleased with the enormous media attention devoted to Nixon's efforts to curtail drug availability at the border. However, because virtually no narcotics were intercepted over a three-week period, Operation Intercept's main purpose was now claimed to be to put pressure on Mexico and make its government more cooperative. Additionally, delays in border crossing by tourists and laborers alarmed both the Mexican government and the State Department concerned of international repercussions that might compromise its Latin American policies. This and increasingly critical press reports led to the quiet withdraw of Operation Intercept.

Now, another country susceptible to U.S. bullying had to be found. CIA information indicated that most of the opium was grown in India, Afghanistan, Pakistan, Thailand, Laos, Burma, and Iran, with Turkey producing less than 10% of the total. India's government, unfriendly to the United States, would likely retaliate diplomatically and in the press to U.S. pressure, and the Shah of Iran, a close U.S. ally, was not to be confronted. Afghanistan, Pakistan, Thailand, Laos, and Burma had central governments incapable of controlling poppy growing clans. That left Turkey by default; a North Atlantic Treaty Organization (NATO) member and recipient of U.S. aid and, it was claimed, the source of most of the heroin reaching Europe. When Ambassador William Handley demanded Turkish officials to drastically reduce the size of the poppy planted area, he was informed that tight distribution controls imposed by the Turkish government precluded much opium finding its way to illegal markets and that farmers from the plains of Afyon, where poppy had been planted for a millennium, depended on it for their livelihood. Indeed, poppy seeds provided cooking oil, protein-rich poppy husks were a source of livestock feed, leaves were used in salads, poppy stems furnished heating fuel, and the gummy juice of the unripened capsule served as a painkiller. Turkish Prime Minister Süleyman Demirel viewed the demand as evidence of American imperialism and of a hypocritical double standard, for no action was demanded from other opium-producing countries. Additionally, he feared his government might be toppled by a surge of popular protests should he comply with U.S. demands. At most, Turkey would redouble its surveillance of poppy production and of its borders. However, Eugene Rossides, a Greek-Cypriot American notoriously unsympathetic to Turkey who was in charge of all law-enforcement activities at the Treasury Department, pressured, with White House acquiescence, the recently created Ad Hoc Cabinet Committee on Narcotics to mount an all-out *crusade* against Turkey. The U.S. Congress and the press were told that Turkey was responsible for 80% of all heroin reaching the United States, a figure pulled out of thin air. Ambassador Handley, under considerable pressure from G. Gordon Liddy and other White House operatives to get quick results, was relieved when the democratically elected Turkish government was overthrown by the U.S.-friendly military. An agreement was quickly reached: the Turks would suspend poppy cultivation after the harvest but ahead of the American presidential election in exchange for a $100 million subsidy over a three-year period offered by the U.S. government to compensate Turkish farmers, which Eugene Rossides managed to reduce to $30 million. The agreement was hailed in the American press as a major victory of President Nixon's crusade against drugs and crime, though its impact on worldwide opium production and on the amount of heroin on American streets was marginal at best. In the end, the ban was short lived, and in 1974, the Turkish government informed the UN it would license poppy cultivation for medical purposes; a program similar to one implemented in India two decades earlier. The UN approved and gave assistance to build a poppy processing plant and to control the program. In 1981, the United States extended special protected market status to both Turkey and India that, to this day, obligates it to purchase at least 80% of narcotic raw materials produced by these two countries.

In the meantime, American intelligence had estimated that most of the heroin reaching the United States came through Marseilles, France, where small labs converted Turkish morphine base into heroin. Hence, when President Nixon appointed former IBM executive Arthur Watson as Ambassador to France he urged him to clean up the heroin problem in France. Upon arriving in Paris, Watson discovered that the French drug enforcement task force was small and nonchalant about heroin, which they considered an American rather than a French problem. He immediately began working to change that perception by planting stories in newspapers and television, as Rockefeller had successfully done in Latin America years earlier, about addiction in the streets and bars of Paris. While his campaign raised drug awareness of the French public, it had little impact on the U.S. State Department, which continued to press for concrete evidence of success, including the seizure of clandestine drug laboratories that, in fact, were little more than a few hard-to-find converted kitchens. The U.S. Embassy science attaché Dr. Edgar Piret conceived the idea of *sniffing out* the fumes of acetic anhydrides, a chemical used in manufacturing heroin. Varian Associates, a California company that had developed a technique to chemically detect the presence of drugs in the urine of soldiers stationed in Vietnam, was given the contract for the *heroin sniffler*, reportedly underwritten by the CIA. Soon, a Volkswagen camper with a conspicuous sniffling snorkel mounted on its roof rolled into Marseilles with an American agent inside charting the beeps signaling the location of drug labs, or so they thought. As it turned out, because acetic acid fumes from vinegar were indistinguishable from acetic anhydride's, the team had pinpointed the location of all the salad-serving restaurants, bistros, and kitchens in Marseilles but detected no drug labs.

Dr. Piret, sent back to the drawing board, came up with another approach, perhaps after reading of Jean Valjean's escape though the sewers of Paris in Victor Hugo's *Les Miserables.* The idea was to test the effluent sewage emanating from drug labs for traces of drug processing chemicals. However, the multitude of sewer lines to be tested and the undesirable working conditions quickly led to another failure. Giving up on Dr. Piret's schemes, Ambassador Watson eventually prevailed on the French drug task force to raid and seize a few drug labs, which was hailed by Washington, by a few touring Congressmen, and by the American media as a major breakthrough. The *French connection* also involved Auguste Ricord, a Corsican *Mafioso* embroiled in the controversial theory about the assassination of President Kennedy.[12] Accused in France of Nazi collaboration, Ricord had fled to Argentina, then settled in Uruguay where he engaged in prostitution and drug trafficking. Obsessed with Ricord, whom he presumed the kingpin of the French connection, President Nixon eventually prevailed on General Alfredo Stroessner, Uruguay's dictator, to arrest and extradite Ricord to the United States to serve a 20-year sentence for heroin smuggling.[13]

How was the Nixon White House able to convince the entire nation and Congress of the imminent dangers of drugs? Having run a campaign platform of law and order, Nixon chose the drug *menace* as his target upon becoming President. He depicted addicts as medieval vampires, each of whom could *infect* at least six unsuspecting innocent victims, including children, and exploited the public's fears to marshal support for his antidrug policies. As part of his strategy to bolster his claim that the nation faced a *national emergency*, his administration disseminated alarming statistics suggesting that drugs threatened every American family. For instance, his 1971 request to Congress for emergency powers to deal with what he described as an *uncontrollable heroin epidemic* was accompanied by official statistics indicating that the number of heroin users had increased from 68,000 in 1969 to 315,000 in 1970 and 559,000 in 1971. Thus, at the stroke of a pen, the Bureau of Narcotics and Dangerous Drugs had managed to increase the number of drug users on American streets by eight-fold over a three-year period; a feat the most enterprising drug traffickers could only dream possible. The method used to generate such statistics was ingenious, albeit deceitful. It was based on the *tagged-fish-in-a-pond* technique used to estimate the fish population in a pond. Briefly, fish caught are tagged and released back into the pond. The ratio of tagged-to-untagged fish caught subsequently is then used to estimate the total fish population before tagging. For example, if 1 in 100 fish caught the second time is tagged, the total fish population is estimated to be 100-fold the number of tagged fish released initially. That approach might be reasonable to estimate the fish populating a pond over a relatively short period, providing no intervening event occurred to disturb the tagged-to-untagged fish ratio. However, the technique is unsuitable for estimating the total number of drug users among the general population. First, users apprehended by police are not randomly distributed over the *drug pond*. Second, previously apprehended users might be more or less susceptible to re-arrest. Third, street conditions vary from day to day depending on drug availability and demand, and from year to year according to changing enforcement procedures.

Interestingly, Nixon's claimed deteriorating drug use statistics between 1969 and 1971, if true, would have been an indictment of his own antidrug policies and a failure to deliver on his campaign pledges, a thought not lost to John Ehrlichman and H. R. Haldeman, his closest advisors. They became concerned that increasing numbers of addicts would hurt Nixon's reelection and ordered all such figures be cleared by White House staff prior to their release to the press. Not surprisingly, subsequent tagged-fish-in-a-pond statistics revealed that after reaching a peak of 559,000 in 1971, the number of heroin addicts unexpectedly and precipitously dropped to 150,000; a clear vindication of Nixon's antidrug crusade and a policy victory quickly trumpeted by his administration. Based on its tagged-fish-in-a-pond statistics, the Nixon administration put a price tag of US$18 billion ($88.5 billion in today's currency[14]) as the annual cost of drug-related street crime in America. The mathematical contortions necessary to arrive at such a staggering figure are interesting to dissect. It was first decided that each heroin addict spent $16,750 annually ($83,400 in today's currency), most of which was raised from two to three thefts (shoplifting, mugging, burglary, armed robbery, and so on) per addict per day. These stunning figures were welcome and obligingly reported by a mass media always bent on unconfirmed hyperbole. Scholarly work did not escape that trend. For instance, in the introduction to his 1972 book *The Politics of Heroin in Southeast Asia*, the author alarmingly warned "AMERICA [original emphasis] is in the grip of a devastating heroin epidemic which leaves no city or suburb untouched, and which also runs rampant through every American military installation both here and abroad. And the plague is spreading into factories and offices (among the middle-aged, middle-class workers as well as the young), into high schools and now grammar schools."[15] A quarter of a century later, in the introduction of his 1998 book *The Truth about Drugs*, the author cautioned, "addiction is a significant threat to civilization. There has never been a time in human history when so many lives have depended on finding the next dose in time."[16] However, a cursory analysis of Nixon's drug costs statistics proves them disingenuous at best or dishonest at worst. First, nowhere is the $16,750 annual cost of heroin to be found from credible sources, except in Nixon's costs estimates included in his June 17, 1971, address to Congress. In it he further claimed, "the cost of supplying a narcotic habit can run from $30 a day to $100 a day. This is $210 to $700 a week, or $10,000 a year to over $36,000 a year."[10] Second, two to three thefts per addict per day would result in over 1 million drug-related crimes each day; a figure that exceeded by at least 100-fold all U.S. crimes reported to police in 1971–1972. It is also interesting to note that no one within or outside the Nixon administration was too concerned about matching numbers being cited. Indeed, at $16,750 apiece, 559,000 heroin users, the highest figure claimed by the Nixon administration would have cost the nation $9.4 billion, not $18 billion, as claimed by the White House.

While these figures were being trumpeted by the Nixon's administration to bolster its claim of imminent national danger, an interagency committee on narcotics and drug abuse contradicted them. It reported that no reliable figures on the number of U.S. addicts or the cost of drug abuse or drug-related crime could be gathered and, "If the misuse of drugs is viewed with proper perspective, it is not in actuality a paramount national problem. . . . However, because of the political significance of the 'Problem', visible, hard-hitting programs must be highlighted to preclude irrational criticism."[8] The report displeased Emil *Bud* Krogh Jr., President Nixon's deputy for law enforcement before he was imprisoned for his role in the Plumbers' operations (mainly the Watergate break-in). He ordered the Office of Science and Technology to analyze all available data on narcotics addiction and crime in the United States. The task was assigned to the Institute for Defense Analysis (IDA). Professional IDA staff, used to the scientific method, first tested the widely spread belief that in order to support their habit addicts commit several thefts each day, which in turn accounted for most crimes in America. As luck would have it, a strike of shipyard workers that interrupted the heroin supply to eastern cities in the summer of 1972 provided the testing ground and an opportunity to assess the validity of the addict–crime link assumption. The strike dried out the heroin supply and quintupled the price of the little that remained. Under these circumstances addicts were expected to either increase their criminal activity in order to afford the higher cost of drugs or to rely on methadone-treatment programs in order to avoid the effects of withdrawal. Yet, crime rates did not increase, nor did enrollment in heroin-treatment programs, suggesting that addicts were able to switch from heroin to other available and less expensive drugs or to simply abstain until heroin became more affordable. IDA analysts concluded: "The little evidence available suggests that during a time of severe heroin shortage, addicts may not be willing or able to increase their crime commensurately with the price increase, and therefore they compensate by reducing their heroin consumption and/or substituting other drugs. Also the data do not suggest that entering treatment is the preferred option."[8]

In that same year, all Washington prison inmates were being routinely tested for opiate, amphetamine, and barbiturate use, providing IDA analysts the opportunity to test the validity of the assumption that addiction is drug-specific. Test results showed that the 20% prestrike heroin use prevalence dropped close to 0% during the strike as amphetamine and barbiturate use levels rose from the single digits to nearly 20%.[8] Similarly, a study assessing the relationship between drug use and crime conducted by the Center for Criminal Justice at Harvard University on addicts enrolled in methadone-treatment programs demonstrated that while drug offenses decreased, robbery, assaults, and property theft actually increased while on methadone. Finally, one of the earliest and most thorough studies on drug use was conducted in 1971 on thousands of U.S. servicemen stationed in Vietnam.[17] Using questionnaire responses and concomitant urine tests the investigators built an objective and reliable database for analysis. Additionally, a three-year follow up of 94% of the studied population enabled them to assess the subjects' drug use status once out of Vietnam and back into civil society. The study revealed that drug use was rampant in Vietnam-stationed servicemen: 90% drank alcohol, nearly 80% smoked marijuana, 38% and 34% used opium and heroin, respectively, and over 25% used amphetamines or barbiturates. The study also found that "the orderly sequence of substance use described as a Guttman scale, in which no one progresses to an illicit drug without having used the legal drugs, alcohol and tobacco, and no one progresses to a 'hard' illicit drug without having used a 'softer' illicit drug, had been turned topsy-turvy in Vietnam."[17] Instead, a history of deviant behavior preservice (e.g., fighting; truanting, drunkenness, arrest, and school expulsion) increased the risk of narcotics use before, during, and after Vietnam and accounted for adverse outcomes (e.g., crime, violence, unemployment, etc.) commonly attributed to drug use. The follow-up data showed that postdischarge, "only 12% of those addicted in Vietnam had been addicted at any time in the 3 years since return, and for those re-addicted, the addiction had usually been very brief."[17] Drug-addicted and drug-indulging U.S. soldiers serving in Vietnam became drug-free as a re-sult of a strict Department of Defense ban on drugs, enforced by compelled urine testing and the threat of more disciplinary action for recidivists, in-cluding an extension of their Vietnam tour of duty, rather than through treat-ment. Indeed, according to the report "only a third of the men addicted in Vietnam received even simple detoxification while in service, and only a tiny percentage of Vietnam enlisted men went into drug abuse treatment after return."[17]

   Four pivotal conclusions can be drawn from these various studies, which dispel key myths underlying many of today's notions about drug use and invalidate misguided policies designed to curb it. First, the stepping stone theory of drug use and the stratifying of drugs from *soft* to *hard*, while in-grained in popular folklore, has no basis in reality and has proven un-founded in large-scale studies. For instance, soldiers serving in Vietnam viewed marijuana as more of a problem than narcotics and were able to abandon either with the same apparent ease.[17] Second, addiction to heroin did not compel addicts to increase their criminal activity in order to main-tain their suddenly more expensive habit. Conversely, supplying metha-done to heroin addicts did not reduce their criminal penchant, except for drug offenses, suggesting that their drug addiction and criminal behavior were not causally related; a prior deviant behavior was, as concluded the Vietnam study. Third, the Vietnam study convincingly refuted the notion that an addict is doomed for life, as popularized by the slogan *once an ad-dict always an addict* and by the notion that drugs "change the average per-son into a slavish addict whose entire existence revolves around his daily dosage."[15] Indeed, tens of thousands of U.S. servicemen in Vietnam, facing stern penalties for continuing to use illicit drugs, were able to give them up by themselves most often without treatment and without relapsing. Fourth, heroin addicts are not inexorably dependent on heroin, as it is alleged. In fact, in the summer of 1972 incarcerated heroin addicts switched to other il-licit drugs in order to ensure continuing pleasure. Conversely, many ad-dicts succeeded in freeing themselves from drugs by devoting themselves to a *normal* activity. For example, a study of 101 self-recovered addicts, after an average of six years of addiction and a seven-year average period of ab-stinence prior to study,[18] revealed that recovery was neither a spontaneous occurrence nor the outcome of a firm underlying resolve to abandon drugs, but a process triggered by a variety of motivations. Motivations ranged from the mundane, such as leaving a drug-using partner, to dramatic life crises when addicts face the uselessness of their own drug-driven lives. A common first step is a break with drugs and the drug scene and filling the void with a substitute endeavor, such as religion, family, work, and the like. For the most drug-dependent and socially cut off addicts, the substitution was crucial for it became their *lifeline,* though alcohol, marijuana, or tranquilizers were often used as a crutch to deal with interim craving. In contrast, addicts less immersed in drugs and those with a network of supportive relatives and friends found it easier to adapt because they were able to rebuild bridges to their own predrug lifestyle. However, completion of the process required addicts to also deal with the social stigma regardless of their drug-dependence level. "Gaining recognition and acceptance from the non-addict world often is a long and difficult process . . . [that requires perseverance in staying off drugs and in pursuing 'normal' activities that ultimately] enable non-addicts to trust the abstainer and, over time, to accept him and respond to him in 'ordinary' ways."[18] In turn, this gives the ex-addict sufficient self-confidence to complete the recovery process. Switching is not limited to illicit drugs and can lead to another addiction when misdirected. The classic example is weight gain following smoking cessation when cigarettes are substituted by food, further arguing against the inherent addictive power of drugs and in support of the view that addiction is behavioral, as discussed in the next chapter.

Unhappy with the IDA report, Nixon thought that, through a new scientific commission of carefully selected like-minded members, he could prove the link between marijuana and crime, despite the fact that neither the Advisory Committee on Drug Dependence and Cannabis of 1968 nor the Canadian LeDain Commission Report of 1970 had found such a link. Nixon appointed Governor Raymond P. Shafer of Pennsylvania, a former prosecutor known as a law and order governor, to head his Presidential Commission on Marijuana and Drug Abuse. The Commission included a congressman and a senator from each party and nine prominent citizens, including the dean of a law school, the head of a mental health hospital, and a retired Chicago police captain. Anticipating the Commission would rubber-stamp his views on marijuana, Nixon continued to denounce it in public speeches and in private conversations and was outraged when he learned his commission might disagree. Recently declassified Oval Office tapes from 1971–1972 reveal that he summoned Shafer to the White House and urged him: "Keep your Commission in line." He also warned him, "You see, the thing that is so terribly important here is that it not appear that the Commission's frankly just a bunch of do-gooders . . . [but] if you're just a bunch of do-gooders that are going to come out with a 'soft on marijuana' report, I'll destroy it right off the bat."[19] However, to his consternation and anger, in its 1972 *Marihuana: A Signal of Misunderstanding* report, the Commission called for decriminalization of marijuana. Its most compelling conclusion was, "The actual and potential harm of use of the drug is not great enough to justify intrusion by the criminal law into private behavior," and suggested "a social control policy seeking to discourage marihuana use, while concentrating primarily on the prevention of heavy and very heavy use."[20] It also recommended that the distinctions between licit and illicit drugs be abandoned, observing that "the use of drugs for pleasure or other non-medical purposes is not inherently irresponsible; alcohol is widely used as an acceptable part of social activities." Expectedly, harsh criticism arose from Nixon and conservative quarters, including Anslinger, who came out of oblivion to claim that enactment of the commission recommendations would result in "a million lunatics filling mental hospitals and a couple of hundred thousands more deaths on the highways."[5] The Nixon tapes also reveal that Nixon's paranoid ideation and bigotry led to a grossly distorted view of history. For instance, in his May 13, 1971, meeting with John Ehrlichman and H. R. Haldeman, he asserted that Aristotle, Socrates, and the last six Roman Emperors were gay, adding "po-po-Popes were laying the nuns, that's been going on for years, centuries . . . it was homosexual. And finally, it had to be cleaned out. Now, that's what's happened to Britain, it happened earlier to France." He concluded his diatribe stating, "You see, homosexuality, dope, immorality in general: These are the enemies of strong societies. That's why the Communists and the left-wingers are pushing the stuff, they're trying to destroy us."[21] Predictably, the Nixon administration ignored the Shafer Report, as it had previously ignored the IDA report, and continued to promote an atmosphere of fear of drugs that ensured congressional passage of extraordinary legislation and appropriations that launched the War on Drugs.

Under subsequent Democratic and Republican administrations, Nixon's antidrug crusade continued to expand and took a global scope. For instance, early in his administration Jimmy Carter (1977–1981) attempted to relax penalties for marijuana use, advising Congress that "penalties should not damage the user more than pot itself." However, his attempt failed in the face of fierce opposition from conservative detractors, parents' groups, opportunistic publications, and the law enforcement community eager to protect its turf. In fact, taking advantage of the outcry against President Carter's proposal, law enforcement was able to convince Congress to increase its War on Drugs budget. This episode suggests that opportunism and its very inability to control the illegal drug trade ensure the drug enforcement establishment's longevity and ever-increasing budgets.

Escalation of antidrug policies and budgets continued under President Ronald Reagan (1981–1989), whose moral conservative mind-set was not unlike President Nixon's and who viewed pot smoking as evidence of moral turpitude and social decay. Reagan emphasized a *zero tolerance* stance on drugs at every opportunity, including White House ceremonies, public speeches, and State of the Union addresses that culminated in the Anti-Drug Abuse Act of 1986. The Act mandated minimum sentences for drug offenses and different penalties for selling powder and crack cocaine. Reagan also signed into law the Anti-Drug Abuse Act of 1988, which created the

Office of National Drug Control Policy (ONDCP). Currently, the principal purpose of ONDCP is "to establish policies, priorities, and objectives for the Nation's drug control program. The goals of the program are to reduce illicit drug use, manufacturing, and trafficking, drug-related crime and violence, and drug-related health consequences."[22] To achieve his goals, Reagan enlisted "the Navy, the Coast Guard, the Customs Service, The IRS, and the U.S. Marshals Service as well as the DEA in his pot campaign."[5] The newly created White House Drug Policy Office, with Carlton Turner at the helm, involved the Forest Service and the Bureau of Land Management with the sole purpose of eradicating marijuana grown in national forests. It is of interest, though unsurprising, that Regan's Anti-Drug Abuse Acts were enacted on the heels of yet another scientific report titled *An Analysis of Marijuana Policy* (1982), conducted by the highly reputable National Acad emy of Sciences, which confirmed the failure of federal policy on drug control. It concluded, "The ineffectiveness of the present federal policy of complete prohibition falls far short of its goal:—preventing use . . . [hence] we believe that a policy of partial prohibition is clearly preferable . . . [though] Implementing such a policy . . . is unlikely to be effective in reducing marijuana use significantly below recent levels."[23] In a replay of Nixon's reaction to his own *Presidential Commission on Marijuana and Drug Abuse* report, Reagan dismissed the findings stating, "We are making no excuses for drugs—hard, soft, or otherwise. Drugs are bad and we are going after them."[5] In a newspaper interview, Turner suggested marijuana to be a *gateway* to homosexuality, prompting Newsweek to proclaim, "Reagan Aid: Pot can make you gay."[24]

Drug repression continued unabated under subsequent administrations, as were the customary distortions of the facts and the hypocrisy involved. For example, William Bennett, the drug *czar* under George H. W. Bush (1989–1993), was a habitual smoker and apparently a closet high-stakes gambler.[25] Ironically, he wrote about personal virtues in books titled *The Book of Virtues* and *The Moral Compass*, which became bestsellers. Bill Clinton's early presidency (1993–2001) seemed to take a more tolerant approach to drug policy, especially marijuana. However, his initial inclination was doomed by rising rates of marijuana use among youth, and soon, under General Jeffrey McCaffrey, his drug czar, the zero tolerance policy claimed more dollars, more arrests, more incarcerations, and longer sentences but no victories. Several additional drug policy initiatives were enacted between 1993 and 1997 that *"extended ONDCP's mission to assessing budgets and resources related to the National Drug Control Strategy"* and assigned it the responsibility of *"developing an outcome-measurement system."* The Reauthorization Act of 1998 gave the ONDCP additional responsibility over drug control policy and over its budget.[22] It is ironic, albeit tragic, that the president who did not *inhale* the marijuana he admittedly smoked in his youth presided over the arrest of 5,144,000 pot-smoking Americans during his eight-year tenure.[26] In fact, during the 1990s, marijuana possession accounted for 79% of the growth in drug arrests.[27] John P. Walters, George W.

Bush's (2001–2009) drug czar, expressed views on drugs that made General Jeffrey McCaffrey's and the President's own sound moderate. For example, Walters "urged Congress for a South American drug policy of shooting down planes suspected of transporting drugs,"[5] resulting in the downing of a plane carrying an American missionary in 2002. Likewise, in *An open letter to America's Prosecutors* dated November 1, 2002, Scott Burns, Deputy Director for State and Local Affairs of the ONDCP, urged them "to take a stand publicly and tell Americans the truth . . . [because] no drug matches the threat posed by marijuana."[28] His recycled old *truths* that marijuana is harmful, addictive, violence inducing, and a gateway to hard drugs ignored the fact that each claim was contrary to scientific evidence, as was his claim that legalization would be a *nightmare for America*. A critic of the War on Drugs, with broad experience as a judge of a state court of appeals, commented, "For Bush and Walters, the government's job is to save its citizens from hell."[5]

Today, "The principal purpose of ONDCP is to establish policies, priorities, and goals for the Nation's drug control program. To achieve this, ONDCP is charged with producing the National Drug Control Strategy (NDCS). The Strategy directs the Nation's anti-drug efforts and establishes a program, a budget, and guidelines for cooperation among Federal, State, and local entities."[29] Through fund allocations, the NDCS involves many U.S. Departments and agencies, at a cost of $13 billion in 2006 (Table 4).[30]

In its 2007 report, the NDCS claims, "The success of the President's National Drug Control Strategy demonstrates that a robust drug control policy can achieve measurable progress in reducing drug abuse."[31] However, in the next sentence it also acknowledges that after six years into the "President's first National Drug Control Strategy, a review of trends in drug use provides important *insights* [emphasis added] into what works in drug control." This is a meager outcome given the enormous effort and cost involved and the needless suffering imposed on large segments of the citizenry.

GLOBAL DRUG CONTROL: INTERNATIONAL CONVENTIONS

> Narcotics police are an enormous, corrupt international bureaucracy . . . and now fund a coterie of researchers who provide them with "scientific support" . . . fanatics who distort the legitimate research of others. . . . The anti-marijuana campaign is a cancerous tissue of lies, undermining law enforcement, aggravating the drug problem, depriving the sick of needed help, and suckering well-intentioned conservatives and countless frightened parents.
> —William F. Buckley, commentary in *The National Review*, April 29, 1983

Global drug control, initially the purview of the League of Nations, is now coordinated by the UNODC, which along with the International Narcotics Control Board (INCB), is under the United Nations Commission on Nar-

Table 4
Drug Control Funding by Agency, FY 2008 Enacted (Adapted from reference 30)

Department of Defense	1,177.4
Department of Education	431.6
Department of Health and Human Services	3,664.8
National Institute on Drug Abuse	*1,0007*
Substance Abuse and Mental Health Services Administration	*2,445.8*
Department of Homeland Security	3,550.1
Customs Border Protection	*2,130.9*
Immigration and Customs Enforcement	*412.3*
United States Coast Guard	*1,004.3*
Department of Justice	2,892.3
Bureau of Prisons	*67.2*
Drug Enforcement Administration	*2,105.3*
Interagency Crime and Drug Enforcement	*497.9*
Office of Justice Programs	*222.8*
ONDCP	421.7
Counterdrug Technology Assessment Center	*1.0*
High Intensity Drug Trafficking Area Program	*230.0*
Other Federal Drug Control Programs	*164.3*
Drug-Free Communities (non-add)	*90.0*
National Youth Anti-Drug Media Campaign (non-add)	*60.0*
Salaries and Expenses	*26.4*
Small Business Administration	1.0
Department of State	1,002.2
Bureau of International Narcotics and Law Enforcement Affairs	*640.8*
United States Agency for International Development	*361.4*
Department of Transportation (*Natl. Highway Traffic Safety Administration*)	2.7
Internal Revenue Service	57.3
Department of Veterans Affairs (*Veterans Health Administration*)	447.2
Total	13,655.4

Note: All figures are in millions of dollars.

cotics Drugs established in 1946. While the UNODC's primary mission is "to educate the world about the dangers of drug abuse and to strengthen international action against drug production, trafficking and drug-related crime through alternative development projects, illicit crop monitoring and anti-money laundering programmes,"[32] the INCB *monitors compliance with the provisions of the international drug control treaties.* Global drug control programs are based on three complementary and mutually supportive drug control treaties. The first, called Single Convention on Narcotic Drugs of 1961, or *Single Convention,* "aims to combat drug abuse by coordinated international action."[32] The second, called Convention on Psychotropic Substances of 1971, or *Psychotropics Convention,* "establishes an international control system for psychotropic substances."[32] The third, called Convention against the Illicit Traffic in Narcotic Drugs and Psychotropic Substances of 1988, or *Trafficking Convention,* "provides comprehensive measures against drug trafficking, including provisions against money laundering and the diversion of precursor chemicals."[32] The three conventions embody the efforts of global governments to cooperate in the field of drug abuse control and provide the framework and the necessary tools for UN member states to address drug production, trafficking, and abuse problems individually and collectively. The three conventions have been supplemented by many drug-related resolutions and decisions, added since 1946.[33]

As is the case for U.S. federal laws and the CSA, international drug control treaties emphasize the principle of maintaining a balance between controlling drug abuse and ensuring that controlled substances are available for medical use and research. To ensure achieving this balance in the United States, the CSA gives the DEA authority to set production quotas for a number of opioids, stimulants, and sedative hypnotics intended for medical use, a stipulation also included in international treaties. Global quotas are arrived at based on each UN member state's quarterly and annual statistical reports on the manufacture, use, import, and export of poppy-based medicines. Nothing in the international treaties should "interfere with ethical medical practice in this country as determined by the secretary of Health and Human Services on the basis of a consensus of the American medical and scientific community."[34] However, DEA policy hangs a Sword of Damocles over prescribing and taking opioids in the United States, and, according to the INCB "most developing countries lack the resources and expertise required for determining medical needs and adjusting drug supply to meet those needs."[35] Hence, on the one hand there is a pain management crisis in the United States despite adequate supplies of opioids, and on the other hand the vast majority of pain-suffering patients in underdeveloped countries have no access to opiates. For example, 7.1 metric tons of morphine were needed in 2005 to adequately treat "end-stage HIV/AIDS and cancer patients in Latin America, but just 600 kg of morphine was actually used, leaving 91% of these patients' pain needs un-met."[35] Likewise, in 1978, the U.S. Congress reaffirmed the principle that the availability of controlled substances *"for useful and legitimate medical and scientific purposes will not be unduly restricted."* However, most American state laws do not achieve this balance. That imbalance and DEA policy implementation tactics interfere with medical practice and with pain management, in clear violation and defiance of congressional intent, is described in chapter 5.

As of July 2007, 140 UN member states out of the current 192 are signatories to each of the three conventions on drug control. Of the 15 East Asia states, 12 are parties to the 1961 convention, 11 are parties to the 1971 convention, and 7 are parties to the 1988 convention.[36] In compliance with the legally binding provisions of the conventions, signatory states assume the responsibility of developing and implementing drug control policies at home and of cooperating with each other and with UN bodies. Hence, public policy is often at odds with public opinion, as is the case in several European countries that favor relaxation of drug laws, drug decriminalization (removal of a conduct from the sphere of criminal law), or depenalization (relaxation of the penal sanctions).[8] However, drug policy changes would require amending international drug control treaties or a unilateral action by a member state, which would be quickly challengeable. For example, when Portugal drafted a law reclassifying drug possession for personal use as an administrative rather than a criminal offense, the INCB opposed the change. It informed Portugal that its action was "not in line with international drug control treaties, which require that drug use be limited to medical and scientific purposes and that States parties make drug possession a criminal offence."[37] In extremis, a signatory state could repeal its adherence to the treaties. However, "unilateral withdrawal from these Treaties would be a very difficult task because like most international treaties they are dominated by political groupings (in particular the United States) which will not, as yet, sanction rational, evidence-based changes in the ways in which the international illicit drug market is regulated. Such constraints make innovation difficult (as experienced by the Dutch) and rational debate elusive."[38] Indeed, any hope for amending international drug treaties requires leadership by American policy makers, whose decisions seem to follow the motto *don't confuse me with the facts; my mind is already made up.* As a result, "criminal law is a 'one-way ratchet': it expands but does not contract."[39]

In the European Union, drug policy is not harmonized, it falls under the responsibility of individual member states, and it ranges from stern to lenient. For instance, while simple use is considered a criminal offense in 7 out of 25 member states (Cyprus, France, Finland, Greece, Luxembourg, Sweden, and Norway), it is handled as an administrative offense in 4 (Estonia, Spain, Latvia, and Portugal).[40] Recent legislation in Belgium, France, Luxemburg, and Portugal have downgraded penalties for personal use. In the Netherlands, a country perceived to have the most liberal drug laws, drug policy is based on two principles: hard drugs (e.g., heroin) are distinguished from soft ones (e.g., cannabis), and drug use is considered a health, not a criminal matter. While under the Dutch *Opium Law,* possession of any drug is punishable; article 11(5) provides that no penalties shall be applied when the quantities of hashish or marijuana in a person's possession do not exceed 5 grams. Moreover, sale, possession, and use of cannabis in coffee shops are not liable to prosecution if the coffee shop does not advertise, sell hard drugs, cause public nuisance, sell to minors, or sell more than 5 grams per person per transaction. The Dutch *Gedoogbeleid* (policy of tolerance), which permits limited and controlled use of marijuana, is designed to depenalize possession and use of soft drugs while also complying with the letter of international drug control treaties.[38,40]

In contrast, the United States has the most repressive drug laws with mandatory penalties, often more severe and lengthier than sentences imposed for the more reprehensible crimes of rape and murder. According to the Sentencing Project, "changes in sentencing law and policy, not increases in crime rates, explain most of the six-fold increase in the national prison population."[41] In fact, incarcerated drug offenders have increased from approximately 40,000 in 1980 to over half a million in 2008, an increase of 1,100%. The following are some of the grim statistics.[42-44] In 2003, the conviction rate (92%) of drug offenders was comparable to that of perpetrators of violent crimes (91%) and of weapons offenses (92%), as was the average length of their sentences (81.4, 97.2, and 83.7 months, respectively).[43,44] Moreover, because in any given year most federal arrests are drug-related, 42.3% of federal inmates at yearend 2003 were drug offenders compared to 5.8% and 6.1% for violent and weapons offenders, respectively.[45] Other incarceration imbalances involve race and education. For instance, 29.6% of federal inmates in 2003 were African Americans, who represented only 19% of the U.S. population, and only 32.0% of them were high school graduates,[46] whereas 80% of African Americans graduated that year.[47] This federal skewed emphasis on drugs applies at the state and local levels. Indeed, out of 14,094,186 Americans arrested in 2005, a staggering 4.7% of the total U.S. population, the largest number (1,846,351) was for drug violations, including 786,500 for marijuana offenses,[26] of which 81.7% was for simple possession.[41] At the end of that year, 2,320,359 Americans were inmates of federal, state, or local prisons. In fact, with 5% of the world population, the United States accounts for 25% of its prisoners. The U.S. Department of Justice said it best in a November 30, 2006, press release; "One in every 32 adults was in prison, jail, or probation, or on parole at the end of 2005."[48] These grim statistics led Humans Rights Watch to conclude, "Putting a person behind bars is so common in the United States and so frequently imposed for minor conduct that it seems the country has lost sight of just how serious a punishment imprisonment is."[49]

In conclusion, the Prohibition era had not yet ended when clamors were already being heard, mostly from the same players, that the new *scourge* of opium and related drugs were destroying American society. The obvious questions are: Why were failed antialcohol policies recycled to combat other mind-altering drugs? What motivates detractors to propose and implement policies to curtail a particular social conduct while others are allowed, independently of their impact on society? Why does society acquiesce to such policies? Why do such policies endure once shown to have failed and been counterproductive? While addressing these issues in detail is the domain of scholars in social and political sciences with greater expertise than my own, a few pertinent thoughts might be helpful. First, it is well documented throughout history that some people do not conform to majority rule or test the legally imposed limits of freedom. Within this group, there are those whose unconventional behavior is objected by the majority. Under such circumstances, objectors' hasty reaction is to stigmatize the behavior, demonize perpetrators, and gather political support to criminalize the objectionable act and demonize the perpetrators. This is especially the case when the targeted activity is easy to stigmatize as being an *out of mainstream* practice of a minority, especially foreigners, dissidents, the poor, the illiterate, and the underprivileged and disenfranchised who do not conform to the moral beliefs or social standards of the majority. Essentially, it amounts to identifying and targeting scapegoats for unrelated societal problems that serves to reinforce a sentiment of self-righteousness or absolve and release inner feelings of inadequacy or guilt.

By portraying a certain category of drugs as *evil, sinful, a plague,* and other intensely evocative names, they became detractors' quintessential targets despite causing less harm to self and society than either alcohol or tobacco. That is, because the recreational use of some drugs by a minority is objectionable to the majority, they were outlawed despite evidence of nonharm to self and society, and since then, users and suppliers are stigmatized and persecuted. In contrast, while tens of thousands of Americans are injured and die in traffic accidents each year, few would advocate banning driving or cars because some drivers drive recklessly or under the influence of mind-altering drugs, potentially endangering themselves and others. For instance, 2.4 million Americans motorists were injured in traffic accidents in 2005, resulting in 33,041 deaths,[50] including 16,885 alcohol-related (or 39%)[50,51] and 7,054 drug-related (or 18%).[52] That leaves 16,897 deaths (or 43%) caused by sober drivers presumably in full control of their mental faculties. The proper response to this carnage on the roadways, adopted in most countries, is to penalize reckless driving whether associated with DUI or DUI-drugs (DUI of drugs), or with neither, rather than outlawing cars. The antidrugs paranoia is such that while penalties for DUI and DUI-drugs are similar in the United States,[53] the DUI penalty does not increase if alcohol is found in the driver's possession whereas drug possession would add a 5-year minimum jail sentence to a first DUI-drugs offender[53] and a possible lifelong incarceration for a recidivist.

As previously described, while self-righteous groups initiated the antialcohol crusade that led to Prohibition, President Nixon spearheaded the antidrug demonization campaign that set in motion the War on Drugs, fulfilling German philosopher Georg Friedrich Hegel's *thesis-antithesis-synthesis* road to power. It consists of deliberately contriving a social problem (*thesis*) and devising a solution (*antithesis*), which leads to the ultimate goal of acquiring more power and control (*synthesis*).[54] Thanks to well-orchestrated disinformation campaigns, both the antialcohol and antidrug movements gained substantial support from large segments of society aided by politicians who, recognizing their ideological, rhetorical, and political usefulness, seized them as their own, misrepresenting facts when needed to fit their political agenda. However, unlike alcohol and tobacco, which are strongly promoted and fiercely protected by powerful lobbies and generate substantial tax revenues for federal, state, and local governments, antidrug campaigns are lobby-orphan, tax-devoid, and nonpartisan issues all politicians can agree and politically afford to support, regardless of their ideological persuasions, accounting for the latter's longevity and the former's early repeal. Moreover, failure to support policies alleged to protect *innocent children* from the *evils* of drugs would amount to political suicide. Hence, after demonization by the Nixon White House came the rhetoric by politicians who outdid and continue to outdo each other depicting the real, imagined, or fictitious *evils* associated with drug use, and portray themselves as *tough on drugs* to please their activist antidrug constituencies. Never mind that numerous American and foreign scientific studies on the effects of drugs conducted between 1894 and 1982 have all disputed or dismissed the vast majority of presumed ill effects of drugs on users and their relationship to crime claimed by supporters of the War on Drugs. Advocates use disinformation, hollow rhetoric, and suggestive clichés in lieu of valid arguments for enacting ever-more punitive antidrug laws and funding ever-expanding antidrug law enforcement, prison infrastructure, and support personnel; all claimed essential to build a utopian *drug-free America.*

This massive governmental infrastructure and the legion of supporting ancillary industries (e.g., training, research, and the like) accumulated over nearly a century of drug prohibition policies is fed by billions of dollars that reward all involved, buy their acquiescence if not their silence, limit debate, and perpetuate the *status quo.* In the meantime the drug-free America, as noble a goal as the one that inspired Prohibition, requires the incarceration of thousands of petty offenders, fosters crime resulting mainly from the criminalization of drugs, and victimizes tens of millions of American pain sufferers. Moreover, in waging its worldwide War on Drugs, the United States has set aside considerations of decency, human rights, and morality enshrined in its constitution and the foundation of its social fabric. Examples include American cooperation with an assortment of dubious regimes around the world, including Mujahideen warlords, Panama's Manuel Noriega, Peru's Alberto Fujimori, Cuba's Fidel Castro, and Burma's military junta, among others. "Such collusion reflects the frustration and desperation [and cynic disregard for the law] of U.S. officials as they have sought to stem the flow of illegal drugs into the United States decade after decade without meaningful, lasting success."[55] To these we must add CIA's involvement, directly or indirectly, in drug dealings in Southeast Asia and Colombia to fund its covert wars against the Marxist regimes of North Vietnam and El Salvador.[56,57]

While drug criminalization and user demonization began in the United States, the movement spread globally as leaders and politicians worldwide recognized the political bonanza associated with antidrug crusades. In fact, drug prohibition was one of the few issues on which capitalist and socialist democracies, German Nazis and Italian Fascists, Communist USSR and China, Latin American dictatorships and anticolonialist Africa could all agree. Moreover, prompted by the United States, the UN forcefully spread and now supervises worldwide drug prohibition, giving antidrug policies legitimacy worldwide and a staying power strengthened by legally binding international conventions that effectively dictate drug policies of 140 signatory countries. Although well intentioned, the UN's current goal of a *drug-free world* is as unrealistic and unachievable as it is inane. In the meantime, the clamor for change is mounting, as evidenced by the voluminous amount of literature arising from a broad ideological spectrum that decries the abject failure of drug policy and condemns the crime and corruption it causes at home and abroad. However, meaningful change will require the emergence of strong leadership from American policy makers with sufficient fortitude and resilience or pressure from an informed electorate to dismantle national and international policies that have raised havoc the world over for several decades and replace them by sound evidence-driven strategies. In the absence of central political leadership and given the expected legislative paralysis in this regard, several state and regional grassroots initiatives are slowly filling the vacuum. For instance, between 2004 and 2006, over half a dozen states initiated or expanded drug treatment programs and other alternatives to incarceration. Perhaps the most revealing grassroots movement was Arizona's Proposition 200, named the Drug Medicalization, Prevention, and Control Act of 1996. The initiative called for probation and treatment for new nonviolent drug offenders instead of incarceration, parole for those already in prison, and for doctors to be allowed to prescribe schedule I drugs. The initiative was approved by 65% of voters, despite fierce opposition by the Governor, the state legislature, the congressional delegation, the DEA, and by President Clinton. Emboldened by such broad-based political support, the Arizona legislature overturned most of the initiative the following year, but voters reversed the changes in subsequent referendums, making it more difficult for legislators to tamper with future voter-approved initiatives. Recent budgetary constraints, aggravated by the 2008 financial crisis, and an awareness that enforcing drug policy overwhelms courts, overcrowds prisons, and diverts dwindling human and financial resources away from real crime, seem to signal a more liberal future drug policy. For instance, in August 2009, Mexico decriminalized possession of small amounts of all drugs in order to concentrate its resources on traffickers, and the Argentine Supreme Court declared unconstitutional that country's law criminalizing drug possession.

In the United States, personal use of marijuana is legal in 14 states (Alaska, California, Colorado, Hawaii, Maine, Maryland, Michigan, Montana, Nevada, New Mexico, Oregon, Rhode Island, Vermont, and Washington), and its cultivation permitted in three (New Mexico, Rhode Island, and Massachusetts). While users in these states are in defiance of federal law and subject to arrest and incarceration, the Obama administration announced on October 19, 2009 that they would no longer be federally prosecuted as long as they conform to state laws. In Europe, seven countries decriminalized drug use, placing it and addiction in the realm of health care rather than under criminal law. Yet, when Professor David Nutt, head of the UK's Advisory Council on the Misuse of Drugs, suggested based on empirical evidence that alcohol was more harmful than cannabis, LSD, and ecstasy, and that the latter was no more risky than riding horses, each claiming a few deaths each year, he was sacked by his country's home secretary.[58] Politicians' dismissal of studies refuting claims of drug harm and links to crime, political opposition to Arizona's proposition 200, INCB's resistance to the relaxation of drug laws by some European countries, and the dichotomy between science and politics in the drug policy debate underlying Professor Nutt's sacking underscore the difficulties that lie in the path of overturning drug policy. However, it will be done. Indeed, as we will learn in subsequent chapters, reform proposals to date, while modest and tentative, are an implicit admission that criminal law is inappropriate to address drug possession and use and an evolving recognition that education and treatment are sensible, less expensive, and more effective responses to what constitutes a nonconforming or deviant behavior rather than a criminal act.

PART II

Medical Aspects
of Mind-Altering Drugs

CHAPTER 4

Current Theories of Addiction

The aim of the wise is not to secure pleasure, but to avoid pain.
—Aristotle (384 B.C.E.–322 B.C.E.)

The term *addiction* derives from the Latin *addicere,* meaning *bound to* or *enslaved by;* a term and meaning that have become synonymous with impaired control over substance use, though non–substance-related disorders are increasingly included as well. Today, the definition of addiction is as varied as the personal or professional interests or biases of its authors. English and medical dictionaries define addiction broadly as a "persistent compulsive use of a substance known by the user to be harmful,"[1] a "psychological or physiological dependence on a drug,"[2] or "the loss of control over drug use, or the compulsive seeking and taking of drug regardless of the consequences."[3] In these and in most common definitions, the recurring theme is still *drug* or *substance,* reflecting a prevailing mindset that explains the focus of current research being centered on drug–brain interactions and viewing addiction as a brain disease. In a broader sense, addiction has been defined as, "a recurring compulsion . . . often reserved for drugs but . . . sometimes applied to other compulsions, such as problem gambling and compulsive overeating."[4,5] However, using words such as *problem* to define addiction adds confusion, though professional organizations' definitions might not be clearer. For instance, the American Psychiatric Association's *Diagnostic and Statistical Manual of Mental Disorders* (4th edition) includes, not the specific term *addiction* but the categories of *Substance Use Disorders, Impulse Control Disorders,* and *Obsessive Compulsive Disorders.* These disorders share some features, including impulsivity and impaired control over use, and it has been suggested that certain impulse control disorders such as compulsive gambling, compulsive shopping, compulsive computer use, and compulsive sexual behaviors are "behavioral addictions or addictions without the drug,"[6] implying that drug addiction is not the only *real* addiction and that all are behavioral.[7] Likewise, the WHO *International Classification of Diseases and Related Health Problems* lists impulse control disorders under "Habit and Impulse Disorders"[8] and includes drug abuse under *Dependence Syndrome*. It defines the latter as "a cluster of behavioural, cognitive, and physiological phenomena that develop after repeated substance use and that typically include a strong desire to take the drug, difficulties in controlling its use, persisting in its use despite harmful consequences, a higher priority given to drug use than to other activities and obligations, increased tolerance, and sometimes a physical withdrawal state."[8] This bewildering array of classifications and definitions of compulsive, impaired use control, reward-seeking behaviors that interfere with major areas of life functioning compound their understanding and management.

Theories on the causes of addiction have been based on moral, biological, sociological, psychological, and social learning models, among many others. Consequently, addiction is said to be the domain of the police officer, the neurobiologist, the psychiatrist, the social worker, the priest, or the policy maker depending on the proponents' points of view. Each stance can affect the income and fate of professionals and organizations engaged in addiction prevention, control, or treatment and the type of support offered to or punishment imposed on addicts. While it is not my purpose to reconcile these viewpoints through a *grand unifying theory*, I subscribe to the view that they can be reduced to two opposing camps: the *disease* vs. the *behavioral* model advocates. In addition to identifying the two core themes underlying all theories and definitions of addiction, these opposite views carry profound clinical, policymaking, and legal implications. Advocates of the *disease* model view addicts as *victims* of an alleged defective neurocircuitry implicated in drug abuse hence promote the development and use of drugs as the basis for its management. On the other hand, proponents of the *behavioral* model consider addiction a *choice* and promote behavior modification methods as the most suitable means to treat substance and non–substance abuse behaviors, at best, or incarceration, at worst. These two diverging views of addiction have divided the scientific community and the public at large to the point that each has become a dogma and, as such, a nonnegotiable polarizing issue to its proponents. In the next few pages, I examine the pros and cons of each model.

THE DISEASE (VICTIM) MODEL

Although references to drunkenness as a disease can be found in ancient Egyptian and Greek writings, Scottish physician Thomas Trotter (1760–1832) is credited as the first to characterize excessive drinking as a disease in mod-

ern times. In America, drunkenness continued to be viewed as a condition
that bridged morality and medicine. For instance, in his "Inquiry into the effects of ardent spirits on the human mind and body,"[9] American physician
Benjamin Rush (1745–1813), considered the *father of American psychiatry*, introduced the idea that the loss of control characteristic of alcoholism was a disease *induced by vice* but caused by the *inherent properties* of alcohol. Likewise,
in his "Six Sermons on the Nature, Occasions, Signs, Evils, and Remedy of
Intemperance,"[10] reverend Lyman Beecher referred to *intemperance* as a *sin*,
an *evil habit*, and *a disease as well as a crime*. However, of greater interest is
Dr. William Sweetser's 1829 insightful argument that "intemperance is a disease produced and maintained by voluntary acts, which is a very different
thing from a disease with which providence inflicts us, though one that
causes a morbid alteration of the body." This view would be resurrected in
support of the disease theory of addiction over a century later, as discussed
later. Likewise, doctor Samuel Woodward described *intemperance* as a
"physical disease which preys upon health and spirits . . . making him a willing slave to his appetite."[11] He also believed that heredity played a role in
drunkenness. Swedish Physician Magnus Huss (1807–1890), who considered the condition as a chronic, relapsing disease, first coined the term *alcoholism*, in 1849.

Hence, the disease concept of alcoholism was already taking shape in the
middle of the 19th century, including the features of impaired control, craving, tolerance, and a presumed predisposition to drinking. Its biological, psychological, and social consequences also were being recognized. However,
New York–born E. Morton Jellinek (1890–1963) was to propel the *science of
alcoholism*, and the disease theory of alcoholism and by extension of drugs
of abuse, to center stage. Jellinek's father, a Hungarian, had taken his family
back to Budapest when young Jellinek was a preschool boy. From his sister's
account[11] we know that he first served as a captain in the Hungarian Red
Cross in World War I before going bankrupt as a currency speculator. He re-
appeared in 1920 working for a steamship line in Sierra Leone under the
name of Nikita Hartmann, then as a banana researcher in Honduras for the
United Fruit Company, before becoming a biostatistician at Worcester State
Hospital in Massachusetts in 1931. In 1939, age 50, he was hired to manage an
alcohol study called the Carnegie Project. According to his sister, he "knew
very little about alcoholism but he was interested so he got some books on
the subject and spent a weekend in bed studying."[12] Jellinek devoted the rest
of his life to the field and earned the respect and admiration of his peers, who
were unaware that he had fabricated his degrees. Indeed, his claim to a Doctor of Science degree from the short-lived University of Tegucigalpa in Honduras was never substantiated, and the *honorary* prefix of a Doctor of Science
degree he claimed the University of Leipzig bestowed upon him soon disappeared from his publications. Yet, he became an Associate Professor of
Applied Physiology at Yale University (1941 to 1952) and subsequently a
consultant on alcoholism to the WHO in Geneva. In 1958, he joined the

psychiatry departments of the Universities of Toronto and Alberta, and in 1962, he moved to Stanford University, where he died a year later.

Because alcohol was the most obvious drug of abuse in Jellinek's time and often ran in families, genetics was suggested as a possible cause, though, according to this criterion, child abuse and religion that also run in families would qualify as addictions. In attempts to separate environmental from genetic factors, cohort studies of adopted children from alcoholic parents were compared to adopted children from nonalcoholic families. Some studies suggested a three- to four-fold increased incidence of alcoholism among the former.[13,14] However, such studies failed to account for nongenetic factors (e.g., ethnicity) that impact incidence rates and could not explain how alcoholism is *inherited*. Subsequently, the focus shifted to the search for predisposing factors that confer the bearer an *inherited vulnerability* to alcoholism rather than a *predetermined alcoholic destiny*. Some of the metabolic defects claimed to predispose to alcoholism included: an inability of alcoholics to discriminate blood alcohol levels, which presumably leads to lesser effects from alcohol and to increased drinking;[15] an altered alcohol metabolism associated with higher levels of acetaldehyde and related symptoms and with decreased drinking;[15] or an aberrant brain circuitry that reinforces drinking.[16] For instance, a mutant ALDH-2 gene protein that metabolizes acetaldehyde, a product of alcohol elimination, reduces its tissue accumulation, inducing flushing, dizziness, and nausea, which is thought to reduce the risk of alcoholism in carriers. Indeed, approximately 50% of Asians born with this mutant gene drink less than their normal counterparts even after migrating to the United States, suggesting that genetics might be the stronger predisposing influence in that population. However, children of immigrant Asian Americans drink more than their parents, and the generational difference in drinking level is greater than that observed between carriers of the mutant and of the normal ALDH-2 gene. These findings conclusively prove that the drinking behavior of first generation Asian Americans is impacted more by environmental factors than by heredity. Likewise, sensitivity to blood alcohol levels, variations in alcohol metabolism, and abnormal brain circuitry in response to alcohol intake do not predict or correlate with alcoholism,[17] nor do they differentiate the occasional or social alcohol user from an alcohol-dependent individual.

Another interesting historical episode on the presumed inheritance of deviant behavior is associated with Cesare Lombroso's now discredited theories described in his influential book *l'Uomo delinquente*[18] (the delinquent man). Born in Verona in 1835, Lombroso studied medicine in Pavia, Padua, Vienna, and Genoa and taught legal medicine and public hygiene at the University of Turin. His interest in psychology and psychiatry along with his studies on brain anatomy and physiology ultimately led to his anthropometric (the study of the measurement and proportions of the human body) analysis of criminals and the mentally disturbed. Years of postmortem examinations and anthropometric studies of criminals, the insane, and normal individuals convinced Lombroso that, contrary to the prevailing view, crime was a characteristic of human nature. He proposed the existence of the *reo nato* (born criminal) that was anatomically identifiable by certain physical stigmata (a mark or characteristic of a disease or an abnormality), such as a sloping forehead, handle-shaped ears, high cheekbones, hawk-like noses or fleshy lips, prognatism (a forward projecting of the lower jaw), and excessively long arms. These physical features, he thought, indicated a throwback to a primitive form of humans whose behavior was inevitably contrary to the rules and expectations of modern civilized society. Not unlike some of today's researchers who seem convinced of the genetic basis of addiction, he reluctantly admitted the influence of the environment in the etiology of crime but continued to believe in the predominant role of *predisposing* organic and genetic factors. While Lombroso's notions gained many adepts throughout Europe, they were eventually discredited by Charles Goring in his book *The English Convict*, published in 1913, where he documented that anatomical differences found in criminals were minimal at best.

Since the decade of the 1960s, when illicit drugs began their ascent, addiction has become synonymous with drug abuse, and its study expanded to include neuroscientists, molecular biologists, pharmacologists, psychologists, geneticists, and even circadian rhythm (recurrent biological patterns claimed to influence drug efficacy, behavior, etc.) theorists. Inevitably, each discipline brings a special one-dimensional approach and conclusions to the study of addiction that confounds the understanding of this highly complex issue involving behaviors that transcend drug abuse. For example, it has been suggested that, "all drugs of abuse converge on a common circuitry in the brain limbic system . . . [especially] the ventral tegmental area (TVA) of the midbrain . . . [and]. their target in the nucleus accumbens (NAc). The VTA-NAc pathway is one the most important substrates for the acute rewarding effects of all drugs of abuse . . . [though] additional brain areas that interact with the VTA and NAc are also essential for acute drug reward and chronic changes associated with addiction."[19] From study results such as this, it is concluded that addiction is "a chronic, relapsing brain disease . . . because drugs change the brain . . . and can lead to the harmful behaviors seen in people who abuse drugs."[4] However, even if drugs of abuse change brain chemistry, reinforcing the reward circuitry that perpetuates the cycle of addiction, the question remains: what leads someone to use drugs in the first place? That is, what is first: behavior affecting the brain or brain changes that affect behavior? Likewise, if drugs *change the brain,* why is the vast majority of drug use transient and sporadic, and why can most drug abusers who *choose to quit* do so, more often than not, without third-party assistance? In fact, no neurocircuits or neurotransmitters can compel anyone to abuse drugs for even the most drug-centered and self-destructive addicts retain a certain degree of control on how much drug they take at any given time, keeping some supply for the next *high.* Moreover, neurocircuitry and chemical reward theories of addiction are unable to account for the wide spectrum of addiction, ranging from

not only licit or illicit drugs, prescription medications, and chemical products, but extending to non–substance-based activities such as gambling and
others that are normal, ordinary, and nonaddictive for most people, such
as drinking coffee, eating, and having sex. Hence, addiction is linked to the
individual, not to any intrinsic *addictive property* of the substance or activity
abused or its effect on the brain. Furthermore, the suggestion that the VTA-
NAc pathway also mediates "the acute positive emotional effects of natural
rewards such as food, sex, and social interactions"[19] does not validate viewing addicts as victims of their brain chemistry.

These arguments suggest that drug-receptor interactions theorized as the
underlying mechanism for a self-reinforcing *reward* pathway blamed for
addiction are at best simplistic, for they reduce behavior to simple neurobio-
chemical processes excluding free choice as a factor, or at worst seek to support preconceived notions intended to absolve drug abusers of responsibility.
In fact, the reward pathway is an evolutionary brain circuit that reinforces
behavior that makes us feel good and ensures our survival. Moreover, no
brain pathways or neurotransmitters need be discovered to confirm what
daily living teaches us: experiences are sought after if enjoyable and avoided
if unpleasant. Seeking to recreate pleasurable experiences is a normal and common reaction of all living creatures from the lowest of worms to rodents to
humans and is therefore incidental to the deviant and often self-destructing
abuse behavior we call addiction. The issue is not whether seeking pleasurable experiences is reinforced through a reward pathway, which it is, but
what factors underlie the type of impaired control behavior that initially
leads to drug seeking and later to compulsive use. In short, because chemical rewards have no power to dictate human behavior, the key question is
what leads some casual users to become addicted whereas the vast majority
doesn't; a pivotal step that neurobiologists cannot explain. Simply put, *our
brains do not make us do it*. Likewise, theorizing that opiates and other drugs
of abuse are inherently addictive or that repeated exposure will inevitably
lead to addiction, while ingrained in popular folklore, have no scientific
basis. Indeed, some of the *most addictive* drugs of abuse induce tolerance
and withdrawal symptoms (e.g., heroin), some induce one but not the other
(e.g., cocaine, fentanyl), and others induce neither (e.g., Levo-Alpha Acetyl
Methadol), suggesting that these properties are not central to addiction as it
is claimed. Moreover, the notion that certain drugs are inherently addictive
ignores solid medical evidence, including: the rarity of addiction among
the millions of Americans taking narcotics round-the-clock for months to
years for pain relief;[20-22] the low rate of addiction among casual drug users,
most of whom eventually give up the habit; and the major drop off into
illicit drugs initiation after age 29.[23] Finally, few would consider ordinary
foodstuff as inherently addictive. Yet, it is undeniable that many individuals
with *compulsive eating disorder* are in fact addicted.

Yet, a most forceful and influential proponent of the disease theory of addiction is the National Institute on Drug Abuse (NIDA), the Federal agency

whose mission is *to lead the Nation in bringing the power of science to bear on drug abuse and addiction*, which it does by steering research on addiction through selective allocation of funds. It defines addiction("as a chronic, relapsing brain disease that is characterized by compulsive drug seeking and use, despite harmful consequences. It is considered a brain disease because drugs change the brain—they change its structure and how it works. These brain changes can be long lasting, and can lead to the harmful behaviors seen in people who abuse drugs."[5] In an August 2007 online educational presentation, the NIDA likened drug addiction to several common *somatic* (related to the body) diseases on the basis that they all exhibit genetic and behavioral components and are not self-inflicted. In that presentation, the claim is made that "Addiction, like heart disease, cancers, and type II diabetes, is a real and complex disease . . . no one chooses to be a drug addict or to develop heart disease . . . sometimes people do choose behaviors that have undesirable effects . . . addictive behaviors have clearly implicated both environmental and genetic influences."[4] These analogies were carefully chosen to convey a sense that if heart disease, cancers, and type II diabetes are acknowledged diseases, despite being the unintended outcome of poor lifestyle choices (e.g., overeating, a sedentary lifestyle, and cigarette smoking, in the case of lung cancer), addiction must also be classified as a disease. The parallel appears strengthened by invoking a genetic link based on the proposition that Apolipoprotein-E (a protein involved in heart disease) and the μ-opioid receptor contribute to heart disease and heroin addiction, respectively. However, the comparison is inappropriate because there is no such a thing as cancer or heart disease but a diverse group of over 200 cancers and a plethora of heart diseases caused or contributed to by factors as diverse as heredity and behavior or lifestyle. Examples include hereditary nonpolyposis colorectal cancer (a type of colon and rectum cancer) and hypertrophic cardiomyopathy (familial thickening of the heart muscle). Examples of behavior- and lifestyle-related diseases include tobacco-induced lung cancer and atherosclerosis (plaques within arteries, commonly know as *hardening* of arteries) linked to obesity. Moreover, the comparison would remain disingenuous even if it were limited to behavior- or lifestyle-related heart diseases and cancers, as it steers the reader's attention toward the potential *outcome* of addictive behavior rather than its causes. The appropriate comparison should be between heavy smoking and heavy drug use, both being addictions albeit to products arbitrarily placed on opposite sides of the law; or between lung cancer and HIV infection, both being *disease outcomes* often associated with the *addictive behavior* of smoking and IV drug use, respectively. Similarly, overeating to the point of developing long-term health consequences, including morbid obesity, atherosclerosis, type II diabetes, or colon cancer, is also a form of addiction albeit one not yet sanctioned by the politically correct medical establishment or acknowledged by the public(To assert that addiction is a disease because drug users do not intend to become addicts is as ludicrous as claiming that heavy smoking is a disease because smokers don't plan to develop lung cancer. Smoking, overeating, and drug abuse are all addictions albeit with a different focus; the major difference being that the latter has been made into an illicit behavior. Likewise, to claim that the very existence of μ-opioid brain receptors proves or supports the genetic basis of heroin addiction is tantamount to suggesting that the human brain evolved such a receptor in anticipation of its usefulness as a mediator of heroin addiction centuries later. In fact, the term *opioid receptor* derives from neurobiological studies on narcotics[24] and is unrelated to the primary function of a receptor humans share with mice, rats, bullfrogs, chicken, cattle, and several fish species,[25] suggesting an evolutionary function that certainly transcends addiction. Finally, it has been reported that, "genetic variants of the μ-opioid receptor OPRM1 play a role in pain perception and in the susceptibility to substance abuse."[26] However, susceptibility does not mean inevitability, and subscribing to this claim requires believing that, out of tens of millions of pain-suffering patients taking opioids on a daily basis for pain relief, only 0.03% of them are endowed with this variant receptor and become addicted;[20–22] an unlikely proposition indeed.

Sorting out the specific and individual effects of a multitude of factors impacting addictive, compulsive, or obsessive behavior, and indeed any human behavior, is a highly complex, uncertain, and daunting process. Moreover, limitations in the tools available for study; flaws in the design, methodology, analysis, or conclusions of many studies; and the mindset and preconceptions of many addiction researchers are further impediments in the search for reliable answers. For instance, the authors of a recent study of the possible genetic bases of nicotine dependence and abstinence concluded "the ability to abstain from nicotine has polygenic genetic components that overlap, in part, with those that contribute to vulnerability to nicotine dependence."[27] In essence, the set of genes that predispose you to smoke also predispose you not to smoke! Hence, this study supports the view that to smoke or not to smoke is the result not of genes but of a conscientious decision—a choice—made by the smoker, albeit one that is influenced by a multitude of psychological, familial, social, environmental, and genetic factors, as are all human decisions. Similarly, a study report on the role of genetics in human sexuality claimed having found the *gay gene.*[28] Given its social, political, legal, and eugenics (the science of improving genetic characteristics) implications, the report and its lead gay author became highly controversial. The report identified a genetic marker in region 28 of the long or "q arm of the X chromosome" (the female gene), shared by 33 (or 83%) of the 40 pairs of homosexual, nontwin brothers in which both members of each pair were gay and concluded that male homosexuality is X-linked. The Xq 28 marker, not itself a gene, is now known as *GAY-1.* The report was initially hailed as the scientific foundation that supported prior claims of inherited sexual orientation. Such claims were based mainly on a prior study showing midbrain size differences of homosexual young men and on several studies showing concordance (sameness with regard to a particular characteristic) in homosexual rates among monozygotic (arising from a single ovum) twins raised apart (100% concordance indicates a 100% inheritance). However, none of these studies are conclusive. First, many of the studied homosexuals with smaller midbrains died of acquired immune deficiency syndrome (AIDS), a condition that affects the brain. Second, concordance rates in identical male twin studies ranged between 0% and 100%, suggesting flaws in subject selection or in the design, implementation, or interpretation of such studies. Finally, a linkage between homosexuality and the Xq 28 region was not confirmed in a careful study of 52 gay male sibling pairs.[29] In contrast to claims that link certain deviant behaviors to hypothetical genetic causes, there are approximately 4,000 diseases directly linked to chromosomal changes or gene mutations (DNA or gene sequence alterations) that can be inherited or acquired. Examples of the former include Ataxia Telangiectasia and Bloom syndrome. Acquired genetic mutations are caused by environmental *mutagens* (agents that cause mutations) and take the form of microscopic structural chromosomal changes such as multi-copy (e.g., Downs syndrome), translocations (e.g., Burkitt's lymphoma), partial deletions (e.g., acute myelogenous leukemia), or point mutations (e.g., sickle cell disease).[30] Hence, it is evident that genetic mutations can and do cause disease, and there are genetic components in everything we are and in everything we do. However, evidence to date shows that behavior is modulated by a myriad of nongenetic factors (e.g., educational, religious, social, familial, psychological, and environmental) superimposed to a nonspecific and nondetermining genetic makeup. Indeed, while genes govern the biological processes of all living organisms in a direct, predictable, and deterministic manner, they have a more circuitous and subtle effect on human behavior that influences rather than eliminates free will through difficult-to-assess gene–brain link. Simply put, *our genes do not make us do it.*

THE BEHAVIORAL (CHOICE) MODEL

While drug addiction is not a disease and is not caused by genetic abnormalities or a compelling abnormal brain reward circuitry, it can be viewed as the outcome of a *process* that begins with an encounter with drugs followed by casual drug-use that can progress to drug abuse in certain individuals, often to the detriment of self.[31] However, this process, which is similar for any *substance of abuse* or *activity of abuse*, is not a continuum, for something intervenes to lead few casual users to become addicted whereas most do not. Perhaps the best-known example is alcohol, the most indulged drug that a large segment of the population (48% worldwide) consumes casually, socially, or daily. While most consumption is moderate and without adverse effects, a minority of users become addicted (approximately 3% of Americans in 2001–2002[32]) and suffer the medical, psychological, economic, and social consequences of their excessive drinking. Likewise, as discussed in chapter 2, the natural history of drug abuse suggests that, following peaks of problem behavior in adolescence and young adulthood, unassisted recovery is the norm for most casual and not-so-casual users. Indeed, while the *30-day* prevalence rate for *any illicit* drug use by the 18- to 26-year-old cohort was approximately 1 in 5 in 2007, it dropped to 1 in 10 by age 45, despite the fact that approximately 80% of them admitted lifetime experience with illicit drugs[33] (see chapter 2, figure 1). Additionally, as discussed in detail in the previous chapter, the prevalence rate of licit and illicit drug use among U.S. servicemen during the Vietnam War was rampant (alcohol, 90%; marijuana, 80%; opium, 38%; heroin 34%; amphetamines and barbiturates, 25% each). However, a strict Department of Defense ban on drugs, enforced by compelled urine testing and the threat of more disciplinary action for recidivists, including extending their Vietnam tour and a negative urine test required to be discharged from service, were the main incentives, rather than treatment, for most users to abandon drugs. A three-year follow-up study showed a relapse rate of only 12%, which in most cases was short-lived.[34] Such extraordinarily high remission rates and continued abstinence contradict the still widely held belief that addiction is essentially irreversible, especially without treatment. These two studies, conducted 25 years apart, and many in between and since, demonstrate that most users *mature* out of their drug dependence or find sufficiently compelling motivations, often associated with love or religion, to override or compensate their cravings for drugs, and do so without professional or other assistance.[35]

Users who become addicted and remain addicted constitute a very small subpopulation within the user population. Most, if not all, are trapped in personal, familial, and psychosocial problems that contribute to placing drug reinforcers (stimuli that increase the strength of behavioral responses) in control of a significant portion of their behavior, which some neurobiologists call the *hijacking* of the reinforcement pathway by drugs.[36] The reinforcing stimulus can be euphoria from drugs, a feeling of satiety from food, an expectation of financial gain from gambling, or an adrenaline rush from high-risk activities. Although such stimuli might not become preeminent while the activities in question remain moderate rather than all consuming, they can progressively escalate to eventually dominate behavior when competing activities within the available repertoire provide less potent reinforcing stimuli, especially in individuals with impaired self-control or with nonsupportive environments. Alternatively, when exposed to reinforcers incompatible with drug abuse (e.g., marriage, drug-free employment, etc.), addicts are able to substitute drugs for the new activity, achieving a more satisfying and often life-changing type of behavior reinforcement. As a corollary, it can be envisioned that the segment of the population that never tries drugs is made of individuals for who *drugs of addiction* or *activities of addiction* do not fit in their value system; a value system based on discipline and self-control that provides one or multiple reinforcers of nondeviant behavior.

Hence, the brain reward circuitry proposed by some neurobiologists as the cause of addiction is only a conduit common to most, if not all, reinforcing stimuli whether resulting from normal or deviant behavior. What determines whether casual or moderate use will become compulsive and eventually all consuming depends on the individual's access to, handling of, or adherence to alternative reinforcers and on his/her level of discipline and self-control. Motivation is pivotal to the type of reinforcement achieved and whether addiction will ensue. Consequently, relief of chronic pain accompanied by a greater sense of well-being and a higher level of functioning are both reinforcers of *opioids-for-pain-relief* seekers, whereas interference with major areas of functioning is the hallmark of compulsive seeking *opioids-for-pleasure*. As a result, pain patients experience no euphoria from taking opioids, have no reasons to continue their use once pain is relieved, and very rarely become addicted.[20-22] Similarly, it has been postulated that addicts who do not *mature* out of their addiction might not have access to alternative reinforcers, might not seek them out, or find them unsuitable replacement for the more potent reward derived from drugs or other deviant behavior. In either case, selection of reinforcers is a choice heavily dependent not on genetics but on personal, familial, and psychosocial factors, all of which contribute to forming an individual's personality, itself made of traits such as self-control, discipline, and willpower.

Self-control is the restraint exercised over one's own impulses, emotions, desires, and actions that are the foundation of behavior. Self-control, which embodies the concepts of character, willpower, and discipline, is a personality trait that is learned mostly from parents but also from family members, teachers, friends and acquaintances, and from a variety of life experiences. Depending on the individual's environment, this learning process can lead to a strong or to an impaired self-control with positive or negative consequences, respectively. For instance, a child well nurtured by dedicated and loving parents in a stable family and social environments is likely to develop robust character traits suitable for making appropriate decisions emulating learned positive patterns of behavior conducive to personal success and to the avoidance of deviant choices later in life. In contrast, a child neglected by uncaring parents, themselves lacking strong character traits, and surrounded by a perfidious environment is unlikely to develop personality traits protective of the many life pitfalls, is less well prepared to face psychosocial challenges, and is therefore more likely to engage in deviant behavior later in life.[37] One pioneering study that supports the importance and predictive value of early development in self-control is known as the *marshmallow* test,[38] conducted in the 1960s by Walter Mischel to examine preschoolers' abilities to forego immediate gratification for a larger but delayed reward. In the study, a group of 4 year olds were given a marshmallow and promised another if they would wait 20 minutes before eating the first one. Following the progress of each child into adolescence, via surveys of their parents and their teachers, the researchers found that ability (self-control) to delay gratification was both predictive of favorable personal outcomes (e.g., higher educational achievements and better social and cognitive competence) and protective against a variety of potential vulnerabilities later in life (e.g., lower drug use). Jellinek first described the concept of *loss of control,* in the context of alcoholism, as an inability to stop drinking leading to binge drinking. However, the concept has evolved to include the inability to refrain from substance use (or from engaging in other deviant behavior) and to terminate use or activity once begun. Yet loss of control is widely believed to be relative rather than absolute. That is, addicts are capable of exercising some degree of control over their behavior, at least some of the time.[39] How loss of control relates to the behavior reinforcing effects of the stimulus, whether drug or activity, or to the addict's expectation of pleasure from a particular impaired control behavior is largely unsolved and hotly debated.

Neurobiologists and electro-physiologists are now searching for neural correlates of self-control and of behavior that might explain how the brain assigns relative value to different incoming stimuli in order to select the most appropriate. For example, alcohol effects on the brain include impaired frontal lobe tasks, as judged by Positron Emission Tomography (PET) scans, by metabolic studies, and by a neuropsychological test battery designed to assess cognitive functions and processes.[40] Frontal lobe dysfunction, whether associated with decreased or increased activity, has also been documented for many psychoactive agents. However, the key question is whether drug-induced frontal lobe dysfunctional changes predate abuse, which would support genetic predisposition, or are the result of abuse, which would not. That is, whether they are the cause or the result of impaired self-control. Partial recovery from chronic alcohol-induced frontal lobe dysfunction following an extended period of abstinence suggests dysfunctional frontal lobe changes to be the result of impaired control and of abuse behavior, not the cause. Hence, biological correlates of abuse are expected to complement our understanding of the neurobiological processes associated with the brain's handling of reinforcing stimuli but are unlikely to account for addiction and other deviant behaviors.

In the meantime, "behaviorists reject the prevalent neuro-scientific notion that drugs themselves are responsible for the development of addiction, and see addiction not primarily as a 'brain disease' but as a behavioral disorder that cannot be separated from the prevailing and historical contingencies of reinforcement."[31] Simply put, like any deviant behavior, addiction is a deliberate choice that, while influenced by genetics, converges and mirrors an individual's formal and informal education and encompasses all previous life experiences. The notion that addiction is a learned behavior born of life experiences is not only common sense but has been corroborated by two decades of research.[40-47] Moreover, the behavioral model transcends the disease theory of addiction in three crucial areas. First, it accounts for the behavior of individuals who seek drugs for pleasure, whether addicted or casual users, and explains why patients who seek pain relief do not become addicted despite repeated or prolonged drug exposure. Second, it provides a foundation for understanding and explaining all forms of addiction, whether substance-

or non–substance-related. Third and most importantly, it lays down medical, social, and legal frameworks for developing prevention and treatment modalities aimed at restoring addicts' discipline and willpower, empowering them to develop self-relying behavioral patterns instead of perpetuating the myth that they are powerless victims, as embodied in the disease model of addiction. Hence, "solutions [for controlling addiction] that do not take into account the basic motivations and propensities underlying addictive behavior are destined to failure."[48]

In conclusion, scientific evidence shows that addiction cannot be blamed on an alleged intrinsic addictive power of drugs, on genetics, or on neuro-circuitry reward pathways and is not a disease or an indication of moral turpitude, as it is often claimed. There are at least three lines of reasoning that support the view that addiction is not substance-dependent but behavior-driven. First, an extensive repertoire of addictive behaviors extends well beyond drugs. Indeed, the addiction spectrum includes not only licit and illicit drugs (e.g., alcohol, narcotics), prescription medications (e.g., painkillers, tranquilizers), and chemical substances (e.g., inhalants, glues) but extends to a variety of dietary products (e.g., caffeine, chocolate), certain activities (e.g., Internet browsing, gambling, exercise, sex), or even ordinary foodstuff, which the vast majority of the population indulges in moderation. Second, no substance or activity is intrinsically addictive. For instance, narcotics and foodstuff are not addictive when taken for pain relief and nourishment, respectively, but can become reinforcers of addiction when indulged for pleasure. Third, the vast majority of casual drug users do not become addicted, and most who do eventually free themselves from their addiction, most often without help. Likewise, no specific genetic mutations or brain pathways have been identified that doom the carrier to addiction, and no chemical rewards have been shown to compel a casual user to engage in substance or nonsubstance abuse and become addicted.

In the words of a noted critic of the disease theory of addiction, "The idea that addiction is a disease is the greatest medical hoax since the idea that masturbation would make you go blind."[49] However, addiction can lead to certain diseases and even to self-destruction as possible outcomes. Examples include liver cirrhosis from alcoholism, lung cancer from smoking, AIDS in addicts who share needles, and death from any of them. Equating cause to effect of addiction has been and continues to be exploited by proponents of the disease theory of addiction in part out of conviction but also driven by personal self-interest and to protect a multitude of highly lucrative businesses that profit from it. However, while addiction is not a disease, addicts are not criminals to be persecuted and incarcerated, as is done the world over, or stigmatized as sinners. Indeed, addiction is not a crime (though certain drugs of abuse have been criminalized worldwide), nor is it a sign of moral or spiritual decay, or a sin (though it is so viewed in most religious circles). Rather, "people take drugs because it makes sense for them to do so given the choices available, rather than because they are compelled by the pharmacology of the drugs they take."[50] Indeed, evidence shows that addiction is a chosen behavior, just as are all choices that addicts and non-addicts make on a daily basis. In fact, everybody makes unwise choices in life that can lead to adverse outcomes such as addiction, a failed relationship, a disease, a financial loss, and even death. As in any decision making, unwise choices most often are based on an analysis of available information that is influenced by personality traits of self-control, discipline, and willpower developed from one's life experiences superimposed to a non-determining genetic background. In this book, the term *addiction* denotes a reward-seeking behavior associated with compulsive or impaired control over use that interferes with life functioning and carries an implied risk of personal harm. Such a definition encompasses all types of addiction, accounts for a virtual absence of addiction among medical users of narcotics, and assigns to users behavioral responsibility and the power to overcome it. That being the case, three key questions arise: Should society enact social policies to prevent individuals from making unwise choices? When individuals make bad choices, should society intervene? When unwise choices lead to addiction, should addicts be held accountable? Abandoned to their fate? Treated and rehabilitated at society's expense? More on this later.

CHAPTER 5

Pain Control:
Narcotics and the DEA

THE SPECTER OF THE DEA

Not only are we here to protect the public from vicious criminals in the street but also to protect the public from harmful ideas.

Robert Ingersoll, director of the Bureau of Narcotics and Dangerous Drugs and first DEA director, quoted by Jack Anderson in the *Washington Post*, June 24, 1972

Today, physicians have at their disposal an array of pain medications ranging in strength from mild to powerful, with the most effective painkillers widely blamed for but rarely found associated with addiction. In the 1980s and 1990s, some of these, especially narcotics, found their way to the black market with the occasional connivance of unscrupulous physicians. The public and Congress became acutely aware of the problem when a barrage of media reports claimed that diversion of OxyContin, an oxycodone-based opioid narcotic, was responsible for an outbreak of overdoses, deaths, and crime. Although many of these reports were exaggerated or unfounded, the DEA responded to critics in Congress and in the Department of Justice (DOJ) by implementing an aggressive program ostensibly designed to eliminate the diversion and illegal use of OxyContin and other narcotics. The DEA "uses familiar law enforcement methods from the War on Drugs, such as aggressive undercover investigation, asset forfeiture, and informers."[1] Its tactics, especially vigorous and broadly publicized when prosecuting physicians suspected of drug malfeasance, have had a chilling effect on legitimate narcotics prescriptions. Consequently, tens of millions of Americans suffer from untreated or undertreated pain on a daily basis.[2] Indeed, the

AMA reported that 97 million patients suffered from unrelenting pain in 1997, and most of them "received inadequate care because of barriers to pain treatment."[3] Additional barriers include inadequate pain management training in medical schools, a shortage of pain medicine specialists, and reluctance on the part of many patients to take what they perceive to be addictive medications. However, it is clear that U.S. physicians are frightened by the prospects of falling victims to federal or state prosecutors eager to indict and convict "licensed physicians for drug distribution, fraud, manslaughter, and even murder for the deaths of people who misused and/or overdosed on prescription painkillers."[1] Likewise, restrictions on the production and distribution of narcotics imposed by international drug control treaties restrict their availability in nonindustrialized countries. According to the WHO,[4] 80% of persons suffering from severe pain worldwide do not receive adequate treatment. The human cost of untreated or undertreated *chronic* pain (pain that persists weeks to months) includes depression, absenteeism, alcoholism, family disruption and violence, and suicide. The economic cost to society, including medical expenses and lost wages, is incalculable, but has been estimated to reach $100 billion per year in the United States alone.[5,6]

Targeting physicians for prosecution is not a new phenomenon born with the DEA. The first federal law that criminalized the recreational use of opium, morphine, and cocaine was the Harrison Act, passed in 1914.[7] This took place within the general thrust toward Prohibition by advocates of the temperance movement, at a time when opiates were widely popular as medicinal and recreational drugs. They were thought to have tranquilizing, antidepressant, analgesic, and other properties that made them ideal for self-medicating a variety of ailments. They were sold at grocery stores as potions and elixirs, alongside beer and wine, and by itinerant salesmen roaming the countryside with a *shill* (an accomplice planted in the crowd) attesting to the astonishing properties of each boisterously promoted concoction. Examples of the most popular medicinal cannabis sold in the 1800s and early 1900s boasted eclectic claims.[8] *Handy Corn Plaster,* manufactured by The Chamberlain Medicine Co. of Des Moines, IA, was formulated "for hard and soft corns and bunions, guaranteed to give satisfaction or money refunded." *Doctor Macalister's Cough Mixture,* produced by John P. Lee of Chicago, IL, was promoted as "the best remedy for coughs and colds of adults and for croup and whooping cough of children." *Dr Poppy's Wonder Elixir* was advertised as "the one bottle cure for Colds, Coughs, Rheumatism, Head tension, Gout, Shingles, Influenza and Arthritis . . . a glass in the morning is guaranteed to relieve symptoms and leaves a pleasant feeling that lasts all day."

A plethora of *nostrums* or *patent medicines,* as these products were called, permeated American society in the mid- to late 19th century as they appealed to a public need left void by traditional medicine in an environment where no laws existed to regulate their content or curb claims of their curative properties. A notorious 19th-century peddler of *patent medicines* containing opium as the active ingredient was William Avery Rockefeller (*Big Bill*), an eccentric man who made a quick fortune that enabled his only son, John Davison Rockefeller, to build an oil empire that made him the richest man in America.[9] However, muckraking journalists such as Samuel H. Adams, the General Federation of Women's Clubs, the AMA, the American Pharmaceutical Association, and others exposed the worthless or harmful ingredients in most nostrums, the unfounded claims of their curative properties, and the manufacturers' deceitful advertising practices. At that time, Upton Sinclair published *The Jungle*, a shocking novel exposing the appalling living and working conditions and hopelessness of immigrant workers in Chicago and the lack of hygiene in meat packing plants. His novel includes episodes of workers falling into meat processing tanks and being ground, along with animal parts, and sold as *Durham's Pure Leaf Lard*. Such exposés quickly captured public and congressional attention and were instrumental in the passage of the first federal Food and Drugs Act in 1906. As could be expected, this act did not put quacks out of business; they still prosper today in myriad new schemes. However, it was the first attempt toward consumer protection legislation in the United States.

Eight years later, the U.S. Congress passed the Harrison Act, the first federal law designed to regulate the medical use of narcotics by criminalizing their recreational use. Given possible opposition on constitutional grounds, the statute was masqueraded as a tax. The Act required all those who "produce, import, manufacture, compound, deal in, dispense, sell, distribute, or give away opium or coca leaves, their salts, derivatives, or preparations, and for other purposes" to register, obtain and fill out forms, and place and retain tax stamps on packages containing narcotics.[7] Registered physicians, dentists, and veterinary surgeons were to keep records for two years "of all such drugs dispensed or distributed, showing the amount dispensed or distributed, the date, and the name and address of the person to whom such drugs are dispensed or distributed . . . subject to inspection, as provided in this Act."[7] Any person who "violates or fails to comply with any of the requirements of this Act shall, on conviction, be fined not more than $2,000 or be imprisoned not more than five years, or both."[7] To facilitate enforcement of the Harrison Act, possession of narcotics in any form other than the official tax-stamped package was sufficient evidence to justify conviction unless the defendant explained the possession to the jury's satisfaction. Over the ensuing 25 years, tens of thousands of people were prosecuted for violations of the Harrison Act, and nearly 25,000 physicians were arrested, 3,000 were convicted and jailed, and thousands more lost their license and livelihood.[8,9] This marked the U.S. government's "aggressive, unprecedented pursuit of physicians and their addicted patients."[1]

In 1970, the Harrison Act was replaced by the Comprehensive Drug Abuse Prevention and Control Act, which included the CSA. The latter was to serve as the foundation for the *War on Drugs* that followed, including unleashing a new wave of prosecutions of physicians accused of drug malfeasance. The CSA, which classifies certain drugs (including all painkillers) into five *Drug Schedules* and establishes guidelines for their use, empowered the DEA to regulate all Scheduled drugs, including prescription analgesics. Scheduled drugs range from Schedule I drugs, which have "high potential for abuse," "no currently accepted medical use in treatment in the US," and "lack accepted safety for use of the drug . . . under medical supervision," to Schedule V drugs, which have "low potential for abuse," "currently accepted medical use," and "abuse may lead to limited physical dependence." Schedule I drugs include heroin, which is used in much of Europe as a powerful pain reliever especially useful for managing terminal cancer patients. Ironically, a drug does not need to have a high abuse potential or be especially harmful to merit placement in Schedule I. This is how the DEA justifies listing *marijuana* alongside heroin,[10] despite it being far less harmful than tobacco and its medical use permitted in some European countries and in 14 U.S. states, as of October 2009. No prescriptions may be written for Schedule I drugs, and nonviolent street peddlers prosecuted for multiple offenses can face life sentences.[1] Schedule II drugs, which include morphine, cocaine, and various formulations of opium among others, are available only by nonrefillable prescriptions, their production is subject to quotas, and their distribution is controlled by the DEA, albeit incompetently.

In 1973, President Nixon created the DEA, under DOJ jurisdiction, as part of his Reorganization Plan No. 2. Early on, the mission of the DEA was to "bring to the criminal and civil justice system substances destined for illicit traffic in the US."[11] But, by the late 1990s and early 2000s, the DEA came under criticism from Congress for having no measurable proof that the illegal drug supply and use in the United States had declined under its watch. In the same time frame, Glen A. Fine, the DOJ inspector general, claimed that a major problem of "prescription drug abuse" existed in the United States, citing suspect statistics regarding the magnitude of the problem and chastising the DEA for having failed to address it.[1] For example, Fine cited the unverifiable figures of 6.4 million Americans having used painkillers illegally in 2001 whereas "just over 4 million used cocaine."[1] The DEA contributed to the disinformation campaign, claiming "people who abuse controlled pharmaceuticals each year equals the number who abuse cocaine: 2 to 4 percent of the US population,"[12] and were responsible for 25% of deaths from drug overdose.[12] The media joined the chorus, contributing to an atmosphere of fear and hysteria about a supposed threat of a massive diversion of prescription painkillers by physicians who they likened to drug pushers. Included in the chain reaction, denouncing the dangers of the potent painkiller OxyContin, were high-profile publications like *Time* magazine, *US News and World Report,* and *The New York Times.*

For instance, on January 2001, *Time* reported, "OxyContin may succeed crack cocaine on the street."[13] On February 2001, *US News and World Report* reported on the dangers of OxyContin, featuring a physician who purportedly supplied illegal narcotics to addicts and was responsible for a rise in crime in his community.[14] The same month, *The New York Times* reported that 59 people had died of OxyContin overdose in eastern Kentucky in 2000 and that the drug had set a wave of pharmacy burglaries, overdoses, and physician arrests.[15] WDSU Channel 6 of New Orleans ran five stories involving OxyContin, with titles such as *Dad arrested in son's OxyContin death,* four of which were printed between April 10, 2001, and May 15, 2001.[16] And, on December 12, 2001, CBS's *48 Hours: Addicted,* anchored by Dan Rather, was followed the next night by MTV News and Docs' *True Life: I'm Hooked on OxyContin,* hosted by Serena Altschul. The theme of both newscasts was, "Dependency on prescription drugs like OxyContin is a mounting problem among young people and the general population, alike."[17] However, the most notorious example of unscrupulous media reporting was the now infamous five-part *Orlando Sentinel* series published October 19–23, 2003, titled *OxyContin Under Fire,* written by Doris Bloodsworth.[18] The articles, citing alarming though dubious statistics[1] and including photographs of *innocent victims* and accompanying editorials, seemed designed to elicit maximum aversion toward OxyContin and sympathy for its victims. However, some of the *victims* had a prior history of drug abuse or addiction, as was discovered when the *Sentinel* stories unraveled and the paper retracted much of the information it had published.[19]

In response to the *Sentinel* series and without further inquiry, Florida Governor Jeb Bush proposed a bill that would create a prescription drug database to track and cross-reference the prescription drug records of all Florida citizens. Moreover, to make it harder for patients to abuse OxyContin, the Florida legislature also passed a law to stop paying for prescriptions exceeding 120 pills without prior approval from Medicaid. Howard Dean, governor of Vermont and a physician himself, also took advantage of the prevailing anti-OxyContin paranoia requiring that all prescriptions for that drug, written for 1,200 out of 128,000 patients enrolled in the State Medicaid and the Vermont Health Access Programs, be approved in advance.[20] Other states that now curb OxyContin distribution to Medicaid recipients include West Virginia, Ohio, South Carolina, and Maine. Whether these state measures had the intended outcome is doubtful. As could be expected, many trial attorneys expecting a wave of lawsuits added OxyContin to the list of drugs their lucrative practices aggressively target. Yet, they appear to have misjudged the financial potential of OxyContin, for "all 1,665 personal injury claims filed by individual plaintiffs have either been dismissed or abandoned," according to Purdue Pharma L. P., OxyContin manufacturer.[21] It is noteworthy that, long after the *Sentinel* and other OxyContin-related stories were exposed as inaccurate, exaggerated, or deceitful, some reporters and their editors continue to pound on a dead horse, unaware or oblivious of the generally accepted notion that the 2001–2003 media blitz on OxyContin was overstated, at best, or designed to increase newspapers sales, at worst. For example, in August 2004, the *Boston Globe* and the *Ottawa Citizen* published reports on OxyContin abuse or deaths, citing statistics out of context, or quoting alarming but uninformed statements by local officials.[22,23] Likewise, a book published in 2004 claims that "whether prescribed by a physician as OxyContin or purchased on the street as 'hillbilly heroin', painkilling drugs are extremely effective in eliminating physical, emotional, and psychological distress. The problem is that these drugs are also incredibly addictive"[24]—a common misconception based more on popular folklore than on facts.

However, it must be observed that many in the media and law enforcement communities will feel vindicated by the plea agreement by Purdue Frederick Co., an affiliate of Purdue Pharma L. P., and three of its executives. They agreed to pay an aggregate of $634 million for "falsely claiming that OxyContin was less addictive, less subject to abuse, and less likely to cause withdrawal symptoms than other pain medications."[25] This was the outcome of a four-year investigation conducted by a consortium of eight state and federal agencies. They included the Virginia Attorney General's Medicaid Fraud Control Unit, the Food and Dug Administration's (FDA) Office of Criminal Investigations, the (Internal Revenue Service) IRS Criminal Investigation unit, the Department of Health and Human Services, the Department of Labor, the Defense Criminal Investigative Service, the Virginia State Police, and the West Virginia State Police. The outcome of the witch-hunt triggered a series of grandiloquent and self-serving pronouncements by law enforcement, such as, "It is unthinkable that purely for greed, addictive drugs were fraudulently marketed to the public, and in so doing threatened the health and safety of our citizens. Among those endangered were soldiers, sailors, airmen, marines, and their families, all of who avail themselves of the military health system. At a time when our military personnel and their loved ones are sacrificing so much, something like this is incomprehensible and grossly reprehensible."[25] The media obligingly applauded the settlement but judged it insufficient, arguing "we were seeing a tsunami of opioid addiction in young people who had recreationally used OxyContin and had become rapidly addicted to this highly potent opioid. Soaring crime rates, multiple medical complications, an epidemic of intravenous drug abuse and Hepatitis C, a harrowing increase in overdose deaths and fractured families, overwhelmed the medical, legal and social systems that simply didn't have the resources to meet the problems."[26] Let the reader judge whether these are responsible and objective statements by law enforcement and the media.

Emboldened by a clamor of public indignation against narcotics and physicians accused of diverting drugs to the black market, the DEA announced its newly deployed "OxyContin Action Plan" of 2001.[12] This plan, like the Harrison Act, equated legal prescription drugs listed under Schedule II with illegal, nonprescription drugs included in Schedule I. This placed physicians on an equal footing with drug dealers, making them legally responsible for the consequences of legitimate prescription drugs diverted by criminal elements. Asa Hutchinson, DEA director from 2001 to 2003, announced that given the threat of the new prescription drug epidemic his agency would reallocate resources to fight illicit prescription drugs and that it would use its Asset Forfeiture Fund to help finance the new plan.[27] His perverse logic was impeccable. Shifting the focus from hard-to-penetrate black markets of illegal drugs controlled by unknown and ever-changing players to a pool of easy-to-track, stable, registered, cooperative, record-keeping, tax-paying physicians with plenty of forfeitable assets would help subsidize their own prosecutions, appease Congress, and validate the DEA's own existence. It must be remembered that in the 1980s, prior to the *prescription drug diversion* scare, drug prohibitionists and the media portrayed crack cocaine as the "the most addicting drug known to man" that was quickly spreading to suburbs and schools and was responsible for most street crime, deteriorating social conditions, and for failing school grades. Politicians quickly adopted and amplified the unsubstantiated claims, using the issue as a rallying point to vote major budget increases for law enforcement, the prison system, and the military to save America's children from the plague of crack cocaine. When the short-lived craze for crack cocaine ended, presumably because its extreme and vicious ups and down are undesirable to most users, politicians, the media, and law enforcement simply refocused their attention and their campaigns on other *most addictive drugs known to man,* mainly prescription narcotics. This new *evil* was an easier target to monitor and pursue and provided law enforcement an opportunity to control narcotics prescriptions, even if the DEA continues to claim not to be in the business of regulating physicians; a state prerogative. However, this claim contradicts its requirement that physicians register and obtain a DEA license for the privilege of prescribing controlled substances that also serves as an agency's tool to monitor prescribing patterns. Moreover, using "all available enforcement tools" to disrupt drug "diversion, illegal sale, and abuse,"[28] where physicians play a *primary* role according to the agency, along with using revenues from license fees to investigate and prosecute targeted physicians, contradict its claims not to regulate and not to target physicians. Another source of revenue for drug enforcement is the DOJ's Asset Forfeiture Fund, which is financed by *Criminal, Judicial, and Administrative* forfeitures.[29] The former is a perfectly transparent legal action invoked during the criminal prosecution of a defendant. It requires the indictment of the property and of its owner, a determination by a jury that the property is forfeitable, and a court order of forfeiture. *Civil judicial forfeiture* is an action brought in court against the property without charging the owner. More ominously, the DOJ's *Administrative forfeiture* "is an *in rem* [against property] action that permits the federal seizing agency to forfeit the property without judicial involvement . . . Property that can be administratively forfeited is: merchandise the importation of which is prohibited; a conveyance used to import, transport, or store a controlled substance; a monetary instrument; or other property that does not exceed $500,000 in value."[29]

However, if some features of the DOJ's forfeiture program appear excessive, the DEA's investigative tactics and *modus operandi* are even more questionable. Indeed, innocent targets are too often the DEA's focus, causing numerous abuses and miscarriages of justice that can wreck patients' lives and destroy physicians' careers. The tools it uses are multiple and all encompassing. They include redefining *addict, drug dealer,* and *drug distributor;* aggressively using the asset forfeiture law at the arrest rather than the conviction stage of an investigation; offering leniency to arrested drug offenders in exchange for information incriminating physicians; character assassination; using Special Weapons Assault Teams (SWAT) indiscriminately; and even disavowing its own guidelines when expedient to convict a high-profile suspect. By defining an addict as, "any individual . . . who is so far addicted to the use of narcotic drugs as to have lost the power of self-control with reference to his addiction,"[30] the DEA blurs the crucial distinction between *addiction* and *physical dependence.* Indeed, while an addict compulsively seeks pleasure from a drug despite adverse health or social consequences that frequently lead to a deteriorated lifestyle, a pain patient is said to be *physically dependent* when taking a drug becomes necessary to relieve excruciating pain and to function with some semblance of normality. Another phenomenon, called *tolerance,* can develop when patients take opioids long-term. In such cases, increasing doses of medication are required to maintain the same level of pain control. Finally, seeking or taking higher than prescribed doses of opioids, a condition that may be associated with tolerance and withdrawal symptoms, characterizes *pseudo-addiction.* This seemingly aberrant behavior is the result of undertreatment of pain, rather than an indication of addiction, and disappears with pain relief. Hence, even if physical dependence, tolerance, or pseudo-addiction develops in patients taking opioids for chronic pain relief, addiction is very rare.[31] In addition, chronic pain sufferers do not experience euphoria, a psychological effect of opioids sought after and experienced by addicts. Likewise, patients do not exceed their prescribed dose of painkillers after reaching adequate analgesia, and they do not engage in aberrant drug-related behaviors that are hallmarks of addiction. Finally, withdrawal symptoms, a phenomenon associated with stopping opioids or missing a dose, occur in addicts unable to get a timely *fix* but not in pain patients and are not life threatening as they can be with severe alcohol withdrawal, called *delirium tremens.*

The DEA also played loose with its definition of OxyContin-related deaths, neglecting to inform the public that most of the 464 deaths it reported for 2000 and 2001 involved at least one other drug, precluding determination of which caused death. Indeed, the *Journal of Analytical Toxicology* reported that out of 919 deaths listed as *oxycodone deaths* over a three-year period, oxycodone was detected alone in the system in only 12 of the deceased.[32] Likewise, because the DEA considers possessing a drug in amounts exceeding a certain limit is a presumption of *intent to distribute*, many patients have been prosecuted as *drug dealers* and their physicians as *drug distributors.* Moreover, mandatory minimum sentences tie judges' hands precluding their taking into consideration special circumstances of a case. Finally, because the DEA has criminalized prescription drugs, it makes no distinction between a homicide committed by a drug dealer in a turf war and an overdose death caused by a diverted prescription drug written in good faith to a legitimate patient. In both cases, the dealer and the physician could face life imprisonment.

With the expanding role of the DEA in the War on Drugs, so has exploded the use of SWAT teams. Today, SWAT teams raid over 100 private homes each day, and most involve drug offenses. "These raids are commonly conducted late at night, or just before dawn, to catch suspects by surprise. Police sometimes deploy 'flash grenades,' then batter down or blow up doors with explosives. They then storm the home, subduing occupants, handcuffing them at gunpoint, sometimes pushing them to the ground."[33] Such aggressive and confrontational raids are justifiable in response to violent crimes, hostage situations, or to threats to the community. However, in the prosecution of drug cases, agents frequently rely on law-breaking informers motivated by leniency for themselves rather than by objectivity. As a result, many SWAT raids "have left a long trail of 'wrong address' frightened innocents, needless injury, and even death."[33] One such episode occurred "on the night of April 23, 1973, [when] Herbert Joseph Giglotto, a hardworking boilermaker, and his wife, Louise, were sleeping soundly in their suburban house in Collinsville, Illinois. Suddenly, and without warning, armed men broke into their house and rushed up the stairs to the Giglottos' bedroom. Giglotto later recalled, 'I got out of bed; I took about three steps, looked down the hall and I [saw] men running up the hall dressed like hippies with pistols, yelling and screeching. I turned to my wife: God, honey, we're dead.' The night intruders threw Giglotto down on his bed and tied his hands behind his back. Holding a loaded gun at his head, one of the men pointed to his wife and asked, 'Who is that bitch laying there?' Giglotto begged the raiders, 'Before you shoot her, before you do anything, check my identification, because I know you're in the wrong place.' The men refused to allow the terrified couple to move from the bed or put on any clothes while they proceeded to search the residence. As books were swept from shelves and clothes were ripped from hangers, one man said, 'You're going to die unless you tell us where the stuff is.' Then the intrusion ended as suddenly as it began when the leader of the raiders concluded, 'We made a mistake.'"[9]

Another favorite DEA tactic is character assassination of arrested physicians through press releases as exemplified by DEA administrator Karen Tandy's reckless portrayal of the 42 physicians arrested in 2004. "Those 42," she claimed without providing evidence, "were not arrested for prescribing too much medicine. They committed egregious criminal acts such as exchanging prescriptions for sexual favors or kickbacks."[28] It should be noted that the DOJ's Asset Forfeiture Fund is financed in part by assets seized from suspects under investigation and is used to complement the funding of the DEA's Diversion Control Program and to reward state and local drug enforcement agencies that cooperate with the DEA.[1] For instance, $220,000 was seized from Dr. Eli Schneider before he was even charged.[1] Of that amount, $50,000 went to the U.S. Department of Health and Human Services, $29,000 to the Cincinnati Police Department, $24,000 to the Ohio Department of Health and Human Services, $14,000 to the FBI, (Federal Bureau of Investigation) and $3,752 to the Ohio Medicaid Fraud Control Unit. Not unlike war practices of yesteryear, the DOJ's forfeiture policy gives the conquering troops the authority to loot the conquered and share the spoils. This perverse financial incentive system contributes to the overly aggressive pursuit of well-off physicians by cash-short state and local police departments leading to numerous abuses. The following are three well-known and often cited prosecution examples[1] arising from the DEA's misguided and overzealous policies.

Richard Paey was a 45-year-old wheelchair-bound patient with chronic pain caused by a car accident and a botched back surgery. After moving to Florida, he elected to have his New Jersey physician mail him signed, undated pain prescriptions, some of which he photocopied and had filled. Although no evidence was presented in court that he sold any of the painkiller pills he purchased, he was charged with "intent to distribute" because the amount of narcotics found in his possession exceeded the statutory limit needed to be charged. Feeling that he was not a criminal, Paey refused a house arrest and probation and later a five-year jail sentence offered by the prosecution to avert a trial. Under the mandatory minimum sentencing guidelines, Paey received a sentence of 25 years and a $500,000 fine.[1,34] "Today, Paey sits in a Florida prison with a morphine pump, paid for by Florida taxpayers."[1]

Dr. William Hurwitz is an example of a physician running afoul of the DEA.[1] He was one of several dozen doctors, pharmacists, and patients caught in the DEA's *Cotton Candy* web. Dr. Hurwitz, who is Jewish, was arrested by a 20-agent strong SWAT team at his ex-wife's house in McLean, VA, while visiting his children on Rosh Hashanah eve. He was jailed on a $2 million bond. All his assets, including his retirement account, were seized, essentially for being duped by some of his patients to write narcotics prescriptions that were later sold on the streets.[35] Dr. Hurwitz was charged with "conspiring to traffic drugs, drug trafficking resulting in death and serious injury, engaging in a criminal enterprise, and health care fraud."[36] At the trial, his attorney was limited to present only five patients' testimonials, whereas the prosecution was allowed 63 witnesses, including Dr. Michael Ashburn, whose testimony was promptly refuted by six past presidents of the American Pain Society in a letter addressed to one of his lawyers on December 10, 2004.[37] These pain experts took this unusual step because they felt "deeply concerned that serious misrepresentations in the testimony provided by the government's expert, Dr. Michael Ashburn, will undermine the welfare of patients who suffer in chronic pain." The letter concluded: "In the past, each of us perceived Dr. Ashburn as a respected colleague and his selection as an expert by the government as understandable. We are stunned by his testimony. As leaders in this field, we feel compelled to correct the errors in his testimony, lest it be used in the future in a manner that worsens the national tragedy of untreated pain. We will try to correct the public record after the trial concludes and sincerely hope that the government and the court will consider this information now."[33] Dr. Hurwitz was convicted of 50 of 62 counts, sentenced to 25 years in prison, and fined $1 million.[38] After the trial, the jury foreman stated to the media that Dr. Hurwitz was "sloppy" and a "bit cavalier" in recordkeeping but not "running a criminal enterprise,"[39] as accused. On August 15, 2006, the 4th U.S. Circuit Court of Appeals ordered a new trial because the trial judge had "effectively deprived the jury of the opportunity to consider Hurwitz's defense" by barring the jury from considering whether Dr. Hurwitz "acted in good faith" in treating his patients.[40] At issue were DEA guidelines that the agency disavowed at the time of the trial in order to prevent their introduction as evidence by Dr. Hurwitz's defense attorney. The disavowed document included specific guidelines for "Health Care Professionals and Law Enforcement Personnel" enunciating what was and was not "legitimate practice."[41] Dr. Hurwitz's retrial beginning on March 26, 2007, was characterized in the press as "a battle over who sets the rules for treating patients who are in pain: narcotics agents and prosecutors, or doctors and scientists."[42] Using a tried and proven prosecutorial approach particularly effective with jurors, Dr. Hurwitz was portrayed as a drug trafficker and "accused of ignoring blatant 'red flags' . . . that some patients were misusing and reselling the drugs."[42] The defense called on Dr. Russell K. Portenoy and Dr. James N. Campbell, two leading pain experts and past presidents of the American Pain Society, who testified that Dr. Hurwitz was a knowledgeable physician and passionate advocate of pain control and that his pain prescriptions were "within the bounds of medical practice." Yet, after deliberating seven days, the jurors found Dr. Hurwitz guilty on 16 counts of drug trafficking, each carrying a 20-year maximum sentence, exonerated him of 17, and were unable to agree on 16, which were then dismissed by the judge. On July 13, 2007, judge Leonie Brinkema dismissed a life sentence sought by the prosecution and sentenced Dr. Hurwitz to a 57-month prison term observing, "an increasing body of respectable medical literature and expertise support those types of high-dosage, opioid medications." Having already served 2½ years in prison, Dr. Hurwitz was released from prison in late 2008.

Another egregious example of the DEA's tactics against pain-managing physicians is that of Dr. Frank Fisher.[1,43,44] Dr. Fisher, a Harvard graduate whose California practice served a poor rural area, was charged in 1999 with multiple counts of fraud and drug diversion and three counts of murder. The latter included a patient who died of an unrelated car accident, a man who died after he took narcotics stolen from the home of one of Dr. Fisher's patients, and a patient who died after her prescriptions had run out and Dr. Fisher was already in prison. According to Dr. Fisher's own account, the car accident victim

was Rebecca Mae Williams, a 37-year-old who had suffered from incurable low-back pain. After exhausting alternative treatments, I had successfully controlled her pain with 80 milligrams of OxyContin twice a day, a dose that had allowed her to enjoy an active life. The day Becky died, she had taken her usual dose before going furniture shopping with her boyfriend. As their small truck rounded a curve, the driver's door flew open, and David, who was driving, fell out. The truck crashed into a tree, and the impact exploded my patient's heart, fractured her skull, broke her neck, and eviscerated her. Yet on the basis of an impossibly high level of oxycodone measured in a blood sample—later found to be contaminated—the county medical examiner asserted that Becky had died of a drug overdose.[44]

More was to come, as Dr. Fisher recalls: "Before the criminal prosecution would conclude years later, I would be accused of murdering nine people, including several I had never even met."[44] Dr. Fisher was described by the prosecutor and by the press as a mass murderer and a common drug pusher, whereas he claimed,

mindful of "drug seekers" I had established a screening procedure . . . that turned away 60 percent of applicants without my even seeing them. Those accepted into the pain management program had access to a multidisciplinary treatment team that included surgeons, physical therapists, chiropractors, and an acupuncturist. Each patient had to undergo regular psychological evaluation. And acceptance into the program didn't ensure continued treatment. Patients who could not follow the program's guidelines were discharged. By the time I was arrested, some 600 former patients were on the ejected list.[44]

His assets were seized, and he was jailed on a $15 million bond. At the preliminary hearings, the medically naïve medical expert for the prosecution stated, "The majority of [his] patients were on doses that we had never seen before. Some of the doses we thought were incompatible with life."[40] Seizing the opportunity, the defense attorney asked her to read aloud from the OxyContin product literature brochure that pure opioid agonists have no ceiling dose, allowing their use long term and in high doses with few risks but constipation, as described in chapter 6. The judge dismissed five murder charges, downgraded three to manslaughter, reduced the $15 million bond to $50,000, and released Dr. Fisher from prison; a bittersweet victory because, with no assets and now 50, he had to move in with his parents. At the trial that began on January 13, 2003, the prosecuting attorneys admitted not to have sufficient evidence to proceed, and the judge dismissed all remaining charges. Yet, California Attorney General Bill Lockyer charged

Fisher for an alleged $150 *up coding* (altering a disease code to overcharge third-party payers) theft from Medi-Cal (California's Medicaid agency). On May 18, 2004, a jury acquitted Dr. Fisher of that charge as well, with one of the jurors describing "the whole thing as a which-hunt." However, "the criminal phase of my ordeal was over, but the state attorney general had one more gambit: to go after me through the state medical board. He failed there as well."[44] Having faced charges ranging from Medicaid fraud to drug diversion to murder for six years, and after loosing his medical practice and all his assets and spending five months in jail, Dr. Fisher has found a new vocation. He is now "working to resolve the flaws in social policy that drive the pain crisis, with the hope that someday I will once again be able to treat patients with chronic pain effectively."[44]

Skeptics might argue that these are anecdotal cases with little relevance to the overall picture that do not justify physicians' fears of the DEA. To reinforce skeptics' arguments and offset its critics the DEA issued a news release on October 30, 2003, titled "The Myth of the Chilling Effect: Doctors Operating Within Bounds of Accepted Medical Practice Have Nothing to Fear from DEA."[45] In it, the DEA asserts that since 1999 "less than one tenth of one percent" of physicians, or "34 of the 963,385 doctors licensed in the US" in 2003, were arrested for illegally prescribing narcotic painkillers According to these data, only 0.0035% of licensed physicians were arrested that year. Eighteen months later, in a published rebuttal to critics, the DEA administrator stated, "last year, DEA cases resulted in the arrest of 42 doctors . . . less than one arrest for every 23,000 DEA-registered physicians,"[33,46] or 0.0043%. These figures are disingenuous, misleading, and largely irrelevant to the issue of physicians' fears of the DEA and its effect on pain management. The reasons are four-fold, as shown by the analysis of the DEA's 2003 number of arrests claim. First, the origin of the DEA's figure of 963,385 *licensed doctors* is unclear. In fact, the number of practicing physicians in 2003 was far lower if only 720,290 physicians were DEA-*registered* two years later, according to the agency's own figures.[47] Second, 90% of physicians do not routinely treat chronic pain patients, and when they prescribe narcotics, it is on a sporadic basis, for short periods, and in low doses for the management of acute (sudden and brief) or subacute (between acute and chronic) pain. Hence, arrested physicians might represent a tiny fraction of doctors in practice or with a narcotics license from the DEA but a large percentage of those who specialize in pain management and prescribe narcotics routinely. Indeed, it has been estimated from three database sources that the number of pain-treating physicians in the United States ranges from 4,278 to 5,869.[46] Therefore, the 34 physicians arrested represent 0.68% or 1 in 147 pain-treating doctors, rather than "one arrest for every 23,000 physicians," claimed by the DEA. Even adding Medical Oncologists (8,397 with valid certificates in 2003[48]) who treat cancer patients, most of whom will suffer chronic pain associated with disease progression,[49] the percentage of narcotics-prescribing physicians arrested (34 out of 14,266) would be 0.24%, or

1 in 412. Third, the number of arrests made by DEA agents, in this case 34 physicians, is but a fraction of all arrests, most of which are carried out by state and local enforcement agencies working in partnership with the DEA. Fourth, as much as they fear arrest, physicians dread the potentially devastating effect of a DEA investigation on their reputations, their finances, their lives, and on the lives of their patients even if an arrest is never made. Indeed, according to one report,[46] "in 2001, the DEA carried 861 investigations of doctors," representing 17% (1 in 6) of 5,869, or 6% (1 in 16) of 14,266 pain-treating physicians. More recent data from the DEA reveals that the agency investigated 595 of "approximately 720,290 Medical Doctors (MDs) and Doctors of Osteopathic Medicine (DOs) registered with the DEA in 2005."[47] Also, in 2005, there were 43 criminal dispositions against physicians; a figure 50-fold greater than the "less than one tenth of one percent" and 150 times the "one arrest for every 23,000 physicians," claimed by the DEA.

Moreover, while these recalculated DEA figures expose the agency's disingenuous handling of its own data, they do not begin to explain the intensity of physicians' deep-seated fear of the agency. Indeed, what physicians dread is falling victim to the terrorizing tactics of the agency in its relentless pursuit of a case and, if arrested, the prospect of losing all their assets, their medical license, their malpractice insurance, and their livelihood, even if eventually acquitted, as was Dr. Fisher. The uselessness and hypocrisy of targeting physicians is revealed by the DEA's own database, which shows that most diverted narcotics destined to the black market in the United States originate from sources other than physicians' prescriptions and that it does little to prevent or control it. In this regard, an analysis of the DEA's "Report of Theft or Loss of Controlled Substances," obtained through the Freedom of Information Act, sets the record straight on narcotics diversion. The report reveals that between 2000 and 2003 "almost 28 million dosage units of all controlled substances were diverted . . . primarily from pharmacies (89.3%), with smaller portions from medical practitioners, manufacturers, distributors, and some addiction treatment programs that reported theft/losses of methadone."[50] The six most stolen or otherwise diverted opiate analgesics were oxycodone (4,434,731 doses), morphine (1,026,184 doses), methadone (454,503 doses), hydromorphone (325,921 doses), meperidine (132,950 doses), and fentanyl (81,371 doses). The authors of the analysis concluded, "pain medications, regardless of schedule, are being stolen from the drug distribution chain prior to being prescribed, contributing to their illicit availability, abuse, and associated morbidity and mortality."[50] They opined, "If we accept uncritically that drug diversion stems only from prescriptions, we risk distorting our view of the medical profession and patients through a lens of substance abuse, which further weakens physicians' desire to treat pain and worsens patient access to pain care."[50] Finally, they advised, "Diversion control efforts must target the correct sources and not subject law-abiding prescribers and patients to unwarranted scrutiny."[50] Therefore, whether stolen from pharmacies or diverted at other points in the distribution chain, the vast majority of diverted prescription drugs have never been prescribed by a physician nor dispensed by a pharmacist. Moreover, diverted prescription drugs represent but a minute fraction of illegal drugs on the streets, as reported by the White House ONDCP. For instance, "between 1988 and 1995, Americans spent $57.3 billion on drugs, broken down as follows: $38 billion on cocaine, $9.6 billion on heroin, $7 billion on marijuana, and $2.7 billion on other illegal drugs and on the misuse of legal drugs."[51,52] "Other illegal drugs" referred to in the study included depressants, stimulants, inhalants, rohypnol, ketamine, PCP, GHB, MDMA or ecstasy, LSD, and scores of other illegal agents. The "misuse of legal drugs," which referred to diverted prescriptions drugs, accounted for only 4.7% of the $2.7 billion cited, or $60 million, or 1% of the 57.3 billion total; hardly justifying being the DEA's favorite antinarcotics drug enforcement target.

In conclusion, through the DEA, the U.S. government is conducting an aggressive and unjustifiable campaign against pain-treating physicians. This is achieved by a multifaceted approach. It includes redefining the terms *addict*, *drug dealer*, and *drug distributor*; criminalizing opioid prescribing patterns coupled to a disinformation campaign to convince the public that, contrary to evidence, physicians are responsible for a "major prescription drug problem in the US"; and aggressively using the asset forfeiture law at the arrest rather than at the conviction stage of an investigation. Using drug dealers and other unreliable informers is the rule, as is reliance on *no-knock* SWAT raids of targeted physicians' and patients' homes. More ominously, SWAT incursions into the homes of innocent citizens, many of which botched,[33] are often unauthorized or misrepresented and in clear violation of the 4th amendment of the U.S. Constitution. Indeed, the 4th amendment affirms, "The right of the people to be secure in their persons, houses, papers, and effects, against unreasonable searches and seizures, shall not be violated, and no Warrants shall issue, but upon probable cause, supported by Oath or affirmation, and particularly describing the place to be searched, and the persons or things to be seized." It also disavowed its very guidelines on narcotics when judged crucial to convict a suspect.

The DEA's methods and tactics, coupled with its probably unconstitutional position that "the Government can investigate merely on suspicion that the law is being violated, or even just because it wants assurances that it is not,"[1] suggest that abuses and miscarriages of justice are the norm rather that the exception and that most of them never come to light. In prosecuting physicians, the DEA is not bound by the usual rules of evidence and frequently thwarts the expectation of having expert medical testimony as protection against allegations that the physician's actions were "outside the scope of legitimate practice." In fact, the DEA has brought charges against doctors even when prescriptions were not actually filled, leading to the conclusion that "there seems to be no evidentiary standard at all that doctors can rely on to thwart a conviction."[1] By heavily publicizing physician arrests, indictments, and convictions usually accompanied

by character assassination, the DEA ensures high visibility that fosters a
public and congressional perception that it is successfully addressing and
protecting the public from a *major drug problem*. Never mind that the War
on Drugs is being waged at enormous economic and human costs to the
nation. According to the NIDA, "More than half of the estimated costs of
drug abuse [$181 billion in 2002] were associated with drug-related crime.
These costs included lost productivity of victims and incarcerated perpetrators of drug-related crime (20.4 percent); lost legitimate production due
to drug-related crime careers (19.7 percent); and other costs of drug-related
crime, including Federal drug traffic control, property damage, and police,
legal, and corrections services (18.4 percent). Most of the remaining costs
resulted from premature deaths (14.9 percent), lost productivity due to
drug-related illness (14.5 percent), and health care expenditures (10.2 percent).[51] Never mind that, despite these enormous costs and the involvement of an army of *DEA special agents* (5,296 in 2005) and countless state
and local agents, drugs on American streets, including narcotics diverted
from production facilities, warehouses, and in transit to distribution outlets
rather than from physicians' offices, have increased year after year since the
DEA was created. Never mind that by making physicians scapegoats of its
failed War on Drugs the DEA has managed to frighten them by the prospects of falling victim to overzealous federal or state enforcement agents
and prosecutors eager to convict.

While most practitioners are familiar with legal restrictions regarding
prescribing controlled substances, most are unaware or rightfully skepti-
cal of legal provisions intended to ensure that drug law enforcement not
interfere with medical practice. Consequently, the number of pain-treating
physicians has dwindled, and those that remain err on the side of caution,
prescribing what they perceive to be acceptable to the DEA rather than
what's medically appropriate for their patients. As a result, tens of millions of Americans suffer from untreated or undertreated pain on a daily
basis. It seems clear that solving the pain crisis in America requires first
acknowledging that pain control is a fundamental human right[53] and that
millions of American pain sufferers must not be held hostage to an irrational drug policy based on misconceptions, self-serving attitudes, or outright deceptions regarding the *dangers* of illicit drug use to self or society.
Acknowledging these truths is a prerequisite and first step toward ending
drug prohibition.

DEA'S INFRINGEMENT ON STANDARD OF CARE

> The interim policy statement "Dispensing of Controlled Substances for the
> Treatment of Pain" is an unfortunate step backward largely because of the
> tone in which it is written, which promotes a return to an adversarial rela-
> tionship between registrants and the DEA.
>
> —National Association of Attorneys General:
> Letter to DEA administrator Karen P. Tandy, January 19, 2005

Standard of care in medicine is defined in general terms as, "primarily a legal concept that refers to the level of practice that any average, prudent, and reasonable physician would provide under similar circumstances. It must reflect the art (consensus of opinion) and the science (peer-reviewed literature) of medicine.[54] It is not necessarily the best or most advanced care available but care that is considered acceptable and adequate under similar medical and geographic circumstances. Thus, providing treatment that is inferior to the norm is unacceptable and unethical and renders the physician guilty of negligence and potentially liable for malpractice. Although intuitively easy to understand, this definition of standard of care must be put in perspective. In primitive worlds, magicians, conjurers, or shamans probably provided an equivalent level of rudimentary care to tribesmen suffering from similar ailments or complaints. However, medicine has evolved to become a highly complex, multifaceted discipline with thousands of diseases, each with variations and permutations, giving rise to specialties that group, study, and treat diseases classified by organ or type. For example, while gastroenterology deals with diseases of the gastrointestinal tract, the liver, and the pancreas, medical oncology addresses all types of cancers regardless of the organ or tissue of origin. Hence, the *level* of practice will depend on the physician's training and level of expertise and the type of disease under treatment. For example, the level of practice exercised by a generalist treating a minor gastrointestinal ailment might be equivalent to that of a gastroenterologist. On the other hand, because most generalists lack sufficient training and expertise in treating cancer, the level of practice expected from a medical oncologist treating a cancer patient will be considerably higher than that anticipated from a generalist and, for standard of care purposes, should be compared only to that of other medical oncologists. Hence, when referring to the specialists, the standard of care is defined as the level of practice provided by any average, prudent, and reasonable gastroenterologist, oncologist, and so forth. Additionally, standard of care must be "acceptable and adequate under similar circumstances."[54] That is, it must be based on the *art* and *science* of medicine in order to attain the outcome expected under similar circumstances, which might be as definitive as the cure of a disease or as modest as the control of a symptom.

In pain medicine, standard of care implies that an "average, prudent, and reasonable pain-treating physician" must prescribe analgesics in doses and for periods of time sufficient to ensure pain relief, always, and pain control whenever possible. Hence, the determination of which analgesic drug to use, in what doses, and for how long to achieve pain control is not the DEA's prerogative. Rather, it is the physician's responsibility, indeed duty, based on each patient's pain characteristics (type, cause, severity), adjusted according to personal, familial, and psychosocial factors and the presence and type of comorbidities (concurrent diseases) and their treatment. The history of medical malpractice in the United States confirms that physicians enter into an unwritten but legally enforceable contract to provide standard of care to each patient; a contract that, in the case of pain management, is thwarted by DEA policy on narcotics.

How does the DEA interfere with the standard of care delivery by pain-managing physicians? As described earlier, the DEA has created an atmosphere of fear among pain-treating physicians that prescribing medically appropriate doses of opiates might attract the DEA's attention and wrath. Under these circumstances, most physicians opt to bypass opiates altogether, to prescribe them in doses acceptable to the DEA though insufficient to ensure adequate pain control, or to use other analgesics with inferior efficacy and greater toxicity (more on this in chapter 6). The DEA uses a variety of methods to alter the prescribing patterns of pain-managing physicians. For example, the DEA claims to distinguish between a prescription written for a "legitimate medical purpose" and one that is "beyond the bounds of medical practice."[1] However, no guidelines or course of action exist for physicians to observe or for investigators or prosecutors to use as a guide for making that judgment objectively. This is particularly alarming given the fact that drug enforcement agents and jurors with no medical training find themselves the arbiters of what constitutes *legitimate* medical practice in a complex field of medicine that involves biological, psychological, behavioral, familial, and social components they do not comprehend and transcend enforcement policy.

Moreover, the DEA seems intent on blurring the legal–illegal boundary of what it deceptively calls *legitimate practice*. This is strongly suggested by its disavowing its own document titled, "Prescription Pain Medications: Frequently Asked Questions and Answers for Health Care Professionals, and Law Enforcement Personnel,"[41] when it got in the way of Dr. Hurwitz's conviction, cited earlier. This document, compiled in collaboration with noted pain specialists and pain control advocates, offered reasonable pain management guidelines while curtailing drug diversion. Perhaps the DEA objected most to one of its guidelines that stated, "For a physician to be convicted of illegal sale, the authorities must show that the physician knowingly and intentionally prescribed or dispensed controlled substances outside the scope of legitimate practice."[41] Or, to the assertion that prescribing narcotics to a patient with a history of drug abuse or not reporting patients suspected of abusing pain medications was not a violation of Federal law.[41] Because of these and other "misstatements of law and other statements" the DEA repudiated the document, deleted it from its own website "pending review," and pressured the Pain and Policy Studies Group of the University of Wisconsin to do likewise.[55] The DEA's reversal prompted the Liaison Committee on Pain and Addiction representing the American Pain Society, the American Academy of Pain Medicine, and the American Society of Addiction Medicine to send a joint letter of protest. After refuting each of the arguments given by the DEA for its reversal, the letter concluded "The interim policy statement 'Dispensing of Controlled Substances for the Treatment of Pain' is an unfortunate step backward largely because of the tone in which it is written, which promotes a return to an adversarial relationship between registrants and the DEA."[56] Significantly, on January 19, 2005, 30 state attorneys of the National Association of Attorneys General sent a joint letter to the DEA complaining that the document withdrawal occurred without consultation. In part, the letter stated "the Interim Policy Statement, 'Dispensing of Controlled Substances for the Treatment of Pain' . . . emphasizes enforcement, and seems likely to have a chilling effect on physicians engaged in the legitimate practice of medicine."[57] In a sharp rebuttal of DEA policy, the attorneys general affirmed the group's position on pain control. It stated, "As Attorneys General have worked to remove barriers to quality care for citizens of our states at the end of life, we have learned that adequate pain management is often difficult to obtain because many physicians fear investigations and enforcement actions if they prescribe adequate levels of opioids or have many patients with prescriptions for pain medications."[57] They also highlighted the DEA's tunnel vision stating, "There are many nuances of the interactions of medical practice, end of life concerns, definitions of abuse and addiction, and enforcement considerations that make balance difficult in practice. But we believe this balance is very important to our citizens, who deserve the best pain relief available to alleviate suffering, particularly at the end of life."[57]

Other indications of possible *illegitimate medical practice* according to the DEA are *red flags*, which include, among others, "patients who are poorly dressed or are seen without appointments . . . doctors licensed in various states or who dispense large amounts of narcotics from one office . . . or visits lasting less than 25 minutes."[58] Each of these red flags is without merit because poorly dressing and being seen without an appointment might be more an indication of patients' limited means and physicians' benevolence rather than indications of illicit activity by either patients or physicians. Likewise, being licensed in various states and prescribing large amounts of narcotics relate to physicians' evolving geographic practice preferences and to the needs of their patient population, respectively, rather than attempts to evading or braking the law, as assumed by the DEA. Finally, the DEA's arbitrariness and disregard of available statistics in flagging office visits shorter than 25 minutes are highlighted by two large surveys conducted in 1998. Indeed, according to the National Ambulatory Medical Care Survey of the National Center for Health Statistics and the American Medical Association's Socioeconomic Monitoring System, the average office visit lasted 17 and 21 minutes, respectively.[59] Hence, based on this criterion, the DEA would consider suspect most office visits in this country.

Moreover, not only are DEA's red flags egregious in themselves but also the means used to elicit them. For instance, seeking whatever information to build a case, investigators conduct surreptitious video surveillance of targeted physicians' offices, search through their office and home trash, and often confront patients on their way to the physician's office.[1] Posing as pain patients, undercover agents befriend office employees in hopes of uncovering incriminating evidence against the physician. A frequent practice is to analyze physicians' billing practices and prescribing history by painstakingly searching databases from Medicare and Medicaid and from insurance and pharmaceutical companies. The DEA also has established a hotline for anyone to report anonymously doctors suspected of overprescribing. While such a tool is unlikely to be used by legitimate patients seeking pain relief, it is certainly useful to disgruntled patients and employees or rejected addicts. As a result, an atmosphere of distrust has emerged between patients and physicians. Patients must not appear too eager for more medication, a sure sign of addiction, according to the DEA, that must be reported by the physician, and physicians must be distrustful of every pain patient for fear of prosecution should a legitimate narcotics prescription be sold on the street. The latter is especially worrisome because prosecutors are not bound by the presumption of innocence principle and need not prove a doctor's malicious intent or desire to profit from narcotics diversion to secure a conviction.[1]

In conclusion, the DEA has introduced arbitrary and pliable rules of evidence to secure convictions. It includes intentionally blurring the boundary between "the scope of legitimate practice" and what it arbitrarily considers "beyond the bounds of medical practice" and applying unjustifiably aggressive investigative and prosecutorial tactics, including invoking the forfeiture law that effectively ruins targeted physicians and doing so at the pretrial stage. This climate of intimidation and of uncertainty, where presumption of innocence is not assured, has frightened many physicians out of pain management altogether. Those who remain in the field prescribe narcotics in amounts that, deliberately or not, are designed more to protect themselves from falling afoul of the DEA even if adequate pain relief is not achieved. Physicians who ignore these self-preservation precautions do so at their own peril, as the cases of Drs. Hurwitz and Fisher eloquently demonstrate. Likewise, many patients opt not to disclose to their physician the severity of their pain so they can avoid arousing suspicion and running the risk of being reported as suspected addicts. Additionally, the DEA withdrawal of its consensus document drafted by law enforcement representatives, health care practitioners, and patient advocates designed to "achieve a better balance in addressing the treatment of pain while preventing abuse and diversion of pain medications"[41] brought back the dark days of the Harrison Act of 1914 when every narcotics-prescribing physician was viewed as a potential law breaker and every pain sufferer as a drug addict. Under these circumstances, where the DEA acts as a wedge between patient and physician and each is suspicious of the other's motives and intentions, standard of care delivery to chronic pain sufferers has been the casualty. The DEA's interference with standard of care, combined with the terror its aggressive prosecutorial tactics cause among pain-treating physicians, has triggered an unprecedented pain-management crisis where tens of millions of Americans suffer from untreated or undertreated pain on a daily basis.[2,3]

Can enforcement of drug laws by the DEA and standard of care delivery to pain patients be reconciled? It could be envisioned that the pain management crisis in America would be solved if the DEA targeted criminal elements within the drug culture and physicians engaged in activities truly "beyond the bounds of medical practice," according to clear and objective guidelines established by their peers. However, targeting physicians is easier and more financially rewarding and conveys to the public a sense of success and accomplishment through heightened media attention difficult to match by prosecuting drug dealers and drug peddlers. Moreover, the DEA shows no inclination to set legitimate medical purpose guidelines, preferring instead to keep physicians guessing. This is clearly the DEA's intention as demonstrated by its recent (2006) *Policy Statement.*[60] It states, "However . . . it is not appropriate for DEA to address these questions in the form of a guidance document (or to endorse such a guidance document prepared by others)."[60] Another potential solution could be changes in or stern controls over DEA rules, procedures, and modus operandi to ensure fairness and adherence to the rule of law. However, adding layers of bureaucracy to an already bloated agency would compound rather than solve any problem, whichever it might be. A definitive solution to the pain crisis must take into account the political power and vested interests of diverse groups associated with the War on Drugs and the fact that the DEA has evolved into a nearly independent entity accountable for its acts only in retrospect and through court action. Hence, I contend that the pernicious status quo resulting from the DEA's very existence will endure until the U.S. Congress, cognizant of the DEA's failures and abuses and of its unachievable national and international mandates, musters the political will to abolish this ill-conceived, wrongly focused, and socially harmful federal agency. Repeal of the 18th amendment provides a historic precedent for reversing similarly misguided policies intended to protect us from ourselves that brought havoc to our nation instead.

CHAPTER 6

Painkillers

Pain is a more terrible lord of mankind than even death itself.
—Albert Schweitzer, *On the Edge of the Primeval Forest*, 1931

The International Association for the Study of Pain (IASP) defines *pain* as "an unpleasant sensory and emotional experience associated with the actual or potential tissue damage,"[1] which emphasizes the nature of pain and its often ill-defined source. Pain can also be characterized by its severity, as *mild, moderate,* or *severe;* its duration, as *acute, sub-acute,* or *chronic;* its character, as *sharp, dull,* or *throbbing;* its anatomic basis, as *nocioceptive* (arising from inflammation, injury, or trauma) or *neuropathic* (arising from the peripheral or central nervous system); its pathological origin, as *cancerous* or *noncancerous;* and by many other criteria. However, while the medical literature is saturated with a bewildering array of articles addressing a multitude of pain-related issues in a variety of conditions and patient subsets, two overriding concepts emerge in the context of pain management and pain policy: *Acute* versus *chronic* and *mild-to-moderate* versus *moderate-to-severe* pain. Pain is said to be *acute* when it has a clear and time-definable onset arising from a sudden pathological event, such as a toothache, a bone fracture, a myocardial infarction, and so forth. Hence, it is a symptom of disease or injury that disappears once the underlying cause is gone. In contrast, *chronic* pain, whether caused by cancer or by a noncancerous illness, often persists for months or years beyond the period of healing and is considered a disease in its own right by the IASP and increasingly by other medical organizations.

Chronic pain is among the most prevalent, disabling, and costly afflictions worldwide. An analysis of 13 studies published between 1992 and 2002 from countries as diverse as the United States, Israel, France, Turkey, Brazil, Australia, China, Nigeria, and many others showed that chronic pain afflicts between 10.1% and 55.2% of the population.[2] In the United States, it is estimated that "over 20 million American employees miss 433 million work days [each year] due to pain, and indirect business costs have been estimated to be $45 billion. The health care cost . . . has been estimated at $885 billion. In a recent study that surveyed 1.2 million adults, 1 of 5 related that they had some form of chronic pain. Among those with chronic pain, approximately 40% reported that the pain had a 'major' impact on their lives, with half of those noting that they get depressed."[3] As cited earlier, the AMA reported that 97 million patients suffered from unrelenting pain in 1997, and most of them "received inadequate care because of barriers to pain treatment."[4] These grim statistics, and others cited elsewhere in this book, give credence to Voltaire's quip: "Happiness is an illusion; only suffering is real." Two and a half centuries later, we have the means to provide adequate to excellent pain relief quickly and long term to the vast majority (88%) of patients suffering from chronic pain.[5] Our failure to do so is a sad commentary on past policy makers who launched the War on Drugs based on political considerations (see chapter 3) and on current ones unwilling to challenge erroneous notions about the dangers of narcotics, the causes of addiction, and other misconceptions that sustain the status quo. Indeed, until War on Drugs policies are repealed, millions of American pain sufferers will go on suffering day after day, year after year.

This chapter outlines the types of drugs available and commonly used for the treatment of chronic versus acute pain, and it compares their mechanisms of action, efficacy, safety, and side effects. Other approaches to pain management, such as neuroaxial, spinal, or transcutaneous nerve stimulation; acupuncture; cryotherapy; diathermy; physical therapy; and other nonpharmacological modalities, are outside the scope of this book. It must be emphasized at the outset that, contrary to acute pain, the pharmacological management of chronic pain is not a simple matter of prescribing a painkiller and escalating the dose or switching drugs until the desired outcome is achieved. Indeed, chronic pain is a highly complex, multifactorial, and multidimensional symptom that requires a detailed diagnostic workup to uncover its causes and the contributing or confounding impact of comorbidities, as well as the understanding of each patient's psychosocial makeup, which affects pain perception and response to treatment. Hence, it necessitates ample expertise on the part of the treating physician for selecting a management plan best suited to maximize pain relief for each individual patient. A review of the steps leading to a diagnosis and to the selection of an appropriate pain management plan is outside the scope of this book. Suffice it to say that a detailed medical, psychosocial, and pain history complemented by a thorough physical examination and by selective diagnostic testing will expose the source(s) and cause(s) of pain and reveal underlying contributing factors, when present. For example, in certain cases a thorough workup will uncover an unsuspected pain-causing malignancy, whereas in others, particularly in chronic pain cases, an underlying pain-exacerbating depression might be revealed. Hence, a patient feigning pain (a *doctor shopper*) intent on misusing or selling opioids so obtained, will rarely dupe an experienced pain physician even if the pain characteristics are described skillfully because a negative diagnostic work up will raise suspicion. It must be emphasized, however, that the physician's interpretative task is complex because pain is a subjective symptom influenced by personal biological and psychosocial factors, and its intensity often correlates poorly with objective findings. Alternatively, a dishonest patient already on opioids can feign inadequate pain control (a *patient dealer*) in attempts to obtain an additional prescription to be sold. To be effective, any pain management plan must focus on pain relief and function restoration whenever possible and ensure that the patient's expectations be tempered if unrealistic. Benefits and risks of each proposed intervention must be addressed, and means to monitor outcome and to adjust course when needed must be instituted.

Painkillers are the foundation of any pain management plan complemented by antidepressants, neuromodulators, and certain adjuvants (agents that modify the effects of other agents) to treat depression, neuropathic pain, and other comorbidities that often amplify the real or perceived intensity of pain. Painkillers include nonsteroidal anti inflammatory drugs (NSAIDs), favored for treating mild-to-moderate pain, and opioids, best suited for the treatment of moderate-to-severe pain. The WHO has described a three-step ladder as a framework for pain management. It is described as follows: "If pain occurs, there should be prompt oral administration of drugs in the following order: nonopioids (aspirin and paracetamol); then, as necessary, mild opioids (codeine); then strong opioids such as morphine, until the patient is free of pain. To calm fears and anxiety, additional drugs—adjuvants—should be used."[6] In the next two sections, I examine the pros and cons of this escalation ladder and whether it is appropriate and safe for the management of all types of pain. It is my contention that were it not for War on Drugs policies that stigmatize opioid analgesics, restricts their medical use, promotes and perpetuates the fear of addiction, and holds a Damocles sword on all pain management decisions, most patients with chronic pain would be treated with step 3 analgesics (opioids) from the outset, supplemented by adjuvants, when needed. Such an approach, designed to address the currently unmet needs of most chronic pain sufferers, would provide both relief to the millions of patients with undertreated pain and reduce the morbidity and mortality associated with the unwarranted use of nonopioid analgesics in that population. In fact, it is noteworthy that NCI and UN pain experts support this view for treating cancer pain, the most representative and most studied type of chronic pain. For instance, at its 1986 Meeting on the Comprehensive Management of Cancer Pain it was concluded, "In patients with severe pain, morphine—a strong opioid—is the drug of choice."[7] Likewise, a pain management symposium held in 2000 recommended, "It's important to move beyond prescribing opioids for chronic pain and to encourage a comprehensive, interdisciplinary approach to improve patient outcomes."[3] The next section also demonstrates that patients with severe chronic pain should not be exposed to NSAIDs, as contemplated in the WHO's three-step ladder, but should instead be treated with the safer and more potent opioids from the outset and in sufficient doses administered for as long as necessary to provide optimal pain relief and functional restoration. The next 18 pages describe in some detail the mechanisms of action, efficacy, general principals of administration, and side effects of opioids and NSAIDs. Such information is provided to demonstrate the greater efficacy and safety of the former compared to the latter, especially for the treatment of *moderate-to-severe* chronic pain.

NARCOTICS (OPIOIDS)

> Extensive worldwide experience in the long-term management of cancer pain with opioid drugs has demonstrated that opioid administration in cancer patients with no history of substance abuse is only rarely associated with the development of significant abuse or addiction.
>
> —National Cancer Institute:
> Substance Abuse Issues in Cancer

Narcotics can be defined as, "any derivative, natural or synthetic, of opium or morphine, or any substance that has their effect."[8] However, most current definitions of narcotics were developed in the context of drug abuse, oblivious of their analgesic properties and of their medical uses. As a result, most definitions are prejudiced rather than objective using the noun *narcotics* as encompassing all illegally obtained or unlawfully possessed mind-altering drugs, including opioids and nonopioid agents such as cannabis, cocaine, barbiturates, and the like. One definition calls narcotic "an addictive drug, such as opium, that reduces pain, alters mood and behavior, and usually induces sleep or stupor."[9] It is disingenuous to define narcotics primarily as an *addictive drug* listing other side effects (alters mood and behavior, induces sleep and stupor) at par with its major property (reduces pain). Indeed, pain reduction is the hallmark of narcotics taken for legitimate purposes, whereas other properties listed in that definition are side effects affecting only a rare medical user. In fact, as described in chapter 4, addiction and mind-alteration occur mostly in individuals who seek narcotics for their psychotropic effects, whereas pain reduction, without mind-altering adverse effects, is the natural outcome for individuals taking narcotics for pain relief. Another glaringly erroneous definition of narcotics is found in the prestigious Encyclopedia Britannica. It defines *narcotic* as "a drug that produces . . . addiction (physical dependence on the drug),"[10] overlooking the fact that *addiction* and *physical dependence* are entirely different and un-related phenomena, as described in the previous chapter. The WHO addresses the semantics of the nouns *narcotics* and *opioids* stating, "Opioids are classified as narcotics because they have a potential for abuse."[11] This incongruous definition is equally applicable to licit and illicit drugs; to a spectrum of chemical substances, dietary products, and activities; and could even be extended to children and wives, who have *potential for abuse*. The fact that most people do not abuse these agents or activities suggests that potential for abuse originates in the abuser, as elucidated in chapter 4. Hence, from a medical point of view and to avoid pejorative overtones, this class of analgesic agents is best called *opioids* that can be defined as *analgesic agents best suited for the treatment of moderate to severe pain, especially chronic.*

Opioids can be classified according to their origin, as endogenous (e.g., endorphins 1 and 2, which are produced by the body) and exogenous (opium alkaloids). The latter can be derived from the poppy seed (e.g., morphine, codeine, and papaverine) or produced semisynthetically (e.g., oxycodone, hydromorphone, and heroin) or synthetically (e.g., fentanyl, meperidine, and methadone). Functionally, opioids are classified as morphine-like agonists (agents that induce morphine-like effects), partial agonists, or mixed agonist–antagonists, depending on their mechanism of action. In the United States, the medical uses of opioids are restricted to the treatment of very specific clinical entities. In addition to their analgesic and anesthetic use, certain opioids are permitted as cough suppressants (codeine and hydrocodone), to control diarrhea (opium), for the treatment of anxiety due to shortness of breath (oxymorphone), and for the treatment of narcotics addiction (methadone). In contrast, physicians are free to prescribe any nonopioid medication *off-label*. That is, for managing diseases and conditions other than those approved by the FDA. A perverse use of this loophole is prescribing chemotherapeutic agents off-label despite their meager contribution to five-year survival (2.1%–2.3%)[12] and to cure rates (2%)[13] when prescribed for FDA-approved indications.

Mechanisms of Action

Used appropriately, opioids induce prompt and superior analgesia, albeit with a potential for reversible physical dependence and tolerance after chronic administration. Compulsive drug use can occur in a small number of patients with a prior history of addiction. Opioid effects are exerted through their pharmacological actions on cell receptors. There are three major types of opioid receptors (OR): μ (μOR), κ (κOR), and δ (δOR), which are located on neuronal cell membranes of the brain, the spinal cord, and peripheral nerves, mostly of the gastrointestinal tract. When bound to spinal cord or peripheral nerve receptors, opioids interfere with the transmission of peripheral painful signals and block the psychological response to pain at the level of the limbic area (brain structure involved in emotion, motivation, and emotional association with memory), thus diminishing pain perception. When bound to brain receptors, they trigger descending signals that inhibit incoming pain signals. In peripheral tissues such as joints, opioids reduce inflammation. Recent µOR studies on knockout mice (laboratory mice with an inactivated µOR gene that enables studying its function) have shown that the µOR receptor is the molecular target for most morphine effects, including analgesia, sedation, reduced blood pressure, itching, nausea, euphoria, decreased respiration, miosis (constricted pupils), and decreased bowel motility. The presence of µOR is also required for some κOR-mediated analgesic effects.[14] Moreover, antisense mutations (mutations that alter a gene to produce a truncated product) and gene knockout mouse models support µOR receptor functional multiplicity. The latter attribute, plus the dissimilar receptor selectivity and affinity of different opioids, and the varied psychosocial backgrounds among individuals account for the range of side effects observed. κOR is also involved in analgesia, but its activation also produces marked nausea and dysphoria. Hence, opioid receptors are a complex and incompletely understood system of multiple, interrelated, and functionally diverse molecules that mediate all opioid effects, whether therapeutic or undesirable.

Efficacy

Opioids are the most efficacious painkillers for treating moderate-to-severe somatic and inflammatory pain. Because of their efficacy, they offer sufferers of chronic pain, whether from cancer or other chronic illnesses, the best hope for restoring a functional lifestyle. This assertion is supported by my own 30-plus years of clinical practice and by pain experts. For instance, in a recent review article on pain management opioids are characterized as "the most potent and effective analgesics available and have become accepted as appropriate treatment for acute and chronic cancer pain."[15] The critical importance of opioid analgesics is highlighted in the following WHO statement, "Although there are many drug and non-drug pain treatments, the opioid analgesics such as codeine and morphine are **absolutely necessary** [original emphasis] for the management of pain due to cancer. When cancer pain is moderate to severe, there is no substitute for opioids."[11] Likewise, according to educational guidelines from NCI, "Opioids, the major class of analgesics used in management of moderate-to-severe pain, are effective, easily titrated, and have a favorable benefit-to-risk ratio."[16]

Likewise, pain experts also view the use of opioids as a medical imperative to treat chronic noncancer pain. The American Society of Anesthesiologists articulated a widely held view on the subject. It stated, "To deny a patient with chronic pain the right to aggressive, clinically proven treatment using a combination of opioids . . . is simply unforgivable and unacceptable. The argument against the proper use of opioids in chronic pain is debatably a non-argument, which flies in the face of scientifically proven, objective, rational treatment modalities for the chronic pain patient."[17] However, despite forceful endorsements such as this, opioids are unjustifiably controversial, and their medical use is generally inadequate. In too many cases they are used reluctantly and only after exhausting the less efficacious non-opioid painkillers, resulting in undertreatment of pain and needless suffering, morbidity, and mortality, as described in the next section. The reasons for this attitude are multifactorial including: (1) Physicians' cursory knowledge of basic analgesic pharmacology; (2) Poorly informed medical regulators, as revealed by a 1991 survey of state medical board members.[18] Astonishingly, the survey found that most members preferred aspirin and acetaminophen alone or in combination with codeine for managing moderate-to-severe pain and failed to distinguish addiction from physical dependence. Additionally, 14% felt that prescribing opioids for chronic cancer pain was legal but should be discouraged, while 5% believed the practice to be illegal, and 33% stated they would investigate opioid prescribing for nonmalignant pain as an illegal practice. So much for the level of medical and legal erudition of arbiters of medical practice who often are called upon to investigate complaints against their peers' standard of care or medical ethics; (3) Patients' reluctance to take drugs purported to induce addiction at the first contact, fear that acknowledging pain is admitting disease progression, concern of being suspected of drug-abuse behavior rather than seeking pain relief, stoicism, and religious considerations; (4) Drug policy and punitive laws designed to control narcotics diversion to the detriment of pain relief; (5) An inadequate health care system that leaves 40 million-plus Americans uninsured and, for the remainder, focuses primarily on acute disease management, failing to recognize the importance of palliative measures for alleviating chronic suffering and for improving quality of life; and (6) Reimbursement policies that do not cover the cost of prescription drugs or cover the more expensive parenteral administration of analgesics through pumps, blocks, and epidural injections for hospitalized patients, but fail to cover oral analgesics taken at home.

Despite these shortcomings, chronic pain management is slowly improving as revealed by the rise in medical use of opioids since 1990. According to a recent report, "from 1990 to 1996, there were increases in medical use of morphine (59%; 2.2 to 3.5 million g [grams]), fentanyl (1,168%; 3,263 to 41,371 g), oxycodone (23%; 1.6 to 2.0 million g), and hydromorphone (19%; 118,455 to 141,325 g) and a decrease in the medical use of meperidine (35%; 5.2 to 3.4 million g)."[19] Significantly, this rise in the medical use of opioids was not accompanied by a rise in drug abuse. On the contrary, the same report observed, "During the same period . . . reports of abuse decreased for meperidine (39%; 1,335 to 806), oxycodone (29%; 4,526 to 3,190), fentanyl (59%; 59 to 24), and hydromorphone (15%; 718 to 609) and increased for morphine (3%; 838 to 865)."[19] Hence, contrary to unsubstantiated claims by drug policy advocates, increased medical use of opioids does not increase diversion or addiction. Regrettably, palliative care for the terminally ill, especially pain management, remains grossly underutilized in the United States, as illustrated by Medicare expenditures. For instance, out of $210 billion total Medicare payments in 1998, only 1% was spent for hospice care, whereas 28% went for acute care of hospitalized patients and for high-tech interventions during the last year of life, half of it in the last two months.[20] This misguided end-of-life care is but a reflection of Western medicine's focus on aggressive, expensive, excessive, and mostly futile interventions while overlooking cost-effective palliative measures, especially pain relief, that can have the greatest impact on quality of life when it is the most needed.

Mild opioid agonists include codeine, hydrocodone, and the atypical opioid tramadol. Their major disadvantage is a dose-dependent toxicity that severely limits dose escalation. Moderate opioid agonists include meperidine and propoxyphene. Meperidine was the opioid of choice for many years based on its perceived greater safety, lesser risk of addiction, and better antispasmodic effect in treating pain associated with biliary spasm (spasm of bile ducts or the gallbladder) and renal colic (severe ureteral pain caused by passage of a kidney stone). However, it has fallen out of favor in recent years due to its low potency, short duration of action, the unique neurotoxicity (seizures and other neuropsychological effects) of its metabolites (breakdown products of metabolism), and because presumed advantages were proven illusory. Propoxyphene, a relatively weak opioid, is available in the United States as a pure preparation or in combination with acetaminophen. However, both opioids exhibit short action and toxicity that limit their use in the management of chronic pain. In fact, the staying power of propoxyphene is likely due to "concern about oversight and censure [that] may be a factor in the extensive use of propoxyphene (a Schedule IV drug) rather than oxycodone and hydrocodone."[21]

Morphine is the international gold standard opioid for treating moderate-to-severe pain to which all others are compared. It should be chosen from the outset for managing *severe* pain. Morphine was first isolated from opium by Friedrich Wilhelm Sertürner in 1805. Sertürner named the bitter white crystalline alkaloid after the Greek god of dreams, *Morpheus*. Morphine is available as short- and long-acting formulations, as are other narcotics, greatly facilitating chronic pain management. In addition to its efficacy in controlling moderate-to-severe pain, another major benefit of morphine and morphine agonists, such as hydromorphone, codeine, oxycodone, hydrocodone, methadone, levorphanol, and fentanyl, is their lack of efficacy ceiling with increasing doses. That is, their doses can be escalated until adequate pain relief is achieved. Morphine, oxycodone, hydromorphone, fentanyl, and methadone are the strongest and most prescribed opioids in the United States (Table 5).[21] In contrast, partial agonists, such as buprenorphine, are subject to a dose efficacy ceiling, where dose escalation increases toxicity without augmenting the level of analgesia. Opioids with agonist–antagonist activities, such as pentazocine, butorphanol, dezocine, and nalbuphine, activate one type of opioid receptor while blocking or remaining

Table 5
Opioid Analgesics Most Widely Used in the United States (2005)[21]

Generic name	ARCOS[1]	Brand name	Morph Eq[2]	Oral Dose	Parenteral Dose
Morphine	1,297	MS Contin	1:1	15–30 mg Q3–4[3]	2–10 mg
Meperidine	1,267	Demerol	1:10	50–100 mg QD	10–50 mg
Oxycodone	756	Oxycontin	1:1	5–10 mg BID	N/A
Hydromor- phone	53	Dilaudid	5:1	2–4 mg Q3–4	0.5–2 mg
Fentanyl	16	Duragesic	100:1	N/A	25–50 mcg[4]
Methadone		Dolophine	1:2	5 mg TID[5]	2.5–5 mg

[1] Drug amounts (g/100,000 population) flowing from manufacture to sale or distribution.
[2] Morphine equivalent.
[3] Every 3 to 4 hours.
[4] Micrograms.
[5] Three times daily.

neutral to others. Therefore, they can precipitate withdrawal and other symptoms in patients taking opioid agonists concomitantly. Their analgesic efficacy also is limited by a dose-dependent ceiling effect.

General Principles of Administration

Relief of chronic moderate-to-severe pain requires an opioid given in a fixed-schedule, round-the-clock, day after day for as long as necessary.[22] As stated earlier, there is little evidence of the clinical superiority of one opioid over another regarding analgesic efficacy and/or side effects. However, most physicians are more familiar with morphine and tend to initiate therapy with this opioid in its short-acting oral formulation. The analgesic effects of short-acting oral opioids such as morphine, hydromorphone, codeine, and oxycodone begin within 30 minutes and last 4 hours approximately. Hence, they are administered every 4 hours. Oral administration is generally preferred because it is convenient and inexpensive, followed by the rectal or parenteral routes (subcutaneous, transmucosal, intravenous, and intraspinal), which are useful in special circumstances. The initial daily dose, chosen according to pain severity, and the opioid selected can be increased daily by 25% to 50%, if necessary, until pain relief is adequate or side effects become intolerable. Because they have no maximum or ceiling dose, "the appropriate dose of morphine agonists is whatever amount of opioid medication is necessary to control pain with the fewest side effects."[22] As with any pain medication, the goals of opioid treatment are to relieve pain, to enhance functional ability, and to improve quality of life within the context of tolerable side effects. Should tolerance develop, switching opioids becomes an option. Selecting a new opioid is empirical, and the dose equivalence (comparable dose based on relative potencies of the agents) for the new agent should be reduced by 25% to 50% initially to ensure safety. After the switch, patients should be monitored closely as the new opioid dose is escalated for maximum analgesic effect. Contrary to widespread belief, a prior history of substance abuse does not preclude using opioid analgesics but suggests caution when prescribing and careful patient monitoring to prevent abuse.

Once pain relief has been achieved, patients are usually switched to a controlled-release or slow-release formulation. The analgesic effect of controlled-release formulations of morphine and oxycodone, available in the United States, begins in 1 hour, peaks in 2 to 3 hours, and lasts up to 12 hours. Hence, these formulations are usually taken at 12-hour intervals, except for 10% to 20% of patients who require an 8-hour schedule. Fentanyl, a strong transdermal morphine agonist dispensed in patches, is an excellent controlled-release alternative for sustained, long-term pain management. Its analgesic effect begins approximately 12 hours after the application of the morphine-containing patch, peaks in 24 to 48 hours, and lasts for approximately 72 hours. Therefore, patches are replaced every 72 hours except in a small subset of patients who require new patches every 48 hours. Patients who have attained pain relief on a stable dose of a controlled-release opioid can develop occasional pain exacerbations referred to as *breakthrough pain*. Occasional breakthrough pain is easily and rapidly controlled with intravenous or short-acting oral opioids given at a dose approximately 20% of the equianalgesic (equivalent pain-killing power) total daily dose of the controlled-release opioid administered. Frequent breakthrough pains require adjustment of the controlled-release opioid dose or schedule.

Side Effects

Considering the efficacy and potency of opioid analgesics and their usefulness in chronic pain management, their side effects are relatively mild and seldom life-threatening, and addiction is not one of them. Side effects include, in decreasing order of frequency, constipation, nausea and vomiting, neurotoxicity, and less commonly pruritus, respiratory depression, and sexual dysfunction.

Constipation   Opioid analgesics impair gastrointestinal peristalsis (wavelike muscle contractions of the intestinal tract that move food along). Consequently, opioids prolong the gastrointestinal transit time, which promotes dehydration of stools as they slowly move down the intestine, making their evacuation difficult. Hence, constipation in one degree or another occurs in virtually all patients taking opioids on a chronic basis, especially morphine. Unconfirmed reports suggest that fentanyl and methadone might cause less constipation than oral morphine.[23,24] Drinking plenty of fluids is often advised in order to maintain a good level of hydration. However, while encouraging good systemic hydration is reasonable as it reduces stool dehydration, in practice, it is seldom successful in fully reversing opioid-induced constipation. Measures that are more effective include the use of stool softeners (e.g., docusate sodium), mild osmotic agents (e.g., milk of magnesia, 70% sorbitol solution, lactulose), lubricants (e.g., mineral oil), bulk-forming laxatives (e.g., psyllium), or mild cathartic laxatives (e.g., senna). More severe constipation can benefit from stimulant cathartics (e.g., bisacodyl), enemas, or in severe cases the physical removal of impacted stools. Rare cases can advance to a pseudo bowel obstruction, or mechanical ileus (bowel obstruction). Unlike analgesic tolerance, constipation tolerance does not develop, and patients remain constipated for as long as they take opioids. In fact, it is the main reason for patients abandoning opioid therapy.

Nausea   Nausea occurs in approximately one-third to two-thirds of patients taking opioids long term[25] and is related to decreased intestinal motility, dopamine stimulation, or, less frequently, to increased vestibular sensitivity. However, regardless of cause, most patients develop tolerance to nausea after a few days or weeks. Managing persistent nausea requires constipation relief, including measures outlined previously, or the use of agents such as metoclopramide or domperidone, which increase gastrointestinal motility and have antidopamine effects. In cases of motion-induced nausea, antihistamines or antiemetics can be helpful. Patients with refractory nausea might benefit from switching from one opioid agent to another.

Central Nervous System   Opioids can stimulate or inhibit the central nervous system, especially in the elderly. Stimulation, a rare occurrence, can induce hallucinations, generalized myoclonus (repetitive muscle spasm), occasionally hyperalgesia (extreme sensitivity to pain), allodynia (pain evoked by a normally nonpainful stimulus), or rarely delirium.[22] Inhibition can trigger lightheadedness, drowsiness, or confusion. A popular myth is that opioids can cause patients to become *zombies,* unable to function. Experience indicates that neurological side effects are usually rare and temporary, and long-term opioid therapy is usually associated with a normal level of mental function. The risk of developing neurotoxicity is greater in the elderly and in patients taking high doses of opioids, in patients whose opioid dose is suddenly increased, or in patients with chronic dehydration, renal impairment, and other comorbidities. In these clinical circumstances, the culprit appears to be the accumulation of opioid metabolites, a suggestion supported by animal and clinical studies. Neurological symptoms usually subside after three to five days on a constant opioid dose. However, in cases of persisting neurotoxicity, dose reduction, changing the route of administration, or switching to a different opioid agent are strategies worth trying. If this fails, a multidimensional approach might be required that includes managing contributing factors such as interfering drugs and underlying comorbidities, or the pharmacologic treatment of the actual neurological symptoms. The latter includes the use of sedatives (e.g., haloperidol, methotrimeprazine, and chlorpromazine), anxiolytics (e.g., lorazepam), psychostimulants (e.g., caffeine, dextroamphetamine, or methylphenidate), and other psychotropic drugs.

Respiratory Depression   Respiratory depression, a rare event, is more likely to occur when opioid-naïve patients are first started on opioids, when opioids are given parenterally, or when the doses are rapidly escalated, especially in patients whose advanced disease or age make them vulnerable. However, most patients receiving long-term opioid therapy quickly develop tolerance to these agents' respiratory-depressant effects. Additionally,

Table 6
Drugs to Be Avoided for the Treatment of Cancer Pain[22]

Class	Drug	Rationale for not Recommending
Opioids	Meperidine (Demerol)	Short-lived 2–3 hrs analgesia. Risk of CNS toxicity.
Agonists/ antagonists	Pentazocine (Talwin) Butorphanol (Sterol)	Risk of withdrawal in opioid-dependent patients.
	Nalbuphine (Nubian)	Analgesic ceiling. Risk of psychotomimetic effects.
Partial agonist	Buprenorphine (Buprenex)	Analgesic ceiling. May precipitate withdrawal.
Antagonists	Naloxone (Narcan) Naltrexone (ReVia)	Reverses life-threatening agonists complications BUT may precipitate withdrawal.
Combination preparations	Brompton's cocktail	No better than single-opioid analgesics.
	Meperidine, Promethazine, and Chlorpromazine	Lower efficacy than other analgesics. High incidence of adverse effects.
Anxiolytics	Benzodiazepine (e.g., Alprazolam, Xanax; Diazepam, Valium; Lorazepam, Ativan)	OK for some neuropathic pain. Additional sedation to patients on opioids limits neurologic assessment.
Sedatives	Barbiturates Benzodiazepine	Analgesic properties not demonstrated. Added sedation limits opioid dosing.

opioid-induced respiratory depression is easily and quickly reversed by the administration of naloxone, an opioid antagonist (Table 6).

Sexual Dysfunction   Decreased libido and feminizing effects have been known for centuries to occur in men addicted to heroin. Recent studies have revealed low blood testosterone levels in sexually dysfunctional men on long-term methadone treatment of opioid addiction. However, as increasing numbers of chronic pain sufferers are being treated with opioids, sexual dysfunction is being reported more frequently in the context of opioid analgesia. Its management consists of empiric measures such as reducing or eliminating opioids when possible, or adding nonopioid or adjuvant analgesic agents to the pain management regimen. Testosterone replacement therapy, in men, can be beneficial.

Urticaria and Pruritus   Opioid-induced itching and urticaria are usually short-lived and respond to antihistamine treatment or switching to opioids that do not release histamine, such as oxymorphone or fentanyl.

Other Adverse Effects and Precautions   Other adverse effects can occur in patients with comorbidities taking medications that potentiate opioid effects through pharmacologic synergism, the accumulation of opioid metabolites, or patient frailty associated with age and preexisting illnesses. Limitations and cautions to the use of certain opioids, especially for the management of cancer pain, are listed in Table 6.

In conclusion, opioids are strong analgesics best suited for the treatment of moderate-to-severe pain, whether from cancer or from noncancer causes. Their high benefit-to-risk ratio suggests that they are some of the safest drugs on the market despite unjustifiable fears of addiction; a notion that is aggressively promoted by the DEA and state and local drug enforcement agencies, reinforced by detractors and self-serving politicians, and obligingly disseminated by an uncritical media.

Let us sum up the evidence. The incidence of addiction in patients taking opioids long term for analgesic purposes has been reported to range between 0.3%[26] and 24%.[27] The discrepancy is caused by including tolerance and physical dependence, which is listed as criteria for drug abuse in the *Diagnostic and Statistical Manual III-R*, adding pseudo-addictive behavior as true addiction. Today, there is a consensus among pain experts that "aberrant drug-taking behavior from cancer pain management is generally related to a premorbid history of drug addiction."[28] This means that addiction among patients taking opioids long term is similar to that found in the general population adjusted for age. Indeed, drug abuse is less prevalent among older adults and the elderly than among younger population subsets. For instance, in 2004 85.9% of American high school seniors used drugs *within the last 12 months*, compared to 15% for the *older* population.[29] Likewise, 2002 arrests for marijuana possession decreased with increasing age, from 969 (per 100,000) teenagers aged 15 to 19, to 366 for young men 24 to 29, to 162 for men 34 to 39, to 35 for adults 50 to 54, and 7 for the 60 to 64 age group.[30] Finally, according to the latest survey report from the

Institute for Social Research of the University of Michigan,[31] the *30-day* prevalence rate for *any illicit drug* peaks at 17% to 23% for the 18 to 26 age group, falling to 9% by age 45 (chapter 2, figure 1).

Hence, a 5.9% and 3.9% incidence of drug abuse (mainly benzodiazepine) among elderly patients hospitalized or consulting psychiatric services, respectively, reported in a small German study might reflect the true addiction prevalence *expected* in that age population.[32] However, the prevalence of opioid addiction in *chronic pain* sufferers, whether from cancer of other causes, is actually much lower than observed in the population at large regardless of age. In large measure, this is due to these patients' motivation for taking opioids: a desire to obtain pain relief rather than to achieve a hedonistic experience. Therefore, addiction *resulting* from chronic opioid treatment for pain is actually much lower than is being cited, especially by detractors. Indeed, as cited earlier in three large studies involving 24,251 hospitalized patients with no prior history of drug abuse who were administered opioids for chronic noncancer pain, only 7 patients, or 0.03%, showed evidence of abuse or addiction.[26,33,34] These studies established conclusively that when taken for analgesic purposes by patients without prior history of drug abuse opioids are nonaddictive, a judgment endorsed by pain experts, health organizations, medical societies, and other knowledgeable sources.

Hence, perhaps the National Clearing House (an agency of the U.S. Department of Health and Human Services) should justify its uninformed and misleading 2006 guidelines titled "Opioid guidelines in the management of chronic non-cancer pain."[35] It recommends, "prior to embarking on a regimen of opioids the physician must determine, through actual clinical trial or through patient records and history, that non-addictive medication regimens and/or interventional techniques have been inadequate or are unacceptable for solid clinical reasons." In a veiled condemnation of physician practices it also warns, "important issues in opioid therapy for the treatment of chronic pain revolve around the appropriate use of prescription opioids. Consequently, adherence monitoring is crucial to avoid abuse of the drugs and at the same time to encourage appropriate use." Suspecting a potential addict in every patient it suggests, "Adherence monitoring is achieved by screening tests, urine drug testing, and periodic monitoring." Emulating the DEA's anti-physician posture, such *guidelines* hold good pain management hostage to drug policy and coerce practitioners to regard all chronic pain sufferers as potential addicts. The absurdity and capricious implementation of drug policy impose restrictions on the manufacture, distribution, and prescription of opioid analgesics to the detriment of millions of American pain sufferers. Once in place, such policies and repressive laws acquire an inertia of their own that ensures their longevity and the unending violation of individual freedoms and of the fundamental and inviolable human right to pain relief. Only their repeal will give meaning to the maxim "Pain is inevitable; suffering is optional" and empower pain sufferers and their physicians, not the DEA, to exercise that option.

NONOPIOIDS

> If deaths from gastrointestinal toxic effects of NSAIDs were tabulated sepa-
> rately in the National Vital Statistics reports, these effects would constitute
> the 15th most common cause of death in the United States.
> —M. W. Wolfe, D. R. Lichtenstein, and G. Singh (1999)

Nonopioid include all NSAIDs plus acetaminophen because of its similar analgesic properties despite lacking anti-inflammatory effects. NSAIDs
are the most widely used drugs of any kind worldwide,[36-38] the most often
overprescribed, the most misused,[39] and the most frequent cause of iatro-
genic (unintended result of treatment) pathology. Between the mid-1980s
and early 1990s, 70 million prescriptions for NSAIDs were dispensed yearly
in the United States,[36] 20 million in Great Britain,[37] and 10 million in Canada.[38] Aspirin, probably the least expensive and most popular NSAID,
accounts for more than 30 billion tablets dispensed each year in the United
States at a cost in excess of $1 billion. Not bad for a drug derived from
the bark and leaves of the willow tree, used by Hippocrates to treat pain,
whose active ingredient was isolated by Johann Buchner in 1829 and, after
several improvements in extraction, purification, and formulation, was pat-
ented and marketed in February 1900 by Bayer AG. These consumption figures, which do not include over-the-counter self-medicating purchases so
prevalent in the United States, have risen considerably since. NSAIDs are
efficacious and safe analgesics when used for short periods to treat acute
mild-to-moderate pain. However, frequent or protracted use of NSAIDs is
associated with serious and even life-threatening side effects, especially in
frail individuals and the elderly, making them unsuitable for the long-term
management of chronic pain. Aspirin has the distinct advantage of helping prevent heart attacks and colon cancer in addition to its analgesic and
antipyretic properties. Yet, like other NSAIDs, it can cause life-threatening
gastrointestinal side effects and idiosyncratic (peculiar to an individual)
allergic reactions in small subsets of patients that would probably preclude FDA approval of the drug in today's tightly regulated drug environment, according to a former FDA commissioner.[40]

Mechanisms of Action

Based on their mechanism of action, NSAIDs are classified as nonselective and selective (Table 7). Nonselective NSAIDs, the most commonly
prescribed, inhibit prostaglandin synthesis via blocking the activity of both
cyclooxygenase-1 (COX-1) and cyclooxygenase-2 (COX-2). Prostaglandins
are ubiquitous substances involved in inflammation and platelet aggregation and have been implicated in cardiovascular and inflammatory diseases, and even in cancer. COX-1 is present in most tissues, particularly
platelets (blood cells necessary for vascular integrity and clotting), stomach,
and kidney. As a *housekeeper* enzyme, prostaglandins maintain the integrity

Table 7
Common Nonselective and Selective NSAIDs, MRTD or Daily Dose, and NNT

Nonselective NSAIDs	MRTD[2] (or usual daily dose)	Mean NNT[1]
Acetaminophen	50	3.5–3.8
Aspirin	67	4.4
Choline Mg trisalicylate	ND[3] (1,000 mg Q6 hrs[4])	ND
Diclophenac	3.75	2.3
Ibuprofen	40	2.4
Indometacin	ND (25 mg Q6 hrs)	ND
Naproxen	ND (250 mg Q6 hrs)	2.3
Mefenamic acid	21	ND
Meloxicam	ND (7.5 mg QD[5])	ND
Piroxicam	ND (20 mg QD)	2.7
Selective Coxibs		ND
Celecoxib	6.7	2.8
Valdecoxib	Withdrawn from the market	1.6
Rofecoxib	Withdrawn from the market	1.9

[1] Number needed to treat[42] (see text).
[2] Maximum recommended therapeutic dose in mg/kg/day[43]
[3] Not determined.
[4] Every 6 hours.
[5] Daily.

of the gastric mucosa, are necessary for platelet aggregation, and influence kidney function, making their pharmacological inhibition undesirable. On the other hand, COX-2 is a *constitutive* enzyme found in kidney, brain, testicular, and tracheal epithelium, though it is predominantly induced by inflammation with levels rising up to twenty folds, in which case its pharmacological inhibition is desirable and therapeutic.

NSAIDs include more than 30 drugs with slightly different chemical structures, which result in different anti-COX-1 and anti-COX-2 activities, metabolic pathways, and side effect profiles. Studies in guinea pigs have demonstrated a direct correlation between the COX-1 to COX-2 inhibition ratio and side effects of several NSAIDs studied: The lower the COX-1 inhibition the fewer the side effects. For example, in a recent study, meloxicam, an NSAID with a lower-than-average incidence of side effects, exhibited a COX-1/COX-2 inhibition ratio of 0.33, whereas indomethacin, an NSAID with a higher-than-average incidence of side effects, had a ratio of 122.[41] Hence, a new subclass of NSAIDs called *coxibs* was developed to selectively inhibit COX-2 with the expectation of eliminating COX-1-associated side effects. Three coxibs were approved by the FDA: celecoxib, valdecoxib, and rofecoxib. However, rofecoxib was withdrawn from the market on September 30, 2004, after greater-than-expected serious thromboembolic (occlusion of a vessel by a clot originating at a distant site) events were detected in patients taking the drug long term and at higher-than-usual doses as part of a cancer prevention trial. As an aside, this is yet another failed cancer *chemoprevention* study (the use of drugs in attempts to prevent cancer or reduce recurrences) that confirms my view that "the mechanism of action of chemopreventive agents are ill-defined and their long-term side effects can counteract their anticipated cancer preventing benefits."[13] On April 7, 2005, valdecoxib also was withdrawn from the market after the FDA ruled that the drug's overall risks outweighed its potential benefits. Whether celecoxib and other COX-2 inhibitors are safer is a question that must be ascertained given their marginally greater potency and only slightly lower gastrointestinal side effects than nonselective NSAIDs despite their higher cost. As a result, nonselective NSAIDs are still the favored analgesics for acute mild-to-moderate pain, especially combined with agents that protect the gastric mucosa (discussed later).

Efficacy

Ascertaining the efficacy of NSAIDs is complicated by differences in NSAIDs doses, study design, execution, or analysis of the many studies undertaken to gather that information. However, the *Oxford league table of analgesic in acute pain* provides a useful tool to assess relative efficacy of the most common NSAIDs. The Oxford table is based on a meta-analysis (statistical synthesis of data from comparable studies) of multiple randomized, double-blind, single-dose studies in patients taking NSAIDs for moderate-to-severe pain. Each NSAID is ranked according to its "Number [of patients] Needed to Treat" (NNT), or to its inducing 50% pain relief over 4–6 hours.[42] The NNT (Table 7) of several NSAIDs analyzed ranged from 1.6 for valdecoxib (40 mg), to 2.3 for naproxen (440 mg) and ibuprofen (400 mg), to 3.8 for paracetamol (acetaminophen in the United States) (1,000 mg), to 4.4 for aspirin (650 mg), to 5.3 for tramadol (75 mg). It must be stressed that while the NNT provides an indication of the average relative potency of NSAIDs, their efficacy, like that of all painkillers, is influenced by the medical, psychological, and social profiles of each individual patient; the type and severity of the underlying pain-causing disease; and the presence of comorbidities. In addition to NNT, the choice of an NSAID must take into consideration its risks, discussed later under side effects.

General Principles of Administration

According to the WHO's widely adopted "use of analgesic guidelines," patients with mild-to-moderate cancer pain should be treated by the ladder.[6] The sequence is described as follows: "The first step is a non-opioid. If this does not relieve the pain, an opioid for mild to moderate pain should be added. When an opioid for mild to moderate pain in combination with a non-opioid fails to relieve the pain, an opioid for moderate to severe pain should be substituted. Only one from each of the groups should be used at the same time. Adjuvant drugs should be given for specific indications." Implied in the WHO's ladder is the acknowledgment of NSAIDs' low potency relative to opioids, hence the need to add an opioid to adequately treat many cases of mild-to-moderate pain. Therefore, it stands to reason that such agents would be inefficacious for the management of most cases of moderate-to-severe pain. Moreover, as described later, their severe and often potentially life-threatening side effects profiles make them unsuitable for long-term administration required for the management of chronic pain, for which they have proven inefficacious.[44] Consequently, NSAIDS should be restricted to treat acute mild-to-moderate pain.

Acetaminophen is usually favored for the initial treatment of mild pain because, unlike NSAIDs, it is not associated with gastrointestinal complications. However, it can cause liver or kidney damage, especially at doses higher than 4 grams per day. However, NSAIDS have become the drugs of choice for the treatment of all types of pain regardless of severity and anticipated duration. This is confirmed by surveys showing NSAIDs to be the most common analgesics sold both in America, whether over the counter (63%) or by prescription (29%),[39] and worldwide, according to consumption statistics cited earlier. There is wide variation in the way patients respond to the effectiveness and side effects of individual NSAIDs. Likewise, usually recommended doses may be optimal in one case but either too high or too low in another. Hence, physicians must proceed cautiously by trial and error to identify the most appropriate NSAID and the optimal dose for each patient. If the level of pain relief and quality of life outcomes, set by patient and physician, are not met after several weeks of NSAIDs administration, an opioid should replace rather than be added to the NSAID regimen, as advocated by the WHO. All patients should be advised of the risks and monitored closely for signs or symptoms of complications, though ulcers can be asymptomatic at the onset. Finally, great caution should be exercised in patients with a prior history of gastrointestinal ulcers or bleeding, or with a low platelet count.

Side Effects

The most frequent and clinically significant side effects of NSAIDs are gastrointestinal dyspepsia (stomach discomfort), gastric or duodenal ulcer (with or without perforation and bleeding), followed by kidney damage and anaphylaxis (hypersensitivity reaction resulting from prior exposure). Asthma exacerbation and erectile dysfunction occur infrequently.

Gastrointestinal Side Effects   Although NSAIDs are well tolerated generally, gastrointestinal side effects occur in a small but significant percentage of patients, resulting in substantial morbidity and mortality. A meta-analysis of 527 high-quality studies published between 1985 and 2003 involving 5,325 patients receiving NSAIDs for a period of 5 to 1,825 days, put the average relative risk (RR) of NSAIDs-induced gastrointestinal complications compared to controls at 1.54.[45] Indomethacin exhibited the highest risk of the group (RR = 2.25) and ibuprofen the lowest (RR = 1.19), with other NSAIDs ranging between RR 1.43 and 1.83. The risk was time-, dose-, and drug-dependent, with indomethacin triggering side effects as early as seven days, while the others required two to three months of therapy at recommended doses. Patients developing ulcers, bleeding, or perforation, were older on the average than patients with minor or no gastrointestinal complaints. The mechanisms responsible for NSAIDs' gastrointestinal complications have not been elucidated fully but involve both local and systemic factors. Local factors include mucosal injury caused by the acidic properties of NSAIDs and by alteration of the gastric mucus. Systemic factors include inhibition of endogenous prostaglandin synthesis, which leads to decreased epithelial mucus and mucosal blood flow, and epithelial proliferation. Together, these NSAIDs effects impair mucosal resistance to injury,[46] which in turn allows tissue damage by exogenous factors such as gastric acid, pepsin, bile salts, ethanol, NSAIDs themselves, and other noxious agents. Once tissue damage has taken place, COX-1 inhibition of platelet aggregation, which begins the process of plugging vascular leaks, promotes bleeding at the sites of tissue injury.

In the United States, at least 10% to 20% of individuals taking NSAIDs develop dyspepsia, 1% to 2% require hospitalization from serious gastrointestinal complications (e.g., ulcer or gastrointestinal bleeding), and 5% to 10% of these die as a result. Ulcers and gastrointestinal bleeding are often not preceded by symptoms, making these complications the more serious and unpredictable. Older age; prior history of peptic ulcer or of gastrointestinal bleeding; higher NSAID dose; treatment duration; concurrent use of corticosteroids, anticoagulants, alcohol, or smoking; and the presence of comorbidities and their treatment increase the risk of serious NSAID-induced gastrointestinal complications.[47–49] Most deaths from NSAID-related gastrointestinal complications occur in elderly persons, particularly women. Hence, given the seriousness of NSAIDs' gastrointestinal complications, prevention is crucial. It should include avoidance of NSAIDs altogether or choosing an analgesic agent without gastrointestinal side effects (e.g., acetaminophen) for individuals at risk, or the concomitant administration of agents to protect the mucosa from injury. Examples of the latter include H2 receptor agonists (e.g., cimetidine, ranitidine, or famotidine), or proton-pump inhibitors (e.g., omeprazole) to patients not especially vulnerable.

While the incidence of serious NSAIDs-induced side effects mentioned previously is relatively low, it nevertheless translates into very high levels of morbidity and mortality when extrapolated to the entire NSAIDs-medicated population. Indeed, based on the 70 million prescriptions[50] and 30 billion over-the-counter tablets sold annually in the United States, it is estimated that over 100,000 individuals are hospitalized each year for serious gastrointestinal complications, costing in excess of US$2 billion and 16,500 deaths.[47,51,52] The magnitude of the problem has been characterized as follows: "If deaths from gastrointestinal toxic effects of NSAIDs were tabulated separately in the National Vital Statistics reports, these effects would constitute the 15th most common cause of death in the United States. Yet, these toxic effects remain largely a 'silent epidemic,' with many physicians and most patients unaware of the magnitude of the problem. Furthermore, mortality statistics do not include deaths ascribed to the use of over-the-counter NSAIDs."[47] Data from other countries reveal similar statistics. For instance, a recent survey of 83% of the 269 Spanish National Health System hospitals was conducted "to determine mortality associated with hospital admission due to major gastrointestinal (GI) events and NSAID/aspirin use." It found, "the incidence of hospital admissions due to major GI events of the entire (upper and lower) gastrointestinal tract was 121.9 events/100,000 persons/year, but those related to the upper GI tract were six times more frequent. Mortality rate was 5.57% . . . and 5.62% . . . in study 1 and study 2, respectively. Death rate attributed to NSAID/aspirin use was . . . 15.3 deaths/100,000 NSAID/aspirin users. Up to one-third of all NSAID/aspirin deaths can be attributed to low-dose aspirin use."[53]

Other Severe Side Effects   It has been estimated that prolonged exposure to NSAIDs accounts for 11% to 13% of all cases of end-stage renal disease and 26% of all cases of severe drug-induced anaphylactic reactions (a potentially fatal form of allergic shock).[52]

In conclusion, based on WHO's widely adopted "Use of analgesic guidelines,"[6] patients with mild-to-moderate cancer pain should be treated following the three-step ladder. Cancer pain is often used as a benchmark for comparison purposes because many clinical cancer studies, testing numerous variables in a multitude of combinations and permutations, foster greater consensus on its management than that of noncancer pain. Additionally, a diagnosis of cancer conjures up the *finality of death* that *justifies* a presumed risk of addiction to opioids, whereas that risk is felt to be disproportionate for patients expected to recover from the illness causing pain. Hence, the widely adopted ladder approach recommends the use of a nonopioid drug first, adding a mild opioid if this fails, followed by further escalation through stronger opioids plus adjuvant agents, when needed. Using NSAIDs to treat mild-to-moderate pain regardless of cause, particularly if acute or subacute, beginning with the most efficacious and best tolerated (e.g., ibuprofen and naproxen), is indeed appropriate. However, while the unwarranted fear of opioid addiction catapulted NSAIDs to the forefront of chronic cancer and noncancer pain management, the practice is unwise and dangerous. The main reasons are three-fold. First, the relatively weak analgesic potency of NSAIDs usually requires dose escalation or the addition of or switching to an opioid to manage moderate-to-severe pain. Second, most patients with chronic pain are individuals at greater than average risk for serious gastrointestinal side effects given their age, frailty, presence of comorbidities, or the treatment of the latter with medications that contribute to or potentiate NSAIDs' side effects. Thirdly, the frequency of potentially severe and life-threatening side effects increases with NSAIDs dose escalation and long-term administration, both required for the successful management of chronic pain.

Another unwise medical practice is adding NSAIDs to an opioid regimen for managing moderate-to-severe pain, based on an alleged NSAIDs *opioid-sparing effect*. However, reports of opioid sparing[54,55] are based on random effects probably related to variable accumulation of opioid metabolites caused by NSAIDs-induced renal impairment.[56] Likewise, NSAIDs–opioid combinations are ill advised. Indeed, the NSAID component increases the potency of the combination only marginally while reducing side effects of its opioid component insignificantly. Additionally, the potential for increased toxicity from the NSAIDs component precludes escalation of the NSAID–opioid combination. Hence, unless necessary to treat opioid-intolerant patients, a questionable indication, relying on an alleged opioid-sparing effect of NSAIDs or on NSAID opioid combinations is an illogical practice born out of an unjustified fear of addiction to prescription opioids, inexperience, or self-delusion. Indeed, addiction in patients taking opioids for pain relief is extremely rare, μ-agonists (morphine-like) have no ceiling dose and therefore need no sparing, and NSAIDs cause far more frequent and serious complications than opioids they supposedly spare, including thousands of deaths each year. Hence, adding potentially lethal NSAIDs to opioid-based regimens for the purpose of lowering the dose of more potent and far safer opioids seems a bizarre notion that has no place in the practice of evidence-based medicine of the 21st century.

PART III

Geopolitics: Casualties of the Drug War

The War on Drugs has received considerable attention and rightfully generated widespread condemnation over the years. Critics include celebrities ranging from libertarian socialist intellectual Noam Chomsky; to conservative author and commentator William F. Buckley; from financier and philanthropist George Soros; to former U.S. Secretary of Labor, State, and Treasury George Shultz; and economist and Nobel Prize winner Milton Friedman.[1] However, most critics have concentrated on the negative impact of drug policy on American society almost entirely overlooking its geopolitical and socioeconomic impacts at the international level. Therefore, in order to raise awareness on the devastating impact of War on Drugs policies overseas, especially on producer countries, chapter 7 describes in some detail the plight of Colombia, supplier of 80% of the global cocaine demand, and of Afghanistan, provider of over 90% of the worldwide opium market. This stunning concentration of illegal crop production in these two countries is no accident. They both benefit from favorable climactic and geographic conditions and are cursed by inefficient political and legal infrastructures compounded by organized insurgents and criminal groups for which the highly lucrative black market of illicit drugs, initiated and sustained by the criminalization of drugs, is a godsend. Indeed, this irresistible and unmatched road to riches funds guerillas, counter guerillas, warlords, terrorists, and common criminals, often with the complicity of government officials. By supplying consumer countries' insatiable demand for drugs by whatever means, these groups bring devastation to their countries' underclass and corruption to their political and judicial systems. However, while demand drives supply in all commercial transactions, including drugs, placing a large share of blame on consumer countries, producer countries, especially Colombia and Afghanistan, also must assume responsibility for chronically dysfunctional institutions underlying their current precarious sociopolitical and socioeconomic conditions.

Mexico has recently become the center of attention as the main point of illegal drug entry into the United States and as the location of a fierce war on traffickers waged by President Felipe Calderón. However, while the ruthlessness of Mexican traffickers' crimes in bordering towns where they operate and their confrontations with the Mexican Army are locally devastating and cause thousands of casualties, their impact on Mexican institutions and society is so far limited and is not dealt with in this book. Moreover, it represents but the newest chapter in ever shifting players and theaters of operation of a war whose outcome will remain the same: an unmitigated failure.

CHAPTER 7

Colombia

More Colombians die from diseases caused by American tobacco products than do Americans from Colombian cocaine.
—NORML News, New Zealand

We should legalize drugs because we here are providing the dead, and the consumers are there in the US.
—Gustavo de Greiff, former attorney general of Colombia

As the main producer of cocaine destined to supply an unabated demand in countries of consumption, mostly the United States and West European nations, Colombia has been devastated by an unimaginable level of corruption that reaches far and wide and by violence on the rural poor caught between warring factions focused on protecting their turf and illegal sources of income. Social dislocations include 3.4 million peasants, or 13.1% of the rural population, displaced between 1985 and 2004,[2] with over 400,000 in 2002 alone, after being robbed of their land and possessions by guerillas and counter-guerilla groups, creating "the gravest humanitarian situation in Latin America."[3] Political disruptions result mostly from the ongoing collusion with such groups of a large number of conniving congressmen, the Liberal party, and at least two former presidents.[4] From a historical and socioeconomic standpoint, cocaine trafficking was propelled to a business of massive proportions by the *Medellin cartel*, which dominated the trade in the 1970s. After the assassination of its founder and leader, Pablo Escobar, the *Cali cartel* became the predominant cocaine exporter through the 1980s, but its dismantlement in 1995 opened the door for the drug trade to become one of the major funding activities of insurgent guerillas and counter-guerilla groups, along with kidnapping for ransom and extortion. As a result, Colombia is often viewed as a *narco-democracy* where the impact of drugs permeates the economy, the ruling class, the political and judicial systems, and the everyday lives of ordinary Colombians.

Yet, while Colombia is considered today one of the most violent countries in the world, its violent history preceded narco-trafficking. It can be traced back to the period of *La Violencia*, between 1946 and 1965. Characterized by armed confrontation between the two main political parties, La Violencia was the precursor to insurgent left-wing movements of the 1950s and right-wing armies of the 1980s, all eventually funded by drug trafficking that led to drug-related widespread crime and massive human rights violations. However, to pretend that Colombia has brought onto itself all the social and political ills it now faces is tantamount to ignoring the impact of War on Drugs policies and of U.S. foreign policy on its internal affairs. The former has fostered a highly lucrative worldwide black market of illicit drugs that provide guerilla and counter-guerilla armies an irresistible incentive to abandon their initially altruistic goals of bringing social justice to the masses and protection from the rich and powerful, becoming narco-trafficking enterprises instead. In turn, this metamorphosis opened the door for U.S. foreign policy of overt or covert intrusion in Central and South American affairs to become a player in Colombia's 50 year–long internal conflict. Indeed, "U.S. intervention in Colombia [currently through ['Plan Colombia'] is accepted because of its ostensible anti-drug objectives, but its effects extend beyond the sphere of drug control."[5] This chapter describes in some detail major historical and political events that led to the decades-old Colombian conflict and how the drug trade impacted its major players and shaped today's Colombian society.

FROM "LA VIOLENCIA" TO SELF-DEFENSE ARMIES

While Colombia experienced four civil wars between 1895 and 1902, the last one lasting 1,000 days (Thousand-Day War), the period known as La Violencia began in 1946 when Mariano Ospina Perez, candidate for the Conservative party (one of two major political parties) won the presidential election. Over the ensuing decades, La Violencia evolved into a multifaceted armed struggle referred to as El Conflicto.[6] Ospina Perez's electoral victory was due, in large measure, to the split of the Liberal party between a moderate wing, led by the official candidate Gabriel Turbay, and a radical faction headed by populist Jorge Eléicer Gaitán. The assassination of Gaitán on April 9, 1948, ignited the Bogotá Revolution in April 1948 (known as *Bogotázo*) and other major cities and the uprising of disenfranchised peasants, leading to rural violence by guerrilla groups of liberal leaning, especially in the *llanos orientates* (western planes) and in coffee growing areas of the Andes mountains. Conservative counter-revolutionary bands called *los pájaros* (the birds) also roamed the countryside. The polarization intensified under the government of President Laureano Gomez, whose uncontested election had been boycotted by the Liberals. The Gomez regime, supported by the Catholic Church and the United States, viewed uprising peasants as Communist insurgents and intensified their repression, resulting in violent confrontations between Liberal and Conservative camps and between peasants and landowners.

Armed peasant groups of Liberal or Communist persuasion organized themselves mostly for self-defense against the violent incursions of the national Army. For instance, one of the Communist-leaning groups founded *ciudad roja* (red city) in Viotá, one of the first communist-inspired armed communes, with similar settlements soon to follow. In 1953, Gomez was overthrown by a military coup led by General Gustavo Rojas Pinilla, who first dispatched the Army to reclaim lands occupied by peasants but later changed tactics, promising an unmet agrarian reform and issuing a general amnesty with government aid for belligerents willing to lay down their arms. Thousands accepted the offer. However, many of the demobilized men were subsequently killed in an escalating cycle of revenge, and Gomez sympathizers, released from prison, renewed their hostilities against peasants, forcing them to take up arms again. In 1955, Rojas Pinilla responded by launching a massive Army offensive against armed peasants that became known as the *Guerra de Villarica*. This caused a massive exodus of armed peasants towards Marquetalia, Ríochiquito, El Pato, Guayabero, El Duda, and El Ariari where they founded new settlements, loosely called *independent republics*. Like Viotá, these settlements were more a means of self-defense (*autodefensas*) than a prelude to overthrow the central government. Hence, La Violencia was a combination of political interparty fighting for power and a peasant revolt for social justice. In 1957, the two major parties entered into a pact called *Frente Nacional* (National Front) to alternate the presidency and high-level governmental positions as a means to end the political conflict. However, by failing to address inequities and injustices toward the peasant population, the pact was unsuccessful in ending the armed conflict in rural areas.

In the meantime, while leftist *autodefensas* had accepted Rojas Pinilla's amnesty, their Communist counterparts under the leadership of *Charro Negro* and Manuel Marulanda Vélez refused. Theirs remained a minuscule *autodefensas* with little relevance to the national life or politics for several years. However, on May 27, 1964, the government of President Guillermo León Valencia launched a massive assault, by 16,000 infantrymen backed by airpower, on the independent republic of Marquetalia where Marulanda had retrenched with his 48-armed *self-defense* peasants. Their instructions were to destroy the insurgents within three weeks. In response to the attack, Marulanda's *autodefensas* became an outright revolutionary army that two years later would be renamed *Fuerzas Armadas Revolucionarias de Colombia* or FARC (Revolutionary Armed Forces of Colombia), this time with the stated aim to overthrow the government. While the FARC evolved into the largest Colombian insurgent force, it lost its early political ideology, becoming instead a guerilla group caught up in a vicious cycle of narco-trafficking, kidnapping for ransom, and extortion with the tacit compliance of a terrorized rural peasantry.

An additional four insurgent groups emerged during this period: *El Ejército de Liberación Nacional* (National Liberation Army or ELN), inspired on Communist and Cuban ideology and on *liberation theology; El Ejército Popular de Liberación* (Popular Army of Liberation or EPL), a Marxist-Leninist insurgency that was demobilized in 1991; *El Movimiento 19 de Abril* (Movement April 19th or M-19), an insurgent group that gained notoriety through a series of daring urban raids, including the infamous Dominican Embassy occupation in 1980 and the ill-fated takeover of the Palace of Justice in 1985 where more than 100 people died, including 11 Supreme Court judges (in exchange for a full government pardon, the group laid down its weapons in 1989 and joined the country's political system); and finally, *Las Autodefensas Unidas de Colombia* (United Self-defense Forces of Colombia or AUC), better known as *paramilitares*. As the name indicates, these armies were organized with overt or tacit support of the Colombian Army to provide protection against guerilla attack, kidnappings, and extortion. In contrast to the FARC and ELN, the AUC are not a unified organization with a central command, as its name implies, but a collection of semiautonomous regional groups that are infamous for their gratuitous and brutal violence, massive violations of human rights, and for their close connections with many local and national politicians.

GUERRILLA AND COUNTER-GUERILLA ARMIES: ORIGINS AND EVOLUTION

In addition to a host of criminal gangs and hired guns, Colombia confronts two Marxist guerilla movements that remain operative today: the FARC and the ELN, and their sworn enemy, the AUC. The first two groups rose in the mid-1960s in reaction to the state's neglect of the underclass, abuses by the ruling elite, and the desperate socioeconomic conditions of Colombian peasants abandoned to live a subsistence-level existence without access to education, health care, sanitation, electricity, or even running water.

Yet, 50 years later, the plight of most Colombians has changed little. Indeed, "in the year 2000 no more than 0.4 percent of the landowners owned 61.2 percent of the arable land, while 57.3 percent of landowners were small-scale peasants owning just 1.7 percent of the land."[7] In the same time frame (2002), unemployment in the seven largest cities averaged 15.6%, and 48% of Colombians in the *workforce* were street vendors or held sporadic menial jobs.[8] More recently (2006), official figures indicated that nearly 50% of

Colombians still lived below the poverty line (US$3.30 per person, per day),[8,9] ranking Colombia the 34th poorest country in the world,[10] a slight improvement from 2002 levels. The same sources indicated that nearly 15% of Colombians lived in misery in 2006, surviving on less than US$1.50 per person, per day.[9] Today's Americans and Europeans, used to high living standards and minimum hourly wages ranging from US$7.25 to up to 11.00 Euros (US$16.00 at 2009 exchange rates), respectively, will find such appalling living conditions difficult to comprehend.

The AUC, whose original purpose was to protect wealthy landlords from the FARC and the ELN acting as surrogates of the Colombian Army, were demobilized in March 2005 (see caveat under AUC heading). However, although the FARC's and ELN's original commitment to social justice was justifiable and their motives altruistic, and the AUC's defensible at the outset, these groups became decidedly criminalized, which along with their abhorrent *modus operandi* has undermined their credibility and support in Colombia and internationally. Indeed, they engage in wanton violence and massive human rights violations, mostly against the segment of the population they claim to represent, supporting their *cause* through narco-trafficking, kidnapping for ransom, and extortion of businesses and of individuals. As a result, all three have been branded *terrorist organizations*, by the United States, the European Union, and other nations.

Fuerzas Armadas Revolucionarias de Colombia (FARC)

Origins Following the carnage at Marquetalia by the Colombian Army in 1964, Communist *autodefensas* dispersed only to regroup as the *Bloque Sur* (Southern Bloc) later renamed FARC, under the joint leadership of Manuel Marulanda Vélez (real name, Pedro Antonio Marín) a.k.a. *Tirofijo* (Sureshot), its commander, and Jacobo Arenas, its Communist ideologue. Arenas chronicled the attack in a book titled *Diario de la Resistencia de Marquetalia* (Diary of the Marquetalian Resistance). The FARC's initial force of 350 armed men grew slowly until 1982 when, at the *Seventh Guerrilla Conference*, it developed its first *Strategic Plan*. The plan outlined incremental goals to be reached through the *Ejército del Pueblo* (The People's Army), meant to seize power "sometime in the 1990s" using legal and illegal means of struggle. The conference was a turning point in the FARC's struggle, as it provided a forum to focus on policies and plans to achieve their dual goals of seizing power and of creating a Socialist state.

At its peak, the FARC reached an estimated 12,000–18,000 fighters, including 20% to 30% of children as young as 9 years of age. They were organized into five *bloques* and two joint commands that operated throughout Colombia's territory though, as of late, they have been both plagued by desertions and pushed back to southeastern regions by the Colombian Army. Some children-fighters are forcibly recruited, but 3 in 4 join voluntarily, not for ideological reasons, but as a means to escape poverty and unemployment, the lure of the uniform, or in response to parental rejection or abuse.[11] A typical case, described by Amnesty International, reveals these children's tragic lives, "My father abused me [sexually] from the age of five. He didn't want me to study or talk to anyone. Just work milking the cows. My mother knew nothing. He gave the orders. My father came looking for me but I didn't go back. The FARC gave me an AK-47 with three ammunition magazines, clothes and boots. He [the father] couldn't hurt me any more."[12] Recruits are trained to fight and kill without gender distinctions; women are not spared hardships and have the same opportunities as men to become field commanders, and many do. However, sexual harassment and abuse are the rule, as reported by girl recruits who have managed to escape. For instance, Human Rights Watch reports, "When girls join the FARC, the commanders choose among them . . . the women have the final say, but . . . when you're with a commander, you don't have to do the hard work . . . you get away with stuff [and] enjoy privileges. So, most of the prettiest girls are with commanders . . . you see lots of commanders with young girls. Commander Topo was fifty-two. He had a sixteen-year-old girlfriend. This is typical."[13] As for pregnancies, "Even girls as young as twelve are required to use contraception, often by having an intrauterine device inserted by guerrilla nurses. While the AUC-ELN seem more willing to tolerate pregnancies . . . FARC-EP girls are almost invariably made to have abortions if they get pregnant."[13] Amnesty International quotes Janet, a 12-year-old FARC recruit, "As soon as you get there, they give you coils and injections. Any girl who gets pregnant has to have an abortion."[12]

Manuel Marulanda, the legendary founder of the FARC-EP, led the group for 44 years, assisted by his military commander Jorge Briceño, a.k.a. *Mono Jojoy*, until his cardiac death on March 26, 2008, at age 78. The FARC-EP claims to be an insurgent Marxist-Leninist army that represents the poor in a struggle against Colombia's wealthy elite. Its agenda includes expropriation of multinational corporations, nationalization of natural resources, wealth redistribution, and an agrarian reform to dismantle large estates. It fiercely opposes U.S. interference in Colombia's affairs, particularly *Plan Colombia*. Through decades of operations, the FARC-EP became one of the toughest and most disciplined leftist guerillas in the world, and Marulanda one of the best guerilla commanders and strategists. In the late 1980s, the FARC-EP attempted an insertion into the country's political life through a political party, the *Unión Patriótica* (Patriotic Union). However, right-wing death squads, sponsored by drug traffickers with links to government security forces, decimated the party by murdering thousands of its members, including its 1990 presidential candidate.[14] This convinced Marulanda that the road to power was by force rather than through the ballot box, marking the beginnings of a particularly violent decade.

The FARC-EP operate through military and paramilitary means. Conventional military tactics include hit and run attacks against the Colombian Army using state-of-the-art machine guns, rocket launchers, AK-47 rifles,[15] and land mines. On a recent Web site's *War bulletin,* they declared "On the 16th of the current month, units from the FARC's southern bloc activated mines against six anti-narcotic police cars in the Mirabeles vereda (administrative rural area) of the municipality of Hormiga, in the province of Putumayo (one of Colombia's 32 *Departamentos* or Provinces), destroying two cars, killing two policemen and wounding 19."[16] However, as is the case elsewhere, most land mine victims are innocent civilians, including children unaware of the danger lurking in their own backyards.[17] Paramilitary operations are wide-ranging. They include blowing up economic targets such as oil pipelines and electric and water facilities; kidnapping military personnel for political gain and civilians for ransom; murdering known or suspected opponents, meddlesome journalists,[18,19] human rights activists, and holders of or candidates to public office;[20] and conducting indiscriminate massacres of populations suspected of cooperating with the enemy (mainly the AUC).

Their weapons of choice when attacking towns, police stations, and other paramilitary targets include car bombings and crude but gruesomely lethal mortars made of shrapnel-filled gas canisters that, given their inaccuracy, frequently kill more civilians than enemy fighters, as was the case of a 2002 attack on a church in the Chocó province that killed 119 people, including 45 children. As reported at the time:

Chocó is Colombia's poorest province. A jungle region populated by Afro-Colombian and indigenous communities, it has coasts on two oceans and shares a border with Panama, which obviously places it close to the Canal Zone. This strategic location is particularly attractive to armed groups, who use the area as a corridor for drug trafficking and to smuggle weapons. This has sparked a deadly struggle between the FARC and the AUC. Each of these groups wants to control the area . . . On April 21, 2002 four hundred AUC fighters arrived in Vigía del Fuerte and ousted the FARC . . . At 6.00 A.M. on Wednesday, May 1, approximately 2,000 FARC guerrillas launched an attack . . . to regain control. Finding themselves under attack, the AUC retreated to Bellavista . . . [and] the people of Bojayá [county] took refuge in the church, the parish house, and the health post [the only substantial buildings] . . . [On] May 2, at about 10:15 in the morning, the FARC launched a propane gas cylinder against the church. Full of metal shards and explosives, the cylinder broke through the thin roof and exploded on the altar. Roof shingles and wooden chairs inside the church were converted into shrapnel killing many of the [300] people sheltered in the building. Fighting went on for five days. The bodies of the victims were exposed to the inclemency of the tropical sun and rain for three days, before they could be recovered for burial . . . The stench was so horrible that it was difficult even to approach the church.[21]

President Andrés Pastrana Arango (1998–2002) visited the area on May 9, 2002, promising reconstruction aid that never materialized and, say critics, he exploited this especially gruesome episode at the national and international level. To that effect, he made a number of statements to the Colombian press, radio, and television; asked the Office of the United Nations High Commission for Human Rights to investigate the massacre[22]; and embarked on a vigorous diplomatic offensive especially aimed at the European Union (EU). A week after the incident he met Javier Solana, EU High Representative for the Common Foreign and Security Policy, in Madrid, Spain, to make the case that "omission of the FARC from the EU's terrorist list sent the message that Europe tolerates these terrible and cowardly attacks."[23] A few days later, the Foreign Ministers of the then 15 EU member nations meeting in Luxembourg added the FARC to its terrorist list. The initial EU reluctance to act was more pragmatic than philosophic or political. Indeed, "stigmatizing a group or an individual as 'terrorist'—as Ariel Sharon does with regard to the Palestinians, as Russia does with the Chechens, and as Turkey does with the PKK—is an effective means of excluding it from the political arena. You use the term with groups with which you do not want to negotiate."[23] Five years later, awaiting reconstruction, electricity, and running water, the townspeople rebaptized their town *Se verá* (we'll see). Questioned about the lack of progress, the nonchalant project manager disdainfully declared, "we know they can live without electricity as they didn't have it before. As for water, they have tanks to fill with rainwater."[24]

The FARC favors collective over individual kidnappings for obvious financial reasons. An example with a deadly outcome occurred on April 11, 2002, when a FARC *commando* (squad) disguised in military uniform entered the regional assembly of the Valle del Cauca province and evacuated the building under the pretext of a bomb threat, kidnapping 12 *diputados* (municipal officials).[25] They became part of a group of high-profile hostages the FARC hoped to exchange for hundreds of their comrades held in Colombian prisons. Six years later, on June 18, 2007, the FARC announced "11 assembly members of the Valle del Cauca that we had retained in April 2002 died as a result of crossfire when a non-identified military group attacked the camp where they were held."[25] Yet, a forensic investigation of the 11 cadavers, conducted by the *Cuerpo Técnico de Investigaciones* (technical investigational group) of the Fiscalía General de la Nación (Nation's Attorney General) under the watchful eye of the Organization of American States (OAS)'s International Forensic Commission, revealed a very different picture. The 11 diputados had been shot 4 to 15 times each, some at short range and from behind. Ninety percent of the bullets recovered from cadavers were from Russian-made AK-47s, the rifle favored by the FARC, and 10% were from Israeli-made *Galils*, also in the FARC's arsenal.[26]

Sources of Income   Funding a large organization such as the FARC requires substantial and steady revenues. Initially, the FARC was able to get political and financial assistance from the Soviet Union. However, in 1985, Carlos Lehder, a notorious Colombian *narco* (drug baron), introduced them to the booming drug business, marking a shift in their source of income. More recently, some FARC financial and logistical support comes from

Venezuela's leftist President Lt. Col. Hugo Chávez facilitated by a long, unprotected 1,375-mile border with Colombia. Evidence cited includes Chávez's leftist leanings, his virulent attacks on U.S. policy in Latin America, especially *Plan Colombia* also opposed by the FARC, and his choice of Diego Serna, a FARC member, as bodyguard during his May 2001 visit to Colombia. Serna disclosed to *Cambio* (a magazine published by Nobel laureate Gabriel García Marquez) that Chávez was in frequent and secret contacts with the FARC leadership. The Venezuela–FARC connection acquired credence when the Colombian Air Force captured a Venezuelan plane loaded with munitions destined to the FARC;[27] by accusations of collusion between the Chávez government and the FARC made by retired Lt. Col. Jesús Urdaneta, Venezuela's former secret-police chief; and by a video recording of meetings between Venezuelan military leaders and FARC commanders. Eventually, the Chávez–FARC connection was confirmed by a wealth of electronic documents discovered in Raul Reyes's computers, which were retrieved after the March 1, 2008, bombardment of a FARC camp concealed in Ecuadorian territory, by the Colombian Air Force. However, the FARC derives most of their income from the drug trade and extortion. They are involved at all levels of drug production, transportation, and exportation from areas under their control. They also tax every stage of the drug business, from the chemicals needed to process coca leaves into cocaine and poppy into heroin. Extortion takes the form of kidnapping for ransom, which they have turned into a fine-tuned business, and of taxing individuals and businesses presumed to making more than a million dollars a year.

Total revenues from these criminal activities make them probably the richest guerilla group in the world. It is estimated that in 2003 their total income was 2,100 billion pesos (over US$1 billion at the 2003 exchange rate), 88% of which was drug related, more than the ELN's and AUC's combined. Total outlays for that year were 546 billion pesos, including a measly 2,000 pesos (approximately US$1.00) daily to feed each combatant and each hostage.[28] Although ransom money accounts for less than 10% of the FARC's revenues, the enormity of that crime, the family and society disruptions it causes, and the appalling conditions in which hostages are kept day after day, year after year attract international attention and condemnation of its practitioners, mainly the FARC and the ELN. For instance, a recent article titled *Colombia: Secuestros S.A.* (Colombia: Kidnappings, S.A.) reports, "Extortion of rich and poor alike has grown to become one of the most lucrative practices of the FARC and the ELN, where the amount of the ransom is assigned based on the apparent worth of the kidnapped."[29] Accurate figures on the number of kidnappings are difficult to come by, as are other Colombian crime statistics. This is because victims' families do not report many such cases, guerillas or criminal gangs do not boast of their criminal activities, official statistics can be of dubious accuracy,[30] and data gathering nongovernment organizations (NGOs) have their own sources, ways of investigating, and focusing interests. However, it is generally agreed that until recently Colombia had the dubious distinction of holding the world record on reported kidnappings, reaching 3,706 in 2000[31] (3,572 according to another source[32]), or approximately 10 each day, more than 50% of them committed by the FARC-EP and the ELN.[31]

Kidnappings take two forms: *secuestros* and *pesca milagrosa* (miracle catch). While the former usually takes place in urban settings against preselected civil or political targets, the latter consists of blocking major roadways and selecting targets whose vehicle, physical appearance, or dress denotes wealth and therefore a potentially sizeable ransom. Until recently, the fear was such that people traveling by car anywhere in the countryside paid particular attention to traffic fluidity because more than a few minutes without incoming traffic might indicate a roadblock ahead and an ongoing *pesca milagrosa*. A variant of the *pesca milagrosa* follows commando-style attacks on apartment buildings, restaurants, and other places where people gather. A particularly reprehensible form of kidnapping involves minors, as young as 4 years of age as was a case reported by the Colombian and international press on December 4, 2007. Common criminals also engage in kidnappings either directly or as informants. In the latter case, they identify potential targets and sell that information to their guerilla contacts for a fraction of the ransom charged by guerilla captors. Once a kidnap occurs, euphemistically called *retención* (retained), a ransom is demanded from relatives accompanied by a threat of execution should the demand not be met within the specified deadline, or the police be contacted. Victims of political kidnapping are held hostage not for ransom but for political gain or to pressure the government into a prisoner exchange.

Ingrid Betancourt was the most famous hostage held by the FARC. A Colombian politician, Ms. Betancourt was a former senator, anticorruption activist, and founder of the *Green Oxygen* political party. She was kidnapped on February 23, 2002, along with Clara Rojas, while attempting to enter the demilitarized FARC stronghold of San Vicente del Caguán in the Caquetá province against President Pastrana's warning that the government could not guaranty her safety. Because of her dual Colombian–French citizenship and her book *La rage au Coeur* (*Until Death Do Us Part* in the English version), a bestseller in France, she became a *cause célèbre* and the focus of efforts toward her release by French Prime Minister, Dominique de Villepin, a personal friend, and by French President, Nicolas Sarkozy. In her book, she denounced corrupt Senate colleagues and the partial funding of Ernesto Samper's presidential campaign by the Cali cartel, which triggered an investigation that landed Fernando Botero, his campaign manager and son of the celebrated *fat motifs* painter and sculptor, in prison. Ms. Betancourt remained captive over six years, a fate endured by hundreds of hostages held in the jungles of Colombia, until her liberation on July 2, 2008, by Colombian intelligence units in a spectacular, meticulously planned and executed rescue operation that freed 11 hostages, including 3 Americans, without firing a single shot.

Yet, until recently Colombia had shown impotence against the hostage tragedy. In efforts to fill the void several radio stations offer airtime for hostage relatives to send messages of hope to their captive love ones. *Voces del Secuestro* (Hostage Voices), the oldest such program, was founded in 1994 by Herbín Hoyos Medina, a former kidnap victim himself. As of December 7, 2007, the Web site of the program's parent company listed, alphabetically, 4,200 hostages,[33] along with dates and circumstances of their kidnapping. During a TV interview held on December 4, 2007, Mr. Hoyos indicated that 14,000 Colombian families have participated in his broadcast since its inception. How do the FARC justify kidnappings as a source of revenues? The answer was provided by Rodrigo Granda, a leading member of the FARC released from a Colombian prison, in an interview dated October 2, 2007.[34] Of course [he said], a war requires funding . . . a war imposed on us by wealthy Colombians . . . hence they have to finance the war they set off. That is why the FARC retains people and charges a reward [for their freedom] that is in fact a tax." He also justified extortions as follows, "the New State that we are building has decided on a tax for peace. That means that any person or enterprise conducting business in Colombia with profits in excess of a million dollars annually must pay a tax equivalent to 10% of their profits . . . if they fail to do so, of course they are retained and imprisoned until they comply with their obligations." As for kidnappings of politicians and military personnel, he explained, "in the conduct of military operations, some officers or soldiers fall in our hands and are currently retained as prisoners of war . . . as some of ours fall in the hands of the enemy . . . prisoners of war are kept for humanitarian exchange that we hope will take place shortly." Finally, after a protracted and hesitant preamble, Granda explained the FARC's drug involvement as follows, "we are not, in any way, shape, or form, narco-traffickers. We don't get involved in the production, transport, of exportation of narcotics. Our organization has implemented charging a tax to buyers of coca paste in the areas . . . where we operate . . . retaining [non-complying] persons also helps, it must be said, to finance the FARC but is not decisive."[34]

FARC–Government Tug of War: 1998–2002   During his presidential campaign, Andrés Pastrana pledged to end the decades-old internal conflict and met with Manuel Marulanda in June 1998; a tactic that won him the election. Shortly after taking office, he granted the FARC, unilaterally and without preconditions, a Switzerland-size *Zona de Despeje* (demilitarized zone) in the Caquetá province that was to last 90 days. The negotiations had an inauspicious beginning. They were carefully planned by the government "as a spectacle that ranked the FARC at par with the government where President Pastrana was to sit at the negotiating table side-by-side with Manuel Marulanda, head of the FARC. The diplomatic corps and

high-profile personalities were invited to the event and each received a
white hat. A band was contracted for the occasion . . . [but] Marulanda did
not show up."[35] Eventually, negotiations began between both sides in the
town of San Vicente del Caguán only to break up 10 days later on FARC
accusations that the government had not clamped down on the AUC. From
that point on, accusations, counteraccusations, and provocations by each
side characterized the mutual posturing that led to multiple interruptions
and the final collapse of the negotiations. For instance, the government
established military checkpoints around and surveillance flights over the
demilitarized area, while the FARC hijacked a civilian airplane on January 30, 2001, and kidnapped and executed Consuelo Araujo Noguera, the
attorney general's wife. The *coup de grâce* came when the FARC hijacked
a civilian airplane in order to abduct a congressman, leading Pastrana to
end the negotiations in January 2002.

In the interim (between late 1998 and early 2002), the FARC exerted control over the political, judicial, educational, and security affairs of a 42,000
square kilometer territory, an area larger than Massachusetts and New
Jersey combined. The FARC used this safe haven as a springboard for guerilla activities and as a hostage hideout. They used the truce to acquire
weapons and to recruit and train combatants in the manufacture and use
of sophisticated explosives, with the assistance of three Irishmen known in
Colombia as *los tres monos* (the three blond men). *Los tres monos* (Martin
John McCauley, James William Monaghan, and Niall Connolly) were Irish
Republican Army explosives experts who, according to Interpol, had entered Colombia under the names of John Joseph Kelly, Edward Joseph
Campbell, and David Bracken, respectively. On February 15, 2002, they
were charged with entering the country with false passports and with
training the FARC and were sentenced to 17-year prison terms along with
fines in excess of US$200,000 each. However, they managed to flee Colom-
bia on September 15, 2005, and, despite an international arrest warrant,
are back in Ireland claiming their innocence pending a Colombian government extradition request.[36] The FARC also renewed their weaponry
with the cooperation of Vladimiro Montesinos, Peru's spymaster during
Alberto Fujimori's Presidency (1990–2000). As disclosed at his trial, "skim-
ming off money that the CIA intended for use in Peru's anti-drug trafficking efforts, Montesinos set up a major arms deal in the Middle East that
funneled 10,000 AK47 rifles to left-wing FARC guerrillas in Colombia,
thereby fomenting the very uprising that America has pledged $1.3 billion
to stamp out."[37] The rifles had been parachuted into the FARC's *Zona de
Despeje*, in 1999.[38] On June 24, 2001, Montesinos was arrested in Venezuela,
extradited back to Peru, and convicted of arming the FARC and other
crimes. On September 21, 2006, he was sentenced to several multiyear
prison terms to be served consecutively. Hence, aided by foreign rene-
gades, the FARC was able to withstand the larger, better-equipped, and
American-backed National Armed Forces. In 2005 alone, they conducted

attacks in Iscuandé and La Cruz, Nariño province; Mutatá, Antioquia province; Tame, Arauca province; Teteyé, Putumayo province; Atánquez, César province; Sipí and San Marino, Chocó province; San José del Guaviare, Guaviare province; and Vista Hermosa, Meta province, killing, maiming, or kidnapping hundreds of soldiers, policemen, and civilians.[39]

Canjes Humanitarios (Humanitarian Prisoner Exchange) Saga: 2002–2007
The inauguration of the newly elected rightist President Álvaro Uribe Velez, on August 7, 2002, was greeted by the FARC with gas canisters full of dynamite and mortar attacks against the *Casa Nariño* (Presidential palace) and the *Capitolio* (seat of Congress). Several grenades had been launched earlier that day against the Military School, and two unexploded car bombs and assorted explosives were found in Bogotá. One of the canisters exploded in *El Cartucho*, a grisly area of tin-houses inhabited by mendicants and drug addicts located near the targeted buildings, where most of the 16 deaths, including 3 children, and over 30 injuries occurred.[40] This marked the inauspicious beginnings of a thorny relationship. It has been characterized by a never-ending barrage of communiqués from both sides about *canjes humanitarios* that captured international attention thanks to Ingrid Betancourt, the FARC's most *canjeable* prisoner, and to the involvement of two foreign presidents. On one side was Hugo Chávez, the leftist President of the *República Bolivariana de Venezuela* and a FARC supporter, and on the other Nicolas Sarkozy, the newly elected rightist President of France, seeking Betancourt's release. Although endless posturing by both sides raises questions about their willingness to negotiate, history shows that even in the mayhem of Colombian politics such exchanges are possible, if infrequent.

For instance, the 1997 *Acuerdo de Remolinos del Caguán*, under President Ernesto Samper, freed 60 policemen and 10 infantrymen held by the FARC. Likewise, the *Acuerdo de los Pozos* of 2001, under President Andrés Pastrana, led to the exchange of 310 policemen and soldiers, including 42 in poor health, for 15 imprisoned FARC guerillas. More recently, on Christmas day of 2006, 29 policemen, 10 soldiers, and 3 intelligence agents were released by the ELN. Since 1996, 4,152 of the 6,790 persons kidnapped by the FARC were freed through prisoner exchanges or payment of ransom, albeit after years of captivity.[32] The most priced hostages, such as Ingrid Betancourt, are held the longest and without giving evidence of life in expectations of extracting the most concessions from the government or the largest ransom from relatives. In fact, there is little of humanitarianism in these exchanges, especially as it concerns the FARC. For instance, until the rescue of Ingrid Betancourt and the Americans, the FARC claimed 47 politicians and members of the military or police forces as *canjeables*. This excluded 700-plus hostages held for ransom until the extortion process plays out, regardless of duration and the physical and psychological suffering inflicted onto the hostages and their families. Shortly after Álvaro Uribe became President, the FARC demanded that any prisoner exchange would have to take place in a demilitarized zone in Colombian territory, where 47 political and military *prisoners of war* would be exchanged for several thousand FARC fighters held in Colombian prisons. The Uribe government ruled out a demilitarized zone but countered by demanding a cease-fire, the freedom of all hostages, and assurances that freed FARC members would not rearm; preconditions that were promptly rejected by the FARC. A year later, a failed military rescue attempt led to the assassination of several *canjeables*, including the Governor of the Antioquia province, an ex-minister of Defense, and nine military personnel. Hence, the FARC's insistence on being acknowledged as an insurgent army confronting an unjust and oppressive Colombian government, rather than a terrorist organization, is hollow.

The year 2004 was marked by the capture of Ricardo Palmera, a.k.a. *Simon Trinidad* and of Nayibe Rojas, a.k.a. *Sonia*, both prominent members of the FARC, and by attempts by the Colombian Catholic hierarchy, national and international organizations, and hostage families to pressure both sides of the conflict. Throughout the year, the Colombian government offered to release groups of imprisoned guerillas with certain preconditions that were rejected out of hand by the FARC, insisting on a demilitarized zone to conduct the negotiations and demanding the release of Simon Trinidad who had been extradited to the United States. In late 2005, President Uribe extended an olive branch to the FARC by proposing a meeting along with assurances that, during the negotiations, all FARC representatives would be guaranteed safe-conduct nation-wide and that the government would refrain from any military or police action in the negotiation area. At his request, the Embassies of Spain, France, and Switzerland initiated an exploratory mission to the municipalities of *Florida* and *Pradera*, Province of Valle del Cauca, an area the FARC wanted demilitarized. The group formulated a proposal guaranteeing safety for all negotiators, which was quickly approved by the government but rejected by the FARC as another of Uribe's pre-electoral ploys. In early 2007, the escape first of ex-minister Fernando Araujo, during a military rescue attempt, and later of police officer Jhon Frank Pinchao, who gave grim accounts of the fate of his captive comrades, galvanized hostage families and the international community into pressuring the Colombian government for a humanitarian exchange. As a good will gesture, President Uribe released a group of imprisoned FARC members and, at the request of the French government, Rodrigo Granda, the highest ranked FARC prisoner. Once again, the FARC dismissed the government's overtures and made additional demands ironically coinciding with their own communiqué announcing that 11 of the 12 assembly members of the Valle del Cauca that they held hostage, "died as a result of crossfire when a non-identified military group attacked the camp where they were held." President's Uribe's response was predictable: prisoner exchanges would take place at a nondemilitarized site, and military rescue missions would continue, which unsurprisingly incensed hostage families fearing botched attempts, especially Yolanda Pulecio, mother of

Ingrid Betancourt, who redoubled her high profile international campaign in favor of humanitarian exchanges. Eventually, President Uribe agreed to a 42 square kilometer (16.2 square miles) demilitarized zone in the municipality of Pradera instead of the 802 the FARC demanded.

In the meantime, a video[41] of an emaciated and visibly dejected Ingrid Betancourt, seated on a rudimentary stool, was intercepted by Colombian intelligence and released to the press, along with a 12-page letter addressed to her mother and children, dated October 24th, 2007. In it, she wrote "Mamita, I am tired, tired of suffering . . . I have tried to escape on several occasions . . . I have tried to maintain hope . . . but mamita, now I have given up . . . life here is not life . . . It is a gloomy waste of time. I live, or survive, in a hammock hanging from two poles, covered with mosquito netting and a canvas overhead, which serves as a roof, allowing me to think that I have a house. I have a shelf where I keep my equipment, that is my backpack with clothes, and a Bible that is my only luxury."[42] Her despondent look and heart-wrenching account of what constitutes the hopelessness of a kidnapped victim held in the Colombian jungle caused international consternation, many headlines and expressions of support worldwide, but no results. Predictably, outsiders exploited the government–FARC standoff for political or personal gain. For instance, on December 9, 2007, the FARC announced it would release Ingrid Betancourt's old running mate Clara Rojas, her 3-year-old son Emanuel born in captivity, and Consuelo Gonzalez, a former Congresswoman kidnapped in 2001, to Venezuela President Hugo Chávez or his designee. This was orchestrated as a gesture to Chávez for his acrimonious firing by President Uribe as a mediator of prisoner exchange negotiations. Eager to reclaim his status as mediator and as a champion of human rights, Chávez organized *Misión Emanuel*. This obscene media circus, based on the exploitation of suffering hostages and their families, involved presidential emissaries from Argentina, Brazil, Cuba, Ecuador, France, and Switzerland, the International Committee of the Red Cross, and Oliver Stone, an American filmmaker. Wearing the red beret and fatigues of his paratrooper days, Chávez and his international entourage arrived at Villavicencio, in the Meta province, along with two Russian-made MI-172 helicopters, where they were greeted by a barrage of reporters eager to make the most of such a high-profile international media event.

After three days of high expectations and widely broadcast pronouncements by Chávez, Nestor Kirchner, former President of Argentina, and others, the FARC called off the release, claiming insufficient guarantees for the safe transport of the hostages. The same day, President Uribe exposed the FARC's duplicity. Emanuel could not possibly be released for, separated from his mother in 2005, he had been handed over, at 11 months of age, to child welfare workers in San José de Guaviare in a FARC-dominated zone, by José Gomez, a peasant farmer claiming to be the child's great-uncle. The malnourished infant, given the name Juan David Gomez, had been rushed to the *Instituto Colombiano de Bienestar Familiar* (Colombian Institute for Family Welfare), in Bogotá, for fracture-reduction surgery and treatment of leishmaniasis, a tropical parasitic disease produced by leishmania, a protozoan organism transmitted by sand flies. The child had been then referred to foster care. Chávez promptly accused Uribe of "dynamiting a rescue mission that involved observers from five leftist Latin American governments." True to form, the FARC declared that they had placed Emanuel in the care of *honest persons* in Bogotá, but he had been kidnapped by the Colombian government before the hostage release could be finalized.[43] The following Thursday, Clara Rojas and Consuelo Gonzalez were finally released by the FARC and promptly flown to Caracas to meet Chávez, their *savior*. In a video taken at the time of the hostages release and broadcast by *Globovisión*, a TV station, Venezuela's Justice Minister, Ramón Rodriguez Chacín, is heard expressing encouragement to the rebels and support for their struggle. Consuelo Gonzalez had brought letters from eight cohostages to their families. In one, Ingrid Betancourt was said to be so weak at one time that she had to be carried in a hammock during a routine move from one camp to another. In another, Colonel Luis Mendieta, held hostage since 1998, described his weakness to be such that he had to drag himself through the mud to relieve himself in privacy.

In his televised annual *Informe de Gestión* to the National Assembly (equivalent to the U.S. President's State of the Union address), delivered one day after the hostage release, Chávez took full credit and urged the governments of Colombia and of all nations to remove the FARC and the ELN from their terrorist list. In his view, "The FARC and the ELN are not terrorist groups; they are armies, real armies that occupy a space in Colombia. The FARC and the ELN must be given recognition. They are insurgent forces that have a political and Bolivarian project, and that is respected here." Then on January 13, 2008, 48 hours later, *Frente 57* of the FARC kidnapped six tourists in the town of Nuquí, Chocó province.[44] Four days later, the overwhelmingly pro-Chávez Venezuelan National Assembly declared the *belligerent* nature of the *insurgent* groups FARC and ELN, which the bill characterized as "Liberation movements or States unwilling of [foreign] domination," and rejected the "unilateral [terrorist] lists imposed by the government of the US." On February 5, 2008, coinciding with a Gallup poll showing a 96% disapproval of the FARC, hundreds of thousands of Colombians held protest marches in 115 cities around the world demanding "No more kidnappings," "No more violence," "No more FARC." This was Oscar Morales's brainchild, using Facebook to launch a virtual community he called "un millón de voces contra las FARC" (a million voices against the FARC) that Carlos Andrés Santiago converted into a march.[45] Such a massive condemnation of the FARC by the Colombian citizenry shows that they have lost all public support.[46] And although a negotiated settlement is viewed in some quarters as the only road to peace, President Uribe's firm policies for reclaiming his nation from terror have already changed Colombia's security landscape.

Neighbors' Complicity Confirmed   A few minutes into March 1, 2008, the Colombian Air Force bombarded and Army units later raided a FARC camp setup on Ecuadorian territory, less than two miles from the Colombian border. The attack was made possible by eavesdropping on a conversation from a mobile phone known by intelligence units to belong to Luis Édgar Devia, a.k.a. *Raul Reyes,* a member of the FARC *Secretariat* in charge of finances and public relations. In the attack, Raul Reyes and 17 of his comrades were killed, triggering a diplomatic crisis between the two countries. When President Uribe informed Rafael Correa, President of Ecuador, of the bombardment of the FARC camp in a telephone call broadcast on TV, the latter seemed at a loss on how to react, not unlike President George W. Bush's blank stare when informed of the 9/11 attack while he was visiting the Emma E. Booker Elementary School. However, the next day Correa broke diplomatic relations with Colombia in unison with President Chávez who, although not involved in the dispute, deployed approximately 6,000 of his 57,800 men-strong army along the Northeastern Colombian border and threatened war should Colombia violate Venezuelan sovereignty. Five days later, Daniel Ortega, President of distant Nicaragua and another of Chávez's political allies in his global crusade against *El Imperio* (The Empire, as Chávez calls the United States), also broke diplomatic ties with Colombia. A mere 24 hours later, Ortega, Chávez, and Correa agreed to close the chapter and re-establish diplomatic ties at the *Grupo de Río* meeting held in the Dominican Republic on March 6, 2008; a swift about-face that is worth a Guinness Book of World Records mention. At the meeting, President Uribe defended the attack, arguing sarcastically, "I reject the portrayal of our legitimate right to fight a terrorist organization as a massacre of angels clad in pajamas that [certainly] were not preparing [to celebrate] Easter."[46] He also disclosed information mined from Raul Reyes's computers (three laptops, two external hard disks, and two USB memory sticks) that corroborated Chávez's and Correa's support of the FARC.[47] Yet, Uribe failed to convince his Latin American peers that attacking the FARC camp in Ecuadorian territory was justified by Correa's allowing the use of its territory by a foreign terrorist organization as refuge and as a springboard from which to wage war against Colombia. That justification is implicit in UN Resolution 1373 of 2001, which requires all member states to cooperate in the fight of terrorism and to deny support of any terrorist organization. In the end, Colombia was condemned almost unanimously but for one supporting vote from the United States and one abstention from Canada, forcing Uribe to pledge to never again "violate his neighbors' sovereignty," thus averting a potentially serious diplomatic crisis.

The episode served to bring the international community's attention to Venezuela's and Ecuador's complicity with Colombia's terrorist groups. Raul Reyes's computers exposed the complicity's extent and duration.[47] For instance, the FARC appears to have held secret meetings with representatives of the Chávez and Correa governments, to have received

financial support from Chávez, to have been considering business transactions and investments in Venezuela with Chávez's approval, and to
have contributed US$100,000 to Correa's presidential campaign, violating
Ecuador's laws. More ominously, if confirmed, is the revelation that the
FARC were apparently negotiating the purchase of uranium from an in-
termediary offering 50 kilos "but who can deliver a lot more." Reyes's computers also contained instructions on how to build a *dirty bomb*. It is up to
President Uribe to play these cards adroitly and, if the weight of the evidence warrants it, seek UN support to declare Chávez's Venezuela and
Correa's Ecuador as terrorism-sponsoring states, which would isolate the
FARC and cut-off their vital lifelines. Once isolated, dwindling resources
and relentless pressure from the Colombian Armed forces would acceler-
ate the current rate of desertions from its ranks and eventually destroy the
myth of the FARC's *invincibility* that attracts and sustains its combatants.
Some experts already see evidence of implosion in the assassination, three
days after the camp attack, of Iván Ríos a.k.a. *Darío*, the youngest member
of the FARC Secretariat, by his security chief, *Rojas*, who collected the bulk
of the US$2.5 million reward for his boss's head. Hence, within a week
and for the first time in its 40-year existence, the FARC lost two of its nine-
member high command. More ominously for the FARC's negotiating
power and survival, was the July 2, 2008, rescue of Ingrid Betancourt and
three Americans, in a meticulously executed, bloodless, and cunning operation conducted by Colombian intelligence units. These severe blows in
quick succession, the incriminating contents of Raul Reyes's computers,
and the increasing defections among its ranks suggest that the FARC's
demise can finally be contemplated.

Ejército de Liberación Nacional (ELN)

Despite a slow beginning, the ELN eventually became the second largest
guerilla group in Colombia, with approximately 4,000 to 5,000 combatants
at the height of its power. In its 42 years of existence, the ELN has sur-
vived murderous infighting, hostile encounters with the FARC, relentless
attacks by the AUC, and a near obliteration by the National Army. The ELN
is viewed more as an insurgent group than the FARC, with a nationalist,
anti-imperialist, and anti-oligarchic political agenda. For instance, in August 2002, Colombia Vice President Francisco Santos declared, "The ELN
is an armed party and not an army, as the FARC describes itself, which
facilitates the negotiating process with this guerrilla group."[48] Likewise,
the ELN is said to have adopted Che Guevara's *foquismo doctrine;* a theory
that a nucleus of dedicated revolutionaries can awaken a critical mass
within the population sufficient to succeed in its power struggle toward a
just society. Yet, not withstanding the Colombian Vice President's rhetoric
designed to assuage ELN leaders in anticipation of peace negotiations and
ELN claims to look after the welfare of the poor and disenfranchised, its

activities and tactics parallel the FARC's. Like the FARC, it uses kidnapping for ransom, extortion, and to a much lesser extent drug money as the main sources of revenue. It also engages in the murder of opponents and in indiscriminate massacres to intimidate populations it wants to subdue and exploit. For instance, out of 23,401 kidnappings between 1996 and 2008 , 5,407 are attributed to the ELN against 6,863 to the FARC,[49] despite a combatant force one-fourth FARC's size. Homicides and massacres committed by the ELN through the years have also been disproportionate to its size. The following section reviews the evolution of the ELN along the four major periods of its history: rise and expansion (1964–74), crisis (1974–80), restructuring (1980–90), and strategic adaptation and peace talks (1990–2002), before assessing its present status.

   Rise and Expansion   Left-wing students and intellectuals, labor activists, and Catholic radicals founded the ELN in 1964, inspired by Fidel Castro's revolution that overthrew Cuba's dictator Fulgencio Batista in 1959. In fact, Fabio Vásquez and Víctor Medina, ELN's first leaders, trained in Cuba in 1962 along with 60 Colombian university students. Hence, the choice of *San Vicente de Chucurí* in the Santander province as its first camp is not surprising given that province's history of Communist upheavals, it being the seat of one of the country's earliest leftist *autodefensas* during La Violencia period and its sympathetic leftist oil sector trade unions bent on insurrection. From 30 initial members, the ELN grew very slowly to only 350 combatants 20 years later. From the beginning, its *cri de guerre* was *Liberación o muerte* (liberation or death). On January 7, 1965, the ELN launched its first attack against the police station of *Simicota,* a town in Santander province, from which emerged the *Manifiesto de Simicota* and later the *Declaración Programática* (Declaration of Programs). The latter delineated the ELN's political platform. In essence, it contemplated a democratic government by and for the people, elimination of large estates and allocation of private land to peasants, protection of national industries, the development of a communications infrastructure, a popular credit system, affordable housing, and free education and health care for all. It also called for separation of church and state with freedom of worship and of expression, an anti-imperialist foreign policy based on mutual respect, and the establishment of a people's army. However, early Cuban-style Marxist leaning was tempered when Camilo Torres Restrepo, a Catholic priest and university sociology professor from an elite Colombian family, joined the group in 1965. Torres, who had gained national attention as the leader of *Frente Unido* (United Front), a popular left-wing movement opposing the *Frente Nacional*, was a believer in the radical new ideas of liberation theology calling for a Christian–Communist solution to Colombia's rampant corruption, extreme poverty, and social inequity. Although Torres died in February 1966 during an Army ambush, he remained a symbol for the group, inspiring like-minded priests, including Domingo Laín and Manuel Pérez, two Spanish priests who went to Colombia in 1969 to join the ELN. The former was killed in combat in February 1973. The latter, nicknamed *El cura Pérez* (Pérez the Priest) was at first sidelined by Fabio Vásquez who followed a strict foquismo doctrine, but he eventually steered the group's ideology and direction.

From Crisis and Decline to Resurgence   The 1970s marked a period of decline marred by ideological, political, and leadership crises and by counterinsurgency campaigns launched by the Colombian Army, which severely reduced the ELN's military capacity and political relevance. Additionally, in September 1973, ELN commanders committed the serious tactical blunder of stationing 100 fighters near Anorí, Antioquia province; an area where the Army was very active. Quickly encircled, 28 fighters were taken prisoner and 21 killed, including two brothers of Fabio Vásquez, the ELN commander-in-chief. Shortly after Vásquez abandoned the group and fled to Cuba, in November 1974; El cura Pérez assumed joint leadership of the ELN along with Nicolás Rodríguez Bautista, a.k.a. *Gabino*, until his death of malaria in 1998. From his leadership position, El cura Pérez was able to reshape the ELN ideology along Camilo Torres's goal of fusing revolutionary fervor with Christian values of social justice, introducing a new sense of purpose and direction. Hence, after a decade of stagnation in size, funding, and political relevance, the 1980s witnessed a resurgence led by the shared leadership of El cura Pérez and Nicolás Rodríguez Bautista. Together, they reorganized the group, giving it a more dynamic and responsive decentralized command structure, better relations with trade unions, and new sources of revenue extorted from domestic and multinational oil companies exploiting oilfields in the provinces of Arauca, Norte de Santander, and César. Their new strength and confidence was demonstrated by several high-profile operations, including the assassination of José Ramón Rincón Quiñones, the Army's Inspector-General and a driving force against counterinsurgency groups.

In 1983, the ELN held its first national conference named *Reunión Nacional de los Héroes y Mártires de Anorí* (National Meeting of the Heroes and Martyrs of Anorí), where they decided to recruit more fighters and expand operations beyond the northeastern and northwestern territories. As a result, the group grew to over 2,000 combatants and, by 1990, was conducting operations in more than 20 *Frentes de Guerra* (War Fronts), including urban areas. Sabotage of the country's electrical and oil infrastructures remained its main strategy. Yet, they continued to suffer numerous casualties at the hands of the Army, which it sought to counterbalance by merging with other insurgent groups and by trying to join the political process. For instance, they merged with the M-19 and the EPL, a dissident FARC faction. When that failed, they spearheaded the creation of the larger *Simón Bolívar Guerrilla Coordinating Group* and later launched a political movement called *Union Camilista* (UC-ELN) integrated by ELN with *MIR-Patria Libre* members. Both attempts at consolidation failed.

Strategic Adaptation and Peace Talks   Since the mid-1990s, the ELN was confronted by an increasingly powerful and militant AUC, especially in the coca-producing Bolívar province, an area controlled and used as a trafficking base by the AUC *Bloque Central Bolívar* (Central Bolivar Bloc). In contrast, at its Second National Congress of 1989, the ELN had adopted a stance of *Deslinde categórico con las mafias del narcotráfico* (definitive disengagement from narco-trafficking mafias) vis-à-vis illicit crop cultivation, processing, and trafficking. It rightfully viewed involvement in illicit drugs as fostering corruption, impunity, violence, the growth of paramilitarism, and the emergence of a *narco-bourgeoisie* that was taking control over leading political positions at the regional and national levels. In the interim, the M-19 and the EPL had signed peace agreements with the government and were either demobilizing or already fully participating in Colombia's democratic politics. The defection of the dissident FARC member of the Simón Bolívar Guerrilla Coordinating Group in 1991 weakened the coalition, forcing the ELN to seek negotiations with the government that began in Caracas, Venezuela, moving later to Tlaxcala, Mexico. Discussions never went past procedure, and the government ended contacts. This, and the increasing confrontations between the FARC and the ELN, led to the collapse of the Simón Bolívar Guerrilla Coordinating Group.

In 1996, the UC-ELN held its Third National Conference, where it proposed the creation of a *National Convention* to unite "all sectors of national opinion, social movements, political organizations, economic associations, the Church, intellectuals, the Left, democrats, and patriots."[50] The convention would serve as a forum to discuss political, social, and economic issues of concern to all Colombians, especially the underprivileged. In addition to the Convention, the ELN demanded a demilitarized *Zona de Encuentro* (Meeting Zone) of approximately 7,600 square kilometers (and area equal to Delaware and Rhode Island combined) in the municipalities of Santa Rosa, Simití, San Pablo, and Morales as preconditions for peace negotiations. These demands met with fierce opposition by a coalition of politicians, cattle ranchers, and the AUC. Hence, when President Andrés Pastrana initiated peace negotiations with both the ELN and the FARC in October 1998, he rejected the *Zona de Encuentro*, focusing instead on the stronger FARC, apparently assuming the ELN would be a militarily easy prey after reaching an agreement with the FARC. While preliminary contacts were taken place between the ELN and the National Peace Council and the National Conciliation Commission, in Viana, Spain, and Würzburg, Germany, the ELN continued its policy of hostage taking and extortion. In 1998 alone, the ELN is said to have collected US$84 million in ransom and US$255 million in extortion money.[51,52] It also continued the so-called *gramaje;* a protection tax levied from coca and poppy growers. Hence, the government suspended peace talks. In retaliation, the ELN bombed an oil pipeline in Antioquia province on February 1999, killing more than 70 people, and launched a series of mass kidnappings in quick succession. The latter included the hijacking of an Avianca commercial airliner, on April 12, 1999, that was forced to land in Simití, Bolívar province, with its 46 passengers and crewmembers who were promptly hidden in the jungle, and the kidnapping of 140 parishioners attending mass at Cali's La María church the following month. Eighty parishioners were released within a few hours with the help of the Army, but 63 were retained and held hostage for ransom.

These audacious operations, which far exceeded acceptable guerilla behavior even in a country regularly shaken by violence, brought strong national and international condemnation, including the excommunication of participants in the La María assault by Cali's Archbishop, Monsignor Isaías Duarte. On July 30, 1999, an eclectic group of citizens called the *Civilian Facilitating Commission* was formed to negotiate the release of the remaining Avianca and La María hostages and to seek a peace settlement. However, meetings held in Colombia, Cuba, and Venezuela between 2000 and 2002 got nowhere, as did efforts by the *Group of Friends* (Cuba, France, Norway, Spain, and Switzerland) chosen jointly by the ELN and the government as *facilitators*. Despite the *Agreement for Colombia*, signed on November 24, 2001, to implement a transition agenda designed to bridge negotiations with the upcoming new administration, President Pastrana announced the collapse of the negotiations on May 31, 2002. In the meantime, the ELN and representatives from various sectors of Colombian society had signed the *Convention of Geneva*, which banned kidnapping children, the elderly, and pregnant women; a ban that was ignored by the ELN.

The ELN and Uribe   During the mandate of President Uribe, massive spraying of coca plantations in the Caquetá and Putumayo provinces and successful Army assaults against the FARC forced the group to redeploy to the southern provinces of Cauca and Nariño where the ELN had a strong presence. This caused increasingly frequent confrontations between the FARC and the ELN. While the ELN antidrug stance allowed a negotiated nonbelligerent coexistence between the two guerillas in the beginning, economic necessity forced the ELN to increasingly rely on drug revenues to sustain itself; a change in tactics that triggered a fierce competition for coca growing territory and trafficking routes and open warfare with the FARC. At one point, Mono Jojoy instructed his troops that the ELN was as much an enemy of the people as was the government. As a result, increasingly frequent armed confrontations in shared territories led to hundreds of casualties on each side. In the meantime, President Uribe reinitiated negotiations with the ELN as part of his strategy to end the half-century-old conflict and to integrate the various guerilla groups into the political process. To this end, he submitted to Parliament a constitutional reform proposal that, among others, would create additional seats at the municipal and provincial levels to be reserved for defecting guerilla members *committed to peace* and several seats to Parliament intended for *special representatives for peace* appointed by the President.

Exploratory talks began in Havana, Cuba, in December 2005. Negotiators for the ELN included Antonio García, Ramiro Vargas, and Francisco Galán, released from prison for that purpose after serving 13 years of a

20-year sentence. Spokesmen for Colombia included Carlos Restrepo, Colombia's High Commissioner for Peace, and Julio Londoño, Colombia's ambassador to Cuba. International observers from Switzerland, Norway, and Spain were also present. High on the government's agenda were bilateral ceasefire, cessation of hostilities, and the release of all hostages. The ELN sought legal political status, amnesty for its imprisoned members, and integration of the group into the national political process. As a counterbalance to his belligerent policy toward the FARC, President Uribe's offer of an olive branch to the ELN was predicated on his desire to show flexibility, especially to a Democrat-controlled U.S. Congress unlikely to rubber-stamp Plan Colombia without evidence of substantive progress. Additionally, the ELN's apparent renunciation of violence made it a better choice than the FARC as a partner for peace negotiations. For instance, at the conclusion of the fourth round of talks in Havana, Nicolás Rodríguez Bautista, ELN commander, declared his intention to continue a political dialogue with the Colombian government. His statement was followed by decreased guerilla activity. However, the talks fizzled when the two sides disagreed on a talks' framework, on details of a cease fire, and on the terms of a hostage–prisoner exchange. Nevertheless, talks were to restart in late December 2007 under the auspices of Venezuelan President Hugo Chávez as facilitator. Peace talks were rekindled by the arrest in Bogotá, on January 7, 2008, of peace talks opponent Carlos Marín Guarín, a.k.a. *Pablito*, an ELN commander responsible for the 1992 murder of a Catholic bishop in the Arauca province and for more than 200 attacks on the U.S.-owned Caño Limon oil pipeline in northern Colombia. According to Defense Minister Juan Manuel Santos, "on various occasions [Guarín] prevented the ELN central command from signing a peace treaty with the government."[53] On April 3, 2008, President Uribe invited ELN Spokesman Francisco Galán to meet at the presidential palace for new peace talks. However, in a press communiqué hours after the meeting the ELN disavowed Galán as their spokesman. A few weeks later, the ELN's Central Command issued a communiqué proposing a three-point plan toward a *National accord* that included their old standby call for a *Constitutional National Assembly* previously rejected by the government.[54]

Autodefensas Unidas de Colombia (AUC) or Paramilitares

The use of civilian armies by local chieftains, wealthy landlords, political parties, and the Armed forces has a century-long tradition in Colombia. Today, such groups are known as *autodefensas* or *paramilitares*. While the name *autodefensas* reflects their initial purpose vis-à-vis guerilla armies, the pejorative designation *paramilitares* exposes the military links of these semiautonomous armed groups that "are among the most brutal human rights violators in the world today."[55] Their origins can be traced back to 1962, but they have evolved through three periods shaped by guerilla activity, inner corruption, and politics: *official paramilitarism, private para-militarism,* and the *AUC* of the last 20 years.[55] This section briefly reviews their history and their collusion with the nation's military and political establishments so profoundly harmful to Colombia's democratic institutions. Their involvement in the drug trade, in massacres of poor rural populations, and in massive violations of human rights also is outlined.

Official Paramilitarism   In 1962, General Alberto Ruiz Novoa, Commandant of the Armed Forces, proposed the adoption and implementation of *Plan Lazo* (Plan Rope) based on recommendations by the visiting U.S. Army Special Warfare unit led by General William Yarborough. The U.S. team recommended the creation of "select civilian and military personnel [groups] for clandestine training in resistance operations."[55] This marked the beginnings of a new alliance between the United States, intent on preventing the spread of communism throughout Latin America, and the Colombian military anxious to neutralize real or perceived *internal enemies.* General Ruiz's Plan Lazo gained legal status when, in 1965, Presidential Decree 3398 authorized "the organization and tasking of all of the residents of the country" to face emerging insurgent groups.[55] The decree gave rise to *Law 48* three years later. Law 48 allowed the Defense Ministry "to support, when it considers convenient . . . [armies] to be considered as being for the private use of the Armed Forces."[55] These armies were charged to "organize the civilian population militarily so that they may defend themselves against guerrilla actions and assist combat operations."[55] Military manuals of the time stressed that they "should remain in military hands at all times."[55] This abrogation of governmental jurisdiction and lack of civilian control that began during the administration of President Guillermo León Valencia continues to this day, giving the Colombian Armed forces virtual autonomy in handling issues considered of public order. From the outset, Official paramilitary groups operated not in self-defense but offensively against guerrillas and *guerrilla supporters,* a stretchable designation that included social protesters, government critics, trade unionists, community organizers, leftist politicians, and human rights activists. However, despite being an arm of the Colombian military, these groups had little impact on the insurgent armies of the 1960s and are viewed as precursors to the more active and more successful private paramilitary armies of the 1970s and 1980s.

Private Paramilitarism   While official paramilitarism was an extension of the Colombian military allowed by law, private paramilitarism grew out of the necessity of wealthy Colombians, especially owners of large estates, to protect themselves and their families from guerilla kidnappings for ransom and extortion. They too benefited from military backing but in a more subtle and covert way. The origins of private paramilitary armies can be traced back to the early 1980s when newly rich *narcos* invested in large estates, especially cattle ranches. These *narco-ganaderos* (narco-ranchers) became the new oligarchs, hence enemies of guerilla groups and justifiable and highly lucrative kidnap targets. The Ochoa family, which dominated the Cali drug cartel after the death of Pablo Escobar, reacted swiftly and decisively after the kidnapping of Martha Nieves Ochoa, a family member, by declaring an all-out war against guerillas, especially the M-19. To that effect, 223 drug traffickers met in Cali, in December 1981, to launch a paramilitary group they named *Muerte a Secuestradores* (Death to Kidnappers), or MAS. It consisted of 2,230 armed men backed by prominent members of the Medellín and Cali drug cartels and by members of the National Army. Their mission was to execute anyone linked to kidnappings.

Over the following decade, "hundreds of paramilitary organizations based on the MAS model were founded"[56] with the tacit support of the Armed Forces. Captain Oscar de Jesús Echandía of the Bárbula Battalion, stationed in Puerto Boyacá, Santander province, launched the first such group in 1982. Funding came from local politicians, businessmen, ranchers, and representatives of the Texas Petroleum Company backed by military logistic support. Another MAS-inspired self-defense organization was the *Autodefensas Campesinas de Córdoba y Urabá* (Peasant Self-Defenses of Córdoba and Urabá), or ACCU, founded by Carlos and Fidel Castaño as a reaction to the murder of their wealthy landowner father by the FARC. The Castaños were heavily involved in the drug trade, marking the auspicious beginning of today's AUC. Many other military-backed groups sprang up throughout the country, reaching 163 in 1988 according to César Gaviria, Minister of Government. They became known collectively as *autodefensas* for their aim was primarily to protect their bosses from leftist guerrilla violence and extortion unopposed by a perennially underfunded, understaffed, inefficient, and corrupt Colombian police and judicial systems, but also to chase them out of their territory. Because *the enemy of my enemy is my friend*, the *autodefensas* were both tolerated by the state and often assisted by the military. In time, these scattered private armies coalesced into the AUC, a loose federation led by Carlos Castaño until he resigned the position in 2001. Like the MAS before them, the AUC were in essence the military arm of the Colombian elite intent on preserving their socioeconomic privileges against guerillas and leftist groups or any other force for change.

The Last 20 Years   The AUC counted with approximately 15,000 fighters before it was demobilized in 2005. At first, they operated in the Magdalena Medio and Urabá regions of the Antioquia province, but their success in expelling guerrillas from these regions encouraged their expansion to virtually the entire Caribbean and Pacific Coasts and parts of the Eastern Plains. Their military structure consisted of army *Bloques* led by autonomous local commanders coordinated through a central Supreme Commander; Salvatore Mancuso being the last. They were most infamous for their cruelty and unspeakable savagery in massacring civilian populations suspected of helping the guerilla. The AUC perpetrated most massacres and were responsible for the majority of displaced populations countrywide: 40% of the total between 1995 and 1997 and 46% between 2000 and 2001, against 28% and 12%, respectively, for the FARC and ELN combined.[57] In 2002, the year with the most displaced population (412,553), the AUC was responsible for 26% of the total against 19% for the FARC and ELN combined.[58] Subsequently, the AUC changed tactics from indiscriminate massacres to selective assassinations. Hence, AUC's murders from massacres, which averaged 886 per year during 1996–2002 and peaked to 2,367 victims from 352 massacres carried out in 2000–2001, decreased to a yearly average of 227 during the 2002–2006 period. In contrast, selective assassinations remained practically unchanged, from a yearly average of 895 in the 1996–2002 time frame, to 833 for the 2002–2006 period. In contrast, they accounted for a relatively small fraction of the total number of kidnappings. For instance, between 2002 and 2005, 4,650 individuals were kidnapped nationwide, of which 2,456 or 52.8% were attributed to the FARC and ELN combined, against 385 or 8.2% to the paramilitaries.[58] It is noteworthy that the Colombian military is implicated in many assassinations, massacres, and human rights violations attributed to the AUC, as described in the following pages. For instance, out of the total number of murders or *forcible disappearances* reported between 2002 and 2006, 74.5% are attributable to the Army; either directly (12.1%, or 752 victims) or indirectly (62.4%, or 3,887 victims), against 25.5% or 1,588 victims attributed to the FARC and the ELN combined.[58]

Modus Operandi Seen from Within   The microcosm of AUC's activities, modus operandi, and coordination with the Colombian Army emerged from the diary of a former AUC commander recovered from the vehicle he abandoned to escape an ambush set up by former allies.[59] His narration begins,

"When I joined the AUC . . . there was no money for food, uniforms, medicines, and much less for munitions. One day we stopped at a farm asking for something to eat. We were told to come back . . . The next day, 'Monoleche' asked the 'Indian' and Germán to fetch some bananas and yucca [tapioca] from the farm . . . When they didn't return, 'Monoleche' entered the farm only to discover a sickening scene: The 'Indian' had been chopped up and the pieces scattered around the yard . . . Germán's beheaded body had been tied to a tree trunk . . . ten FARC men came out of the house and started shooting but Fidel outmaneuvered them killing seven." He then explains how their fortune took a turn for the better, "A rancher was very helpful to us. With his help, most farmers paid us for protection, as did owners of banana plantations, buses, trucks, even banana exporters . . . they brought us weapons on their returning ships . . . One day we were approached by Elías, a man who traded coca from Puerto Raudal and Valdivia, two towns in Antioquia province. He was interested in shipping through the Urabá gulf under our control, and offered a share of the profits [in exchange for free passage]. Business with Elías went well . . . a month later, he brought us 3 million dollars—incredible—we didn't know what to do with so much money!"[59]

He describes how they ran towns under their control to collect taxes, spy on, and discipline townspeople and coordinated operations with local Army and police units to avoid confrontations. "We levied taxes on everyone and everything that made money . . . in urban areas, shops, restaurants, hotels, butcher shops, pool halls, and jewelries paid 50,000 to 100,000 pesos monthly [approximately US$35 to $70 at the then exchange rate]; gasoline stations, between 100,000 and 200,000 pesos; cattle ranches, 500,000 to 700,000 pesos, according to size. Truckers paid 50,000 each time they crossed [our territory] and transporters of merchandise, 1,000,000 but 5,000,000 if they carried coca."[59] Town mayors were forced to assign public works contracts to AUC sympathizers and retain 30% of the contract value: 10% for themselves and 20% for the AUC. Cooperating Army and police commanders were paid 10 million pesos per year.

He also narrates his rise through the ranks, how he made a fortune, and the deadly confrontations within AUC ranks, but is silent about massacres.

I made friends with Miguel Arroyave who, thanks to me, met with Carlos Castaño in Nudo de Paramillo and came back as commandant of the Meta and Guaviare [provinces]. He told me "here are 2 million dollars. You can stay or retire; no problems" . . . [with that money] I bought two ranches: one in El Dorado the other in San Martín, and invested in farms around my hometown. I was a millionaire; enough for the rest of my life, but greed took over. I was used to having subordinates and to be called "sir," and I stayed . . . Miguel infiltrated and manipulated the politics of the Llanos [eastern plains] . . . He informed the Buitragos [local AUC commanders] that all decisions had to be approved by him. In other words, he proclaimed himself commander-in-chief; an unacceptable situation for Héctor Buitrago and his sons "Caballo" and "Martín Llanos" . . . The war began . . . Miguel summoned his allies to San Pedro de Armería . . . from Casanare came 500 men under my command; "Macao," commandant of bloc Central Bolívar, sent 1,500 men; Guillermo Torres added 200 from Meta, and "Cuchillo" came up with another 500 men from Guaviare . . . Daily encounters resulted in scores of dead in both camps . . . While planning "Operación Punto Final," Belisario proposed to bring a witch from San Martín to pray for combatants so that bullets wouldn't penetrate their bodies. We knew of cases where that had been effective . . . The witch began the ritual of praying while sprinkling the men with aromatized herbal water giving each man a bit of graveyard earth to carry in his pocket . . . According to her, no bullet on earth could now penetrate their body . . . The next day, at 6 A.M., "Pólvora" ordered "Voluntario," second in command, to send his men shooting standing up in a formation we call "curtain-like" . . . By 10, we already had 65 dead and 48 wounded . . . I met with Miguel and told him about our losses . . . He replied, "don't worry, tell me where they are for a politician friend of mine has already contacted the Air Force to launch a bombardment" . . . adding "wait and see, those sons of bitches don't know what's coming to them" . . . About forty minutes later two "Tucano" planes and four "Arpía" helicopters began bombing "La Cooperativa" [the farm where Buitragos' men had retrenched] . . . we could see machinegun fire and 500-pound bombs and missiles exploding on the ground . . . At about 4 P.M., Belisario called euphoric announcing, "Commandant, we did it. Nothing remains standing there. They are all dead" . . . Miguel was overjoyed, "we beat those sons of bitches. The General that helped me is the kind of people we need on our side." No sooner had he spoken that "Pólvora" called in frantic, "those sons of bitches of the Air Force turned against us. They dropped a bomb as big as a cow." Miguel immediately called the "General" and the attack promptly stopped. To celebrate, Miguel ordered a party and told me "to those who excelled, give them a girl, a bottle of whiskey, and pay for everything they consume" . . . Wilson found 50 women . . . I said, "50 is too few because it would be one woman to 20 men . . . and, if the Central Bolívar [men] join in, one for 40 men" . . . When the women arrived, there was quite a stir. We had to post a guard to control them and to raffle turns with the girls.[59]

Massacres and AUC-Military Collusion   Though well-known, the AUC-Military links were confirmed by the high command of both organizations and by numerous NGOs. A noted example acknowledged by the military is the massacre (four or more murders at one time, according to the Ministry of Defense) of Mapiripán, Meta province, between July 15 and 20, 1997. The episode began when two planeloads of paramilitaries arrived at the San José del Guaviare airport on July 12, 1997, and marched through several Army checkpoints before reaching the town of Mapiripán. Fighters used chainsaws and machetes to murder, throat-slit, behead, dismember, and disembowel at least 49 civilians, though many bodies were purposely thrown into the river and could not be counted. According to a report,

One massacre occurred in Mapiripan, Meta department, during July 15–20, 1997. When an estimated 200 ACCU soldiers arrived in the town on July 15, among those they searched for were peasants who had taken part in a department-wide protest over the poor economic conditions in Meta. These people, among others, were rounded up and taken to the town slaughterhouse where soldiers tortured them and then slit their throats. One victim, Antonio María Herrera, "was hung from a hook, and ACCU members quartered his body, throwing the pieces into the Guaviare River." Other victims were decapitated. A local judge in Papiripán, Leonardo Iván Cortés, repeatedly contacted the local security forces during the massacre, requesting help. He stated that, "each night they kill groups of five to six defenseless people, who are cruelly and monstrously massacred after being tortured. The screams of humble people are audible, begging for mercy and asking for help." Cortés made a total of eight phone calls to local security forces but neither the police nor the Army made any appearance or investigation until the paramilitaries had left; strong evidence of military acceptance of paramilitary activity.[55]

When summoned by the *Unidad Nacional de Fiscalías de Derechos Humanos* (National Unit of Prosecutors for Human Rights) for his presumed role as author-by-omission in the Mapiripán massacre, retired General Jaime Alberto Uscátegui, ex-commandant of the 7th Brigade, avowed the Army's involvement. He also revealed that the Army knew in advance of the AUC march on Mapiripán and that, after the massacre, it had mounted a massive retaliatory maneuver to crush a FARC unit dispatched to punish the AUC for operating on their turf.[60]

Another indiscriminate and savage massacre perpetrated by the AUC in collusion with the Army occurred in February 2000.[61] At 6:00 A.M. of February 16th, 2000, the *Bloque Norte y Anorí de las ACCU,* led by Emanuel Ortiz, ex-FARC member who had defected to the AUC along with 15 of his men, stopped a car traveling between El Salado and Carmen de Bolívar, Bolívar province. They slit the throat of five passengers, scattering their bodies on the roadway, and *disappeared* the other two. These actions took place in an area controlled by the *Batallón de Fusilleros de Infantería de Marina, Mafim-3* of the First Brigade, led by lieutenant colonel Harold Mantillla. A few hours later, the same group executed 42 peasants in Ovejas, Sucre province, 39 of whom were tortured before their throats were slit. They also burned several houses with the acquiescence of the *Batallón de Fusilleros de Infantería de Marina, Bafim-5,* of the First Brigade. On February 18, 2000, the same AUC group returned to Carmen de Bolívar where they executed 46 more peasants by beheading, hanging, shooting, or beating, often in front of their wives and children. A hooded member of the group pinpointed, one by one, townspeople to be killed. They also raped several women while celebrating their exploits drinking and dancing to *vallenato* music (popular music of African and peasant Colombian roots) through the afternoon of the following day when, according to eye witness accounts, they were informed of the arrival of the *Infantería de Marina* and left town leisurely. Colonel Harold Mantillla, far from admitting involvement, claimed the dead resulted from a confrontation between the AUC and the FARC.

Another instance, reported by Amnesty International, describes,

Between 1 and 7 May 2003, soldiers from the army's Navas Pardo Battalion of the Brigade XVIII, wearing AUC armbands, reportedly entered the indigenous reserves of Betoyes—Julieros, Velasqueros, Roqueros, Genareros and Parreros—in Tame Municipality, Arauca Department. According to reports, on 5 May in Parreros, armed men raped and killed 16-year-old Omaira Fernández, who was pregnant, before ripping open her belly . . . in front of everyone. The bodies of the girl and the baby were thrown in the river. During this incident, three members of the indigenous community were killed. In Velasqueros, three young girls were raped. According to witnesses, a contingent of men had been parachuted into Parreros from [Army] helicopters . . . they were paramilitaries who live in the battalion [Navas Pardo] with the soldiers.[62]

Likewise, during his January 2007 deposition before the Fiscalía General de la Nación, in compliance with AUC demobilization rules, AUC's supreme commander Salvatore Mancuso made shocking revelations. He disclosed his organization's reliance on the Army and police for training, weapons, and transportation and how on many occasions they were given lists of populations to be massacred or the names of individuals to be assassinated.

Foreign Support   The AUC has received training and support not only from the Colombian Armed Forces but also from Israeli, German, and American mercenaries. While public information about German and American trainers is scant, involvement of retired Israeli Lt. Col. Yair Klein and his associate Lt. Colonel Amatzia Shu'ali has come to light in some detail. In the 1980s, Klein founded a paramilitary mercenary firm called *Hod He'hanitin* (Spearhead Ltd.) that trained Medellín cartel members, MAS groups, and the AUC. Hence, both the Colombian Armed Forces and the AUC have received Israeli support whether directly or indirectly. Indeed, while the former have obtained military hardware and antiterrorist training from the official Israeli military establishment, mercenary ex-members of that institution have trained many Colombian death squads. In 1989, Colombian authorities charged Klein, along with several other former Israeli officers, of arming and training drug lords running international cocaine cartels. Supporting evidence included a video Klein used to instruct death quads found in the house of a Medellín cartel drug lord. He is also suspected of involvement in the downing of a civilian airliner in November of 1989. An extradition request was not honored by Israel, but in 1990, an Israeli court convicted Klein to a fine of US$13,400 and a one-year prison term for smuggling arms and military hardware destined to Colombian terrorist groups. In 1999, he was imprisoned in Sierra Leone for smuggling arms to rebels of the Revolutionary United Front. Initial charges were scaled down and eventually dismissed following behind-the-scenes pressure from Israel. Klein has also been active in El Salvador, Guatemala, and Russia, where Interpol arrested him in August 2007. It remains to be seen whether he will escape a new extradition request outstanding for him to stand trial in Colombia. The United States has been accused of aiding the AUC indirectly, through *Plan Colombia,* despite listing it as a terrorist group. Another argument advanced suggesting U.S. support of the AUC is the U.S.-financed aerial fumigation of coca fields that focuses almost exclusively on FARC-controlled areas despite the fact that most of the coca trade is controlled by the AUC, accounting for 70% of their revenues. Additionally, considering that 71% of American aid under *Plan Colombia* ($2.34 out of $3.29 billion between 2004 and 2007) was earmarked for the Colombian military despite well-known AUC–military links, it has been argued that the groups' ideologies take precedence over narco-trafficking in the implementation of American antiterrorist policy, at least in Colombia.

Parapolitics: A Scandal of National Scope   Military support, the cornerstone of official paramilitary armies of the 1960s, is said to have declined to isolated episodes from rogue military units, marking the AUC's fading relevance. That benign self-serving perception was shattered by revelations that AUC influence reached into the deepest corridors of Colombian power, including the legislative and executive branches of government and its intelligence apparatus. Incriminating evidence was found in the confiscated laptop computer of *Jorge 40*, a notorious AUC commander, and was complemented in disclosures by Rafael García, a former informatics chief at the *Departamento Administrativo de Seguridad*, or DAS (Colombia's CIA equivalent), turned informer, describing how the AUC manipulated local and national elections, controlled politicians, and infiltrated the DAS.[63] Yet, the parapolitics scandal acquired national proportions when it was revealed that scores of politicians had met in Santa Fé Ralito in July 2001 to pledge allegiance to the AUC central command. Based on these revelations, a host of Colombian politicians have being incarcerated or are being investigated by the *Corte Suprema de Justicia* (U.S. Supreme Court equivalent), the Fiscalía General de la Nación, and other judicial authorities for colluding with paramilitary forces. At this writing (July 2008), "32 out of 102 senators and 25 of the 166 representatives are suspected of collusion with the AUC (as are numerous governors, mayors, and members of local assemblies and city councilors). Eighteen senators and twelve representatives are incarcerated and four have been sentenced after pleading guilty."[64]

Rodrigo Tovar Pupo, a.k.a. Jorge 40, is the son of a military officer who grew under the tutelage of his uncle, a former governor of the César province. In 1996, he was recruited by an Army General of the first brigade, along with other members of prominent local families, to participate in a plan to fuse all private armies into a unified force. Jorge 40 and the others met with Carlos Castaño and Salvatore Mancuso, who would become supreme commanders of the newly constituted AUC. While Jorge 40 soon became a local leader, his quest for power clashed with Hernán Giraldo's and Jorge Gnecco's, two local AUC leaders who controlled access to the northern seaports from which cocaine was shipped to the United States and Europe. An unrelenting war with the former ensued, leaving hundreds dead. Summoned to a meeting by Jorge 40, Giraldo's naked body was found riddled with bullets on his way to the meeting. Jorge 40 also ordered the kidnapping of six members of the Gnecco family while others fled the country or were barred from office by the Procuraduría General de la Nación. With both rivals out of the way, Jorge 40 was now in control of the northern seaports of the Magdalena and Guajira provinces and hence of the lucrative drug business from these regions. Jorge 40's now famous computer also detailed drug dealings. Surprisingly, most of the thrice weekly cocaine shipments went, not to the United States, but to Europe, mainly Belgium, Holland, and France, hidden within banana crates or furniture, or carried by *mules* [hired couriers of illegal drugs]. "Each banana crate carried up to 200 grams of cocaine and each sea container contained 1,080 crates, which amounts to transporting 140 to 180 kilograms [per container]."[65] At least one furniture exporter was involved in the drug trade; hiding cocaine within furniture destined to Madrid, Spain, and to several U.S. destinations. Shipping clearance required payment of 1,500,000 to 1,800,000 Colombian pesos (approximately US$750 to $900) per kilo of cocaine to antinarcotics agents stationed at the seaports of Santa Marta and Cartagena. Mules traveled thrice weekly in groups of four to Caracas, Venezuela, or Madrid, Spain, carrying 5 to 10 kilos each hidden in their luggage. Upon arrival, members of Venezuela's *Guardia Nacional* and of Spain's *Guardia Civil* on the narcotraffickers' payroll greeted them. "Each kilo [of cocaine] sells for US$2,500 in Venezuela. The mule and the Commandant of the Guardia at each end are paid a percentage."[66] According to the same source, the margin of benefit for cocaine shipped to Spain was 900 to 1,000 euros per kilo (approximately US$1,350).

However, Jorge 40's ambitions extended well beyond the drug trade. He also wanted to control the public purse strings, which required the connivance of politicians and public office holders, a feat that was facilitated by his enormous military and economic power, which kept everybody in check. A meeting was held at Pivijay, César province, in December 2001, attended by ranchers and politicians to carve out a strategy to ensure the election of friendly politicians to the Senate and House of Representatives. It was decided to divide the Province into three sectors: two where only AUC-friendly candidates would be on the ballot box, and a third sector where competition was allowed. Means to ensure compliance ranged from economic assistance to AUC-sponsored candidates, to kidnapping and murdering unfriendly candidates. An example of the latter is the well-publicized assassination of an ex-mayor aspiring to a congressional seat without AUC approval. Because of the manipulation of the electoral process and intimidation, two AUC-sponsored candidates were elected to the Senate and three to Congress from that province that year. Election of provincial Governor the following year was also influenced by the AUC, which led to the withdrawal of two candidates under AUC pressure, leaving Hernando Molina Araújo unopposed to win the governorship in 2003, only to be investigated by the Supreme Court on allegations of malfeasance, as were several other members of the Araújo clan.

Rafael García, a long-standing member of the AUC's *Bloque Norte*, commanded by Jorge 40, became Chief of informatics at the DAS and promptly deleted AUC files from DAS computers. On November 21, 2006, after 18 months of silence following his arrest, García began a deposition before the Corte Suprema de Justicia that would last three days. He accused Jorge Noguera, his former boss and ex-DAS Director, of long-term collusion with the AUC, especially with Jorge 40 and Hernán Giraldo; a scandal now known as *DAS-Gate*. Prior allegations of wrongdoing had forced Noguera to resign from the DAS directorship, and García's revelations forced his resignation from his new post as Colombian consul in Milan, Italy. According to García, Noguera maintained contacts with both José Gélvez Albarracín, a.k.a. *El canoso* (grey-hair man), the political chief of Hernán Giraldo's *Resistencia Tayrona* group, and with Álvaro Pupo, Jorge 40's cousin. The relationship with the former had begun when both worked in Álvaro Uribe's first presidential campaign in the Magdalena province, which was headed by

Noguera. Álvaro Pupo reportedly acted as go-between for Noguera and Jorge 40, and according to García, "on one occasion, through him [Pupo] DAS agents sent to Jorge 40 a list of union members and professors that were subsequently murdered."[65] García also described lucidly and in great detail AUC's widespread infiltration of state institutions, their manipulation of the electoral process, the influence they exerted over many national politicians and local elected officials, and their control over the revenues of many northern cities and municipalities. Many of his accusations were already known or were confirmed subsequently. As a result of García's deposition, "within two weeks, four congressmen and four 'diputados' were arrested, an order of capture was issued against a former governor of the Sucre province, and an ex-Director of the DAS was called to testify."[65]

Yet, more explosive than García's disclosures were revelations of a secret accord signed between Colombian politicians and elected officials and the AUC central command. On July 23, 2001, 11 congressmen, 2 governors, 3 mayors, and an assortment of elected officials, 32 in all, met at the AUC's central command center near Santa Fé Ralito with Salvatore Mancuso, supreme AUC commander; *Don Berna*, its inspector general; and Jorge 40, commandant of its Bloque Norte. The purpose of the meeting was to approve an AUC program designed to *refounding the homeland* through a *new social contract*. At the meeting, Mancuso circulated the secret document for each participant to sign. While the document did not contain seditious statements, it nevertheless sealed a pact between a group of Colombian elected officials and a criminal enterprise already known to be responsible for most massacres of innocent victims and for the displacement of hundreds of thousands of peasants each year. That day, "part of the Colombian State settled its destiny with one of the most terrifying organizations in recent history."[66,67] Hence, far-fetched excuses concocted by participants facing indictment by the Corte Suprema de Justicia five years later were quickly dismissed, and at this writing, except for one that fled the country, most are in prison charged with aiding, supporting, or participating in criminal activities.[64]

AUC Demobilization: Fact or Fancy?   Demobilization of AUC armies, authorized by legislation approved in 2002, 2003, and 2005, is a commendable goal that was designed to Disarm, Demobilize, and Reintegrate (DDR) these groups and to end massive human rights violations and other egregious crimes they committed against defenseless civil populations. The history of DDR of irregular armies in Colombia dates back to Dictator General Gustavo Rojas Pinilla's successful amnesty of 1953, followed by President Belisario Betancourt's *Ley de Amnistía no condicionada en pro de la paz* (Law of unconditional amnesty towards peace), which succeeded in demobilizing 700 guerrilla members from the FARC, the ELN, and the M-19. However, subsequent presidential initiatives were unsuccessful, including Virgilio Barco's (1986–1990) *Iniciativa para la paz* (peace initiative) designed to dismantle guerillas, Cesar Gaviría's (1990–1994) reduced sentences for drug traffickers, and Andrés Pastrana's (1998–2002) peace negotiations with the FARC, mentioned earlier. Soon after Álvaro Uribe took office in August 2002, the AUC leadership announced its willingness to participate in peace negotiations with his government on condition that none of its members would face prison time or extradition to the United States. In view of President Uribe's favorable response, on November 29, 2002, the AUC proclaimed a unilateral ceasefire. In July 2003, the Colombian government and the AUC signed the *Acuerdo de Santa Fé de Ralito para contribuir a la paz de Colombia* (Santa Fé de Ralito accord toward peace in Colombia), with the expectation that the process would be completed by December 31, 2005.

The legal framework for the demobilization of the AUC and other illegal armed groups rests on Law 418 of 1997, extended and amended by Law 782 of December 2002, later revised by Decree 128 of January 2003, and finally complemented by law 975 of July 2005, also known as *Ley de Justicia y Paz* (Justice and Peace Law). Yet, the resulting directive "still failed to meet international standards on truth, justice and reparation."[68] Indeed, Law 782 refers to "atrocious acts of ferocity or barbarism, terrorism, kidnapping, genocide, and murder committed outside combat," which if complied with would have excluded most AUC combatants from participating.[68] After failed attempts to reach a balance between necessary incentives to motivate combatants and justice for their victims, Decree 128 was finally enacted. Decree 128 confers "pardon, conditional suspension of the execution of a sentence, a cessation of procedure, a resolution of preclusion of an investigation or a resolution of dismissal" but only to those that committed political or petty crimes.[68] It also delineates economic and social benefits for demobilized combatants. And, acquiescing to demands from the AUC high command, Law 975 prohibits extradition of members of illegal armed groups accused of "political" offenses such as rebellion and sedition, albeit allowing it for narco-trafficking and other criminal offenses. In their aggregate, these DDR laws represent an alternative approach to conventional justice and are designed to balance truth, accountability, punishment, reparation, and reconciliation in a process of postconflict healing and recovery. Comparable approaches were adopted in El Salvador, Argentina, and South Africa, among others, to confront their past in hopes of establishing the foundations for a better future. By their very nature, alternative justice approaches to national conflict resolution trigger controversy and contentious debate and lead to imperfect outcomes and to numerous abuses, especially when applied unevenly, as in Colombia's case.

Decree 128 cleared the way for the demobilization process to begin, and on November 25, 2003, 874 members of the *Bloque Cacique Nutibara*, an infamous AUC urban unit operating in Medellin, Antioquia province, laid down their arms. Yet, no demonstrable reduction in crime occurred in Medellin the following year, and 160 members of the AUC's Bloque Cacique Nutibara were pardoned in December 2004 despite being actively in-

vestigated by the Office of the General Prosecutor for human rights violations, making a mockery of decree 128. In the first 30 months of the DDR
process, over 30,000 AUC combatants reportedly demobilized collectively,
and over 3,000 demobilized individually, though the AUC force never exceeded 14,000–15,000 combatants. Also, only 17,000 weapons were turned
in. Moreover, procedural flaws and haphazard application of the law have
tainted the entire process, raising questions about each facet of the DDR
and whether justice is being served and the desired outcome is being
reached. According to a recent Amnesty International report,

"since 2003, paramilitary groups, responsible for the vast majority of human rights
violations in Colombia for over a decade, have been involved in a government-
sponsored 'demobilization' process. More than 25,000 paramilitaries have supposedly
demobilized under a process, which has been criticized by Amnesty International
and other Colombian and international human rights groups, as well as by the
OHCHR [United Nations' Office of the High Commissioner for Human Rights] and
the IACHR [Inter American Commission on Human Rights]. The process is lacking in effective mechanisms for justice and in its inability to ensure that paramilitary members actually cease violent activities."[69]

Moreover, the DDR process doesn't record combatants' group affiliation,
precluding ascertaining whether AUC groups are fully or partially demobilized. Additionally, while human rights violators are not eligible to certain
benefits under DDR laws, the General Attorney responsible to make that
determination only checks its records to establish whether the demobilization applicant is under investigation or has been convicted of human rights
violations. Likewise, combatants are not debriefed, which prevents gathering information on AUCs' structures, crimes, financing, illegal assets, and
other critical information and enables murderers and violators of human
rights to escape prosecution and retain illegally obtained property while
depriving victims of just compensation. For instance, only 24,000 out of
5,000,000 hectares seized by AUC groups between 1998 and 2006 from over
3 million displaced peasants have been restituted. Finally, DDR laws do not
incorporate appropriate safeguards to ensure full reintegration of demobilized AUC combatants into civilian society, leading many of them to initiate or join gangs of common criminals and resume criminal activities.

Amnesty International identifies several flaws in the application of Law
975 that have led to several major negative outcomes and undermines the
government's ability to bring the DDR to an equitable conclusion. They
include, "Providing de facto amnesties for paramilitaries and guerrillas
responsible for serious human rights abuses and violations. Perpetuating
impunity for human rights abusers and violators thereby undermining the
rule of law in Colombia. Failing to guarantee the effective dismantling of
paramilitary structures by focusing solely on individual combatants. Failing to expose those Colombian security forces, government officials, and
private citizens who have supported and benefited from the activities of

the paramilitary. Failing to establish a full and independent judicial process to oversee the demobilization process. Neglecting to respect the rights of victims of human rights violations and abuses to truth, justice, and reparation."[69] Another criticism of the DDR process is that "Colombia's paramilitary groups have agreed to dismantle their military arm, but the process is only legitimizing their network of political power and country-wide control of land, as well as the suppression of anyone who threatens their rule."[69] It must be recognized that "with Colombia's transitional justice process scheduled to proceed over the next eight years, this examination [of the DDR process] has only just begun."[70] However, even an impeccable DDR process flawlessly implemented would not eliminate drug-related crime or achieve lasting peace in Colombia as long as the drug trade remains in place.

CHAPTER 8

Afghanistan

The situation in Afghanistan is not acceptable, but not only because of the drug situation—because of the poverty, because of instability, because of the corruption, because of the insurgency.

> —Antonio Maria Costa, executive
> director of the UN Office on Drugs and Crime

As the world's main opium supplier devastated by a quarter-century of civil war and by outside military interventions that wrecked the country's economic and political infrastructures, a weak and corrupt central government imposed by foreign powers, and a resurgent Taliban (plural of *talib* or seeker of knowledge), Afghanistan poses complex challenges to its neighbors and to the world community. It has become the focal point where the War on Drugs and the War on Terror collide. Indeed, many current and former Afghan warlords utilize opium trade income to maintain their hold on power and to enrich themselves and, when U.S.-friendly or allied to the central government, to help anti-Taliban military operations. However, regardless of their current allegiance, many warlords are former Mujahideen or Mujahideen supporters who would not hesitate to realign their loyalties should their source of revenue be threatened, especially by a foreign power. Additionally, many of them are now integrated into the mainstream political process or have developed key political connections that brought about a symbiotic relationship between the illicit drug trade and the government. Likewise, a resurging Taliban exploits the opium trade as a major source of revenue, especially now that it tries to both regain power it lost following the U.S.-led invasion in October 2001 and to expel foreign troops stationed on their ancestral land.

Like Colombia, Afghanistan plays a prominent role in the worldwide illicit drug trade and, like Colombia, is the target of U.S. intervention: in Colombia, to stem the flow of illicit drugs to the United States; and in Afghanistan, first to oust the Taliban from power ostensibly for refusing to hand over Osama bin Laden, the alleged mastermind of the 9/11 attack, and now to sustain its imposed but fragile democracy. However, they differ fundamentally in that in Colombia's case the illicit drug trade has caused massive disruptions in the social fabric of the country, whereas in Afghanistan it has turned the country into a major battlefield of the U.S.-led War on Terror, allegedly to stop the export of terrorism by radical Islamists. Additionally, Colombia's dynamic and decisive current leader, building on long-standing albeit imperfect democratic institutions and enjoying overwhelming approval from the citizenry and U.S. military and financial support, is well underway to regain control over the whole of his country. His ultimate success would end half a century of guerilla and counter-guerrilla conflict that, in the last two decades, has been funded by the drug trade. In contrast, the future of Afghanistan as a thriving democracy looks bleak[1] despite massive financial, military, and logistic support, and good intentions from the United States and NATO-led International Security Assistance Force (ISAF). Factors that contribute to the country's economic, social, and political stagnation include a weak central government with scant authority outside Kabul, the country's capital; a meager Gross Domestic Product[2] that compels reliance on foreign aid; discontent or distrust of its citizenry; and the lack of democratic infrastructures and of a well-functioning civil society that now faces a resurging Taliban. This chapter briefly delineates events that have shaped today's Afghanistan, outlining the role of geopolitical interests, including America's, and sketching Afghanistan's place in today's confrontation between Islam and the West.

THE EARLY DAYS: PRYING BY THE BRITISH EMPIRE

In 1747, Ahmad Shah Durrani unified the Pashtun tribes in what is today Afghanistan and conquered additional territory that, at the height of his power, included today's Pakistan and parts of both India and Iran.[3] Initially, the new country served as a buffer between the British and Russian empires, but as Durrani's domain started to disintegrate, the British took advantage of the wars of succession by installing ex-Shah Shuya as the head of a puppet government in Kabul, replacing Dost Mohammed who was supported by Russia. This marked the first in a series of moves and ploys, used by both Britain and Russia, known as the *Great Game*, that were designed to expand their respective spheres of influence. However, Shuya was unable to gain support from Afghan tribal chiefs who rose up against him and the British, leading to the first Anglo-Afghan war of 1831–1842. The second Anglo-Afghan war (1878–1881) erupted when Lord Lytton,

Viceroy of India and a loyal promoter of the *Forward Policy* formulated by British Prime Minister Benjamin Disraeli (1804–1881), delivered an ultimatum to Emir Sher Ali to accept a British mission in Kabul. Ali's refusal led the British to invade, in November 1878, and nearly unopposed by an ill-equipped and poorly trained Afghan army, they quickly occupied half the country. This led to the *Treaty of Gandamak*, which stopped the British advance and installed a British Regent in exchange for payment of annual subsidies. However, less than a year later 2,000 unpaid Herati mercenaries from the ancient city of Herat stormed the *Residency* (the British seat of power), killing the entire British garrison. In retaliation, Lord Lytton sent an army that massacred hundreds of Afghans indiscriminately, which in turn rallied 10,000 tribesmen to march on Kabul, forcing the British to anoint Abdul Rahman Khan as Emir who, ironically, was backed by Russia. Hence, while the British were able to crush a second-rate Afghan army in both Anglo-Afghan wars, they were ultimately expelled by tribal warfare, as would be the Soviet army a century later.

British Imperial wars were temporarily halted when William Gladstone (1809–1898) regained the position of Prime Minister in April 1880 with anti-war campaign slogans such as, "The sanctity of life in the hill villages of Afghanistan, among the winter snows, is as inviolable in the eyes of Almighty God as can be your own." Yet, in 1893, Abdul Rahman Khan was forced by the British Indian government to agree to the *Durand Line* as the official boundary between Afghanistan and British India; a 1,610-mile line that now demarcates the border between today's Afghanistan and Pakistan. Because the Durand Line was drawn arbitrarily through Pashtun territory, it continues to be a source of tension between Afghanistan and Pakistan. While the growing power of Germany forced an end to the Great Game through the *Anglo-Russian Convention* of 1907, the third Anglo-Afghan War was launched in May 1919 by Amanullah Khan, the new king of Afghanistan, in May 1919 when the British refused to acknowledge Afghanistan's independence. However, hostilities lasted only a month given British reluctance to re-engage in new war, as World War I was ending, and Afghanistan's eagerness to settle given relentless British air bombardments of Kabul and Jalalabad.[4] Under the convention, Afghanistan regained control of its foreign affairs, usurped by the British in 1878, and established diplomatic relations with the Soviet Union, Iran, Britain, Turkey, Italy, and France. King Amanullah Khan attempted to import democratic reforms instituted in Turkey by Kemal Ataturk. They included Western clothing, secular education, the unveiling of women, and a ban of slavery and forced labor. A constitution, civil rights, a legislative assembly, and a court system were established. However, such changes were too much and too quickly instituted for many tribal chieftains and religious leaders, and forced to abdicate in 1929, Amanullah Khan went into exile with his family, vowing never to return.

EVENTS LEADING TO THE SOVIET INVASION

The following five decades were marked by regional power struggles, short-lived attempts to relax censorship and to emancipate women, shifting geopolitical alliances and confrontations, especially with Pakistan, and to a civil war that led to the Soviet invasion. For instance, when Mohammed Daoud Khan became prime minister (1953–1963) he severed diplomatic relations with Pakistan and turned to the Soviet Union to equip and train the Afghan army and to aid in the development of the country's infrastructure.[5] As his economic policies proved disastrous, King Zahir Shah, Daoud's cousin, ousted him and took control of the government. He instituted a parliamentary democracy with a constitution (1964) that enshrined equal rights for women, including the right to vote and to an education. Wearing of the veil was made optional. However, his cousin and former prime minister he had sacked 10 years earlier, supported by officers of the Afghan army and by the *Khalq* (masses) faction of the People's Democratic Party of Afghanistan (PDPA), deposed King Zahir Shah in 1973. Daoud abolished the monarchy, named himself President, and ran a brutally repressive regime with arbitrary arrests and executions. He also lessened the country's dependence on the Soviet Union and squashed the growing Islamic fundamentalist movement *Jamiat-i Islami* (Islamic Society), a Mujahideen party akin to Pakistan's *Jamaat-e Ismali* and Egypt's *Muslim Brotherhood*. His leader, Burhanuddin Rabbani, fled to Pakistan along with Gulbuddin Hekmatyar and Ahmad Shah Massoud, where they received support to fight the Daoud government. These men would become leaders of the Mujahideen (plural of *Mujahid* or a person involved in *Jihad*) forces that evicted the Soviets.[5]

At the time, Afghanistan was one of the poorest and most underdeveloped countries in the world, with a gross national product of $70 per capita, ranking it 73rd among 83 underdeveloped countries, according to the World Bank.[6] Many Afghans became impatient with King Zahir Shah's rule. Discontent was covertly encouraged by Pakistan, where Daoud's doctrine of *Pashtunistan* or unification of all Pashtuns living on both sides of the Durand Line caused great alarm. If ever realized, annexation of Pashtun lands would cut deeply into Pakistan's Northwest Frontier Province, home of millions of Pashtuns.[7] Unrest led to the PDPA seizing power on April 27, 1978, through a military coup d'état spearheaded by a group of sympathetic Afghan soldiers. Daoud, his family, and thousands of ordinary citizens died, and Nur Muhammad Taraki was installed as President, ending two centuries of control of the country by the Durrani clan. Taraki's aim was to *uproot feudalism* in Afghanistan by implementing reforms to expand social services, education, and women's and religious rights and to strengthen Afghanistan ties to the Soviet Union. However, such measures caused violent opposition by wealthy landlords and chieftains and by the Muslim religious establishment, which included many Mullahs holders of large estates. Opposition turned into open rebellion that by early 1979 had spread to 24 of the 28 Afghan provinces.

THE SOVIET-AFGHAN WAR (1979–1989)

In March 1979, a faction of the Afghan army led by Ismail Khan massacred 100 Soviet advisers stationed near Kabul. The Afghani government crackdown was unable to control the situation despite reportedly killing 10,000 Afghan dissidents. President Taraki and Prime Minister Hafizullah Amin repeatedly urged the Russian leadership to send troops and assistance but were initially rebuffed. As revealed by transcripts of the *Russian Presidential Archive*, the *Ministry of Defense Archive*, and from published memoirs of participating Soviet officers and politicians,[8] Union of Socialist Soviet Republics (USSR) leaders were very reluctant to send troops and instead dispatched military equipment in the spring and summer of 1979. However, after repeated requests, 20 in all, from the PDPA and the Afghani government, and alarmed by the overthrow and assassination of President Taraki by his Prime Minister Amin in September 1979, the Politburo decided to send a *Limited Contingent of Soviet Troops* to Afghanistan against the strong objections of the military high command. Arguments raised centered on the wider geopolitical implications of the situation in Afghanistan, the regional impact of the Iranian revolution, and the perceived U.S. ambitions in that part of the world. The latter was based on reported cooperation between Amin and the CIA, an argument promoted by Yuri Vladimirovich Andropov, the Chairman of the KGB (Soviet's intelligence services), who controlled the flow of information to the ailing General Secretary Leonid Ilyich Brezhnev. Regional geopolitical events that also influenced the Soviet leaders' decision included: the overthrow of Mohammad Reza Pahlavi, Shah (from *Shahanshah:* King of Kings) of Iran, in February 1979; the U.S.-sponsored Israel–Egypt peace treaty in March 1979; and the U.S. military support of Saudi Arabia and North Yemen royalists against Communist factions. Soviet ideologues, unacquainted with tribal societies' ways, unaware of the preeminent role of Islam in Afghan society, and believing that all countries were ripe for socialism, were critical in bringing about the Politburo's decision to invade.

In November–December 1979, Soviet troops stormed across the Amudarya River in tanks and armored personnel carriers, and thousands more were flown into Kabul, Bagram, and Shindand air bases accompanied by Babrak Karmal, one of the founders of the PDPA and leader of its *Parcham* (Banner) faction. Within days, Karmal was installed as the new President of the Soviet-backed Democratic Republic of Afghanistan, after Amin's assassination. Early on, the mission of the Limited Contingent, initially made of reservists, was to take control of major urban centers, military bases, and strategic installations. However, it was unable to pacify the country and, contrary of expectations of being viewed as a friendly force, it was seen as an *infidel* foreign invader; a perception that united Afghanis as no local or national issue could, turning a civil war into a war of liberation. Powerless to control the rebellion, President Karmal demanded the Soviet Army to intervene. Hence, Soviet troops "found themselves pulled into the inter-necine war in Afghanistan and began to fulfill tasks related to suppression of the rebel movement, which initially did not figure in the USSR plans at all."[9] Soviet forces were facing guerilla warfare where massive ground–air offensives undertaken periodically proved ineffective against hit-and-run guerilla tactics by myriad small groups of Mujahideen fighters with knowl-edge of the terrain, logistic support from local populations, and armed with sophisticated equipment supplied by the West, mainly the United States. The Soviet Army brass quickly realized that, given their lack of counter-insurgency training and appropriate military equipment to fight guerilla warfare compounded by shifting directives coming from the Soviet Polit-buro, a military solution was not in the cards. Hence, "the issue of troop withdrawal and the search for a political solution was discussed as early as 1980, but no real steps in that direction were taken, and the Limited Con-tingent continued to fight in Afghanistan without a clearly defined ob-jective."[8]

In the meantime, the United States was increasing its support of the Mu-jahideen and other anti-Communist factions.[7] In fact, U.S. involvement in Afghanistan preceded the Soviet invasion, as later revealed by Robert Gates,[10] a 26-year CIA veteran and its Director (1991–1993) under President George H. W. Bush, and by Zbigniew Brzezinski, American National Secu-rity Advisor (1977–1981) under President Jimmy Carter. In a 1998 interview with Le Nouvel Observateur, Brzezinski revealed that the United States began supporting the Mujahideen well before the Red Army invaded Af-ghanistan. He stated,

according to the official version of history CIA aid to the Mujahideen began during 1980, that is to say, after the Soviet army invaded Afghanistan, 24 Dec 1979. But the reality, secretly guarded until now, is completely otherwise. Indeed, it was July 3, 1979 that President Carter signed the first directive for secret aid to the opponents of the pro-Soviet regime in Kabul. And that very day, I wrote a note to the president in which I explained to him that in my opinion this aid was going to induce a Soviet military intervention . . . We didn't push the Russians to intervene, but we know-ingly increased the probability that they would.[11]

When asked if he regretted anything, he replied, "regret what? That secret operation was an excellent idea. It had the effect of drawing the Russians into the Afghan trap and you want me to regret it? The day that the Sovi-ets officially crossed the border, I wrote to President Carter. We now have the opportunity of giving to the USSR its Vietnam War. Indeed, for almost 10 years, Moscow had to carry on a war unsupportable by the government, a conflict that brought about the demoralization and finally the breakup of the Soviet empire." When pressed, "do you regret having supported Islamic fundamentalism, having given arms and advice to future terrorists?" He replied, "What is most important to the history of the world? The Taliban or the collapse of the Soviet empire? . . . Some stirred-up Muslims or the liberation of Central Europe and the end of the cold war?"[11] Indeed, President Carter's July 3, 1979, directive had authorized funding of anti-Communist guerrillas in Afghanistan, enabling the CIA to launch *Operation Cyclone*, which would channel billions of dollars and sophisticated equipment, including 500 to 2,000 U.S.-made FIM-92 Stingers (shoulder-fired surface-to-air missiles), to support the Mujahideen's anti-Soviet struggle using the Pakistani government as a conduit.

Brzezinski's interventionist approach reached much beyond Afghanistan. His grand strategy, adopted by his successors, was to destabilize the Soviet Union by supporting Islamic fundamentalism not only in Afghanistan but also in all predominantly Muslim Soviet republics in Central Asia. This was to be achieved by financing and arming the Mujahideen, especially Hekmatyar, which were conveniently classified as *freedom fighters*, and by broadcasting a daily barrage of anti-Soviet propaganda through U.S.-run and -funded *Radio Free Europe* and *Radio Liberty*. Subsequent U.S. administrations continued to back the Mujahideen in words and deeds. For instance, in his Proclamation 5034 designating March 21, 1983, as *Afghanistan Day*, President Ronald Reagan stated, "The tragedy of Afghanistan continues as the valiant and courageous Afghan freedom fighters persevere in standing up against the brutal power of the Soviet invasion and occupation."[12] In his radio address that day, he invited his audience "to watch the courageous Afghan freedom fighters battle modern arsenals with simple hand-held weapons is an inspiration to those who love freedom."[13] Yet, the CIA went beyond Afghanistan's freedom fighters in its backfired efforts to counter the Soviets. Apparently dissatisfied at infighting between rebel Afghan factions, it recruited anti-Soviet fighters from the wider Muslim world to join the Afghan Jihad and funded them through Pakistan's Inter-Services Intelligence agency (ISI), a program that was approved by CIA Director, William Casey. "So, [Osama] bin Laden, along with a small group of Islamic militants from Egypt, Pakistan, Lebanon, Syria and Palestinian refugee camps all over the Middle East, became the 'reliable' partners of the CIA in its war against Moscow."[14] In time, thousands of Muslim radicals from scores of Muslim countries were trained in Pakistan in bomb making, guerrilla warfare, and other terrorist activities. Ironically, most never took part in the Afghan struggle, and those that did returned to their country of origin after the war where they organized terrorist groups or engaged in individual acts of violence. Though unforeseen or ignored by the CIA, the danger of that policy was not lost to regional leaders. For instance, Pakistani Prime Minister Benazir Bhutto warned President George H. W. Bush, "you are creating a Frankenstein," and Richard Murphy, assistant secretary of State for Near East and South Asian relations during the Reagan administration, opined "We did spawn a monster in Afghanistan. Once the Soviets were gone . . . [people trained and/or funded by the USA] were looking around for other targets, and Osama bin Laden has settled on the United States as the source of all-evil. Irony? Irony is all over the place."[15]

On the Soviet side, mounting casualties, the success of American-made FIM-92 Stingers in neutralizing its air superiority, the staggering economic cost of the war, and the loss of support at home increased the pressure on the Soviet leadership to end the quagmire. In fact, upon becoming General Secretary of the Communist Party in March 1985, Mikhail Sergeyevich Gorbachev proposed ending the Afghan conflict within a year; at the most two.[16] As a result of the initial Politburo deliberations, the size of the Limited Contingent was increased to approximately 118,000 men, and the day-to-day duties of fighting the Mujahideen were transferred to Afghan forces, which were strengthened in manpower and military capability. The PDPA leadership feared the proposed Soviet withdrawal for it was aware of the lack of motivation and of the high level of desertions within the Afghani army. In fact, Gorbachev had made it clear to President Karmal that there was no going back. He informed the Politburo, at its October 17, 1985, meeting, that he had warned Karmal, "by the end of the summer of 1986 you'll have to have figured out how to defend your cause on your own. We'll help you, but with arms only, not troops. And if you want to survive you'll have to broaden the base of the regime, forget socialism, and make a deal with truly influential forces, including Mujahideen commanders and leaders of now-hostile organizations. You'll have to revive Islam, respect traditions, and try to show the people some tangible benefits of the revolution."[16] In May 1986, Karmal was replaced as party leader and was ousted as president six months later. Haji Mohammad Chamkani, the new interim president (1986–1987), instituted a policy of national reconciliation that neither increased support for the new Moscow-backed Kabul regime nor brought about a truce with insurgents. Moreover, the real power behind the scenes was Mohammed Najibulla, who succeeded him as president (1987–1992). In the meantime, Soviet troop withdrawal continued as planned and was completed by February 1989. If the aftermath of the Limited Contingent's troop surge and refocused objectives are harbingers of President Obama's, the orderly end of Afghanistan's current quagmire and the prospects for a self-sustaining and just democracy in that country are indeed bleak, as described next.

THE AFTERMATH OF THE SOVIET–AFGHAN WAR

Aside from the economic and human costs on both sides, the Soviet–Afghan war unleashed serious and long-lasting geopolitical consequences; mainly terrorism and an illicit drug trade that in turn gave rise to ill-conceived policies and counterproductive strategies to combat each. The political scenario of the post-Soviet era is dominated by alliances, dissen-

sions, and confrontations among the numerous Mujahideen factions vying
for power. One of the most notorious players is Gulbuddin Hekmatyar,
leader of the Islamic Party *Hezb-e-Islami,* which he founded in 1975 to oppose
Daoud's rule. Hekmatyar, who allied himself to and fought every other
Mujahideen group over the years, was strongly backed by Pakistan dictator General Muhammad Zia-ul-Haq,[17] Saudi Arabia, and the CIA during
the Soviet–Afghan war, each to further their own country's strategic interests. By some accounts,[18] he was responsible for countless deaths, assassinations, and human rights violations. For instance, after the Red Army's
withdrawal, Hekmatyar's forces fired thousands of scud rockets at Kabul;
nearly 2,000 civilians died and 500,000 fled the city. Given these chaotic
local circumstances, Western analysts expected the PDPA regime to soon
collapse, especially given American and Pakistani support of the Mujahideen, but it was able to survive thanks to its military strength. In fact, the
Red Army had left behind scores of jet fighters and attack helicopters and
thousands of tanks and armored personnel carriers. Additionally, Soviet aid
was renewed thanks to President Najibullah's socialist reforms, reaching
$3 billion in 1990. Moreover, President Najibullah counted with the sup-
port of progovernment militias, especially Abdul Rashid Dostum's 40,000
men-strong *Jozjani* militia. Hence, a military operation planned by Robert B.
Oakley, U.S. ambassador to Pakistan, and by Pakistani General Hamid Gaul,
head of the ISI, to hasten the demise of the PDPA regime by capturing Jalalabad and make it the temporary seat of a provisional pro-Western government was a failure. This ill-conceived campaign that the Mujahideen had
opposed caused the death of approximately 3,000 of its fighters and the
sacking of General Hamid Gaul by Pakistani Primer Minister Benazir Bhutto,
and it revived the Afghani army's morale and the resolve of the Kabul government.

Yet, what foreign plotters could not achieve was accomplished by inter-
necine fighting between the Khalq and Parcham factions of the PDPA and
by a collapsing Afghan economy that became increasingly depended on
Soviet largesse, curtailed in 1991 by Boris Yeltsin, the first President of the
Russian Federation. As a result, food, fuel, and materiel shortages caused
massive army desertions and the eventual defection of *Jozjani* militia and
of a number of government factions to the Mujahideen. In the meantime,
Ahmad Shah Massoud and Abdul Rashid Dostum, later joined by Sayyed
Mansour, had formed a coalition of militias that controlled nine north and
northeast provinces that became known as the *Northern Alliance.* Witness-
ing the disintegration of his fragile government, Najibullah attempted to
reach a compromise with Massoud under the auspices of the UN. However, talks broke down, his government collapsed, and he sought refuge at
the UN compound in Kabul where he lived until he was dragged out of the
compound by the victorious Taliban, castrated, and brutally murdered on
September 28, 1996; his blood-soaked body was hung from a Kabul lamp
post with his genitals stuffed in his mouth.[19] The Massoud-Dostum coalition

came apart, and fighting among different ethnic and religious factions broke out in many parts of the country, leading to thousands of people being detained, tortured, and killed. Warring factions included the Saudi-backed Pashtun Wahabi *Ittehad-e-Islami* and the Iran-supported Shia *Hezb-e-Wahdat* (Unity Party). Hekmatyar again shelled Kabul, which led to a new wave of deaths and destruction. After Burhanuddin Rabbani, leader of the *Jamiat-e Islami* party, became President (1992–1996), his forces and Hekmatyar's engaged each other, resulting in renewed shelling of Kabul by the latter and thousands of new victims before a cease fire, brokered by Pakistan and Saudi Arabia, took hold in March 1993. Under the treaty, which unraveled two months later when new fighting broke out between Massoud and Dostum militia, Hekmatyar became prime minister. As the factional fighting continued unabated, the Taliban, an Islamic fundamentalist and Pashtun Nationalist movement, emerged on the scene in mid-1994. Its stated aim was to liberate the country from a corrupt and warring leadership and establish an Islamic-based society. As the Taliban gained substantial territory and popular backing, Rabbani and Hekmatyar joined forces to face the common threat. Yet, despite their efforts, the Taliban, now strongly backed and supported by Pakistan, seized Kabul, forcing government forces to abandon the capital. Within hours, key government and military installations had fallen into the Taliban's hands, and Massoud retreated to the north of the country where he organized Afghanistan's main anti-Taliban force.

THE RISE AND FALL OF THE TALIBAN

National and International Implications

Soon after Islam arrived in Afghanistan in the seventh century, the Taliban established themselves as an important component of the social landscape: running schools, mosques and shrines and providing social services to the needy. Yet, they could quickly become fierce Mujahideen fighters when needed, as was the case during the Soviet occupation when they fought from their military training bases in Pakistan. They remained loosely connected regional groups for centuries. However, in 1994, the Kandahar-based Taliban were able to capture the city and the surrounding provinces and went on to control 12 of Afghanistan's 34 provinces in a few months. Their commitment to Islamic lifestyle attracted wide public support from a devout Muslim nation weary of the corruption, brutality, and feuding of Mujahideen warlords, enabling their capturing Kabul in the fall of 1996 and winning over 90% of the country land mass shortly thereafter. Yet, the predominantly Sunni and overwhelmingly Pashtun Taliban failed to pacify Northeast Afghanistan where the Northern Alliance, ethnically comprising Tajiks, Uzbeks, Turkmen, and Hazara of predominantly Shiite affiliation, had established their stronghold, enabling them to repel repeated military offensives and to reject repeated offers of truce offered by the Taliban. Likewise, the international community shunned them, and only Saudi Arabia, Pakistan, and the United Arab Emirates recognized the *Islamic Emirate of Afghanistan*, as they named their regime, as the legitimate government of Afghanistan. Under the leadership of Mullah Muhammad Omar, they established a rigid authoritarian regime based on the strictest interpretation of Islamic *Sharia*, the legal framework that, based on Islamic principles, regulates public and private life. That interpretation seems to have derived from ancestral tribal customs mixed with a radical *Deobandi* version of Islam (a revivalist Islamic movement first taught at *Darul Uloom Deoband* school in Utar Pradesh, India) and indoctrination they received in *Madrasah* (a place of learning/teaching) schools while exiled in Pakistan during the Soviet occupation of Afghanistan. Many such schools, supported by Saudi Arabia, taught a conservative *Wahhabi* Islamic tradition; a conservative view of Islam that originated in Arabia and influenced several reform movements.

Implementation of this combined Islamic orthodoxy as public policy led to banning any *modern* or *Western* activities, such as kite flying, applauding at sports events, shaving, watching television and movies, listening to music, accessing the Internet, and to an especially repressive treatment of women. Women were not allowed to attend school after age 8, to work outside the home, to leave home unaccompanied by a male relative, or to wear nail polish or other adornments. These rules, imposed as part of a strict observance of the Taliban's version of *Purdha* custom (physical segregation of the sexes), also included the wearing of the *Afghan Chadri*; the most concealing style of *Burkha* (a long, loose, and all-enveloping outer garment designed to cloak Muslim women in public) that covers the woman's eyes with a mesh. The Afghan Chadri is still used in northwestern Pakistan and in some parts of Afghanistan controlled by unyielding fanatically fundamentalist warlords. Women not in compliance were flogged on site by officers of the *Ministry for the promotion of virtue and suppression of vice* who patrolling the streets of major cities.[20] In contrast to the Taliban's interpretation of the Purdha, the *Islamic Dress Code* is usually described as designed to promote women's modesty. According to a generally accepted interpretation among Muslims, "in Islam, both men and women are expected to dress simply, modestly, and with dignity . . . When leaving the home, a Muslim woman must at least cover her hair and body in loose and unrevealing clothing, obscuring the details of her body from the public; some also choose to cover their face and hands."[21] In fact, Islam does not impose the wearing of the Burkha nor does it dictate lengths of skirts, or whether a bit of hair can or cannot show under the scarf. Hair and skin exposure and using cosmetics and short or colored dresses often are targeted by restrictive Islamic regimes as exemplified by today's annual street campaigns conducted by the Iranian police aimed at emancipated women wearing clothing more appropriate than the *Burkha* to endure hot Teheran summers, when 110°F temperatures are not unusual.[22] Some traditional Islamic celebrations were also banned, including *Nowruz* (New Year celebration observed in Iran and other central and western Asian regions) and *Ashura* (Shia day of mourning). Yet, perhaps the gratuitous destruction, in March 2001, of the 125- and 174-foot tall Buddha statues, carved out of the cliffsides of Bamiyan in A.D. 507 and 554, respectively, attracted the most attention and international condemnation. Theft was punished by amputation of the hand. Murder and rape led to capital punishment, and adulterers were stoned to death. Punishment, especially executions, was carried out at former soccer stadiums as public events with a high dissuasion value.

The Taliban system of government was unorthodox, to say the least. They did not have or believe in a government per se or head thereof or in institutions of governance, they did not hold elections, and they did not communicate with the governed that did not know what their leaders looked like for photography was banned. They rejected ancestral tribal and feudal structures that dictated the provenance of leaders; a policy designed to avoid sharing power with non-Pashtuns that represented well over 50% of Afghan's population. In their view, leaders' legitimacy derived from the ancestral *Bay'ah* (oath of allegiance). In the case of Mullah Muhammad Omar it occurred on April 4, 1996, when wrapped in the cloak of Prophet Mohammed he appeared on the roof of a building in Kandahar while hundreds of Pashtuns Mullahs chanted *Amir al-Mu'minin* (commander of the faithful), as a pledge of support and submission. Their army was little more than an expanded version of the traditional militia force common to Mujahideen warlords, though they maintained training camps that served as recruiting centers. They ruled with a medieval mind and an iron fist. Their brand of radicalism excluded certain ethnic groups, as well the Shia branch of Islam. For instance, upon capturing Kabul, all senior bureaucrats of Tajik, Uzbek, or Hazara stock were replaced by Pashtuns loyal to the Taliban regardless of qualifications. Likewise, their religious zeal and intolerance led to human rights violations and to massacres of certain non-Pashtun ethnic groups. For instance, immediately following the takeover of the city of Mazar-i-Sharif in August 1998, Mullah Manon Niazi, the new Taliban governor, incited violence against the Persian-speaking Hazaras, a Mongol-descendent minority of Shia Muslims, calling them *kofr* (infidels).[23] This was a precursor of subsequent massacres and human rights violations of the Hazaras and other ethnic groups by the Taliban in reprisal of the 1997 massacre of 2,000 of their own by Hazara fighters. According to eyewitnesses interviewed by news media,[24,25] the UN, and human rights organizations,[26,27] the Taliban apparently went street-by-street and house-by-house looking for Hazara individuals (easy to identify by their Mongolian facial features) and went on a frenzy of revenge killings, slashing throats and raping women. By the end of the week, an estimated 6,000 to 8,000 Hazaras had been massacred. Contrary to Islamic precept that the dead be buried immediately, corpses were left on the spot to rot for several days in the summer heat and eaten by scavengers. The anti-Hazara hate was such that Mullah Musa, director of public health, is said to have taken a group of gunmen to the military hospital in order to exterminate Mongol-featured patients and their visitors.

After loosing Mazar-i-Sharif, the Northern Alliance was relegated to approximately 10% of the north of the country, and on September 9, 2001, its leader, Ahmad Shah Massoud, was assassinated by a suicide bomber posing as a reporter, removing the last obstacle to the Taliban taking control of the entire country. Both, the defeat of Mazar-i-Sharif and the assassination of Massoud was aided by al-Qaeda–trained fighters who had been integrated into the Afghani army shortly after Osama bin Laden moved to Afghanistan from Sudan. The bin Laden–Taliban alliance was one of convenience where al-Qaeda provided financial assistance in exchange for protection. For instance, following the al-Qaeda–blamed August 7, 1998, bombings of U.S. Embassies in Dar es Salaam, Tanzania, and in Nairobi, Kenya, bin Laden was indicted in U.S. criminal court and his extradition requested but promptly rejected by Omar on grounds that the United States had provided no evidence of his involvement in terrorism. The connection was also personal for one of bin Laden's sons is said to have married Omar's daughter. Then came the worst attack on American soil in U.S. history, on September 11, 2001, referred to as 9/11. An FBI investigation code-named *Penttbom* (Pentagon/Twin Towers Bombing Investigation) and launched the next day quickly identified 19 hijackers affiliated to al-Qaeda as the perpetrators. In his September 20, 2001, address to a joint session of Congress, President Bush demanded that the Taliban

"deliver to United States authorities all of the leaders of Al Qaeda who hide in your land . . . release all foreign nationals, including American citizens you have unjustly imprisoned . . . protect foreign journalists, diplomats, and aid workers in your country . . . close immediately and permanently every terrorist training camp in Afghanistan . . . hand over every terrorist and every person, and their support structure to appropriate authorities . . . give the United States full access to terrorist training camps, so we can make sure their demands are not open to negotiation or discussion."[28]

Once again, the Taliban's response was that they would turn bin Laden over if the United States provided evidence of his guilt in the 9/11 attack; a refusal used as justification for the U.S.-led attack on Afghanistan. Yet, bin Laden's involvement, which he denied initially, was suspected but never confirmed. A bin Laden videotape conveniently discovered in a house in Jalalabad and aired in the United States on December 9, 2001, suggesting his preknowledge of the attack in its English translation has been called a fake. Indeed, audio and video experts have questioned the identify of the individual shown on the videotape, and experts commissioned by the German TV station Das Erste challenged the translation. They concluded, "American translators who listened to the tapes and transcribed them apparently wrote a lot of what they wanted to hear but that cannot be heard on the tape no matter how many times you listen to it."[29] However, in a videotape aired on October 29, 2004, and an audiotape broadcasted on May 23, 2006, bin Laden claims responsibility for personally directing the 19 hijackers. In the audiotape, he also asserts that Zacarias Moussaoui, the presumed *alternate 20th hijacker* who had been sentenced three weeks earlier to a life sentence for "conspiring to kill Americans as part of the September 11, 2001, terrorist attacks," had " no connection at all with September 11." Yet, despite his apparent confession, the FBI's *Ten Most Wanted* lists bin Laden "in connection with the August 7, 1998 bombings of the United States Embassies in Dar es Salaam, Tanzania, and Nairobi, Kenya . . . [and as] a suspect in other terrorist attacks throughout the world," but no mention is made of 9/11.[30] When asked why, Rex Tomb of the FBI's public affairs unit explained, "the reason why 9/11 is not mentioned on Usama Bin Laden's Most Wanted page is because the FBI has no hard evidence connecting Bin Laden to 9/11."[31]

The lack of unequivocal evidence that bin Laden was involved in the 9/11 attack and the unexpected collapse of the World Trade Center twin towers and of tower 7, together with other disputed 9/11 events, have provided fodder to conspiracy theories. The three most prevalent hypotheses implicate Saudi Arabia, members of the U.S. government, and Israel. Saudi Arabia became a prime suspect as the home country of 15 out of the 19 hijackers and speculations arose that the Saudi Embassy in Washington arranged flights out of the United States for Saudi nationals, including bin Laden's relatives while all commercial flights were grounded. The speculation was refuted by the *9/11 Commission*. Alternatively, based on Arab-Jewish geopolitical considerations, a *false flag* operation (one designed to appear conducted by an entity other that the perpetrator) conducted by members of Israel's Mossad has been suggested.[32] Dismissal of pre-9/11 warnings of impending attacks on U.S. soil raised by low-level intelligence officers are interpreted in some quarters as contributing negligence by higher echelon U.S. officers, at best, or their implication in the attack, at worst. Finally, the total, sudden, and symmetrical collapse of the World Trade Center twin towers is interpreted by *9/11 Truth Movement organizations* (groups that reject the official version of the 9/11 events) and other conspiracy theorists as evidence of a controlled demolition induced by deliberately placed and sequentially detonated explosive charges. The identical collapse of Tower 7, which was not impacted by an airplane, is thought to be more problematic as fire alone has never before caused the demolition-style collapse of a building. In fact, the National Institute of Standards and Technology has yet to publish its final report, and the Federal Emergency Management Agency's initial investigation reported that its "best hypothesis has only a low probability of occurrence." Nevertheless, America invaded Afghanistan, and long-term consequences are to be expected at the national level of both countries as well as globally, which is examined briefly in the following section as it relates to the opium trade, the Taliban resurgence, and their respective role on the War on Drugs and the War on Terror.

Opium Production and the Taliban

While poppy cultivation in Afghanistan is not new, it expanded rapidly when Iran halted its own production in the mid-1970s and again during the Soviet–Afghan war when vast amounts of money destined to support Mujahideen opposition groups were diverted into opium production, which by 1989 reached 800 metric tons. As the flow of foreign aid dried out after the withdrawal of the Soviet army, warlords consolidated their regional power by securing a lasting and reliable source of revenue via opium cultivation and cross-border smuggling and oil smuggling.[33] It was observed during that time that "there was an arms pipeline going in, and a drugs pipeline coming out of Afghanistan."[34] By the mid-1990s, Afghanistan's opium production averaged 2,200 to 2,400 tons annually. The Taliban inherited a cultivation and smuggling network that they continued to expand so that opium production peaked at 4,565 tons or 79% of the global supply by 1999.[35] In 2006, Afghanistan's opium business was said to "sustain a clan-based and crime-ridden society, it impedes Afghanistan's economic growth, hinders reconstruction efforts of the international community, and ultimately fuels instability and terrorism."[36] Since then, the situation has further deteriorated as described in the UNODC's Opium Survey 2007, which concluded, "the Afghan opium situation looks grim, but it is not yet hopeless."[37] This somber assessment derived from detailed statistics that showed continued expansion of the opium trade despite massive antidrug expenditures, notwithstanding official claims to the contrary, uncritically trumpeted by the media.

Under the Taliban (1996–2003), poppy cultivation ranged between 57,000 and 91,000 hectares, which represented 25% to 45% of the global land area dedicated to opium cultivation. The only exception was in 2001 when Muhammad Omar ruled poppy cultivation against Islamic principles, and only 8,000 hectares, producing 185 tons of opium or 12% of global supply, were dedicated to poppy. Since then, poppy cultivation exploded to 193,000 hectares in 2007, representing 82% of global poppy-dedicated land cultivation; more than the total land set aside for coca cultivation in Colombia, Peru, and Bolivia combined. Five southern provinces along the Pakistani border, which are the richest, most fertile, and the breadbasket of the country, now produce an astounding 70% of Afghanistan's opium harvest, with Hilmand province alone producing over 50%. In excess of 3,000,000 Afghans from 509,000 families are involved in opium cultivation, or 14.3% of Afghanis, though it varies from province to province. In the province of Hilmand, for instance, more than 80% of farming families were involved in opium poppy cultivation in 2007. This is not surprising considering that one hectare of opium generates US$5,200 gross yearly income against $546 for one hectare of wheat; a daily wage of approximately $9.30 versus $1.00, respectively, which should give food for thought to those advocating alternate crop growing as a solution to the drug problem in Afghanistan and elsewhere. In addition to a surging poppy-growing landmass, opium yield also increased (to 42.5 kg/Ha in 2007). As a result, 8,200 tons of opium were produced in 2007, which amounts to 93% of the global production and exceeded medicinal global demand by approximately 2,000 tons. Hence, under the U.S. and ISAF's watch Afghanistan has reclaimed its titled as the world's largest drug producer. These statistics demonstrate that poppy crop eradication, the foundation of the international community's efforts to reduce the amount of opium produced, has been an utter failure, as have been attempts to rein Colombia's coca harvest. Indeed, only 19,047 hectares of planted poppy were eliminated in 2007, mainly of marginal fields and "often as the result of corrupt deals between field owners, village elders and eradication teams: as a result poor farmers suffered the brunt of eradication,"[35] and opium production rose 34% between 2006 and 2007. Yet, eradication fueled insecurity and violence resulting in 31 injuries and 19 deaths in 2007 alone.

The value of the 2007 Afghani opium harvest reached US$4 billion or 35% of GDP: $1 billion going to farmers and $3 billion to traffickers and laboratories that, to feed the drug trade, convert nearly 60% of the native opium into morphine and heroin using chemicals imported from neighboring countries. The Taliban largely control the southern poppy-growing provinces, especially Hilmand province, and use the cash crop revenue to fund their insurgency and quest for supremacy. Hence, while "opium is undoubtedly a governance problem across the country. In the south and east, however, it is also strongly related to the Kabul government's most immediate existential threat; the Taliban-led insurgency as well as to the funding of 139 suicide attacks in 2006."[37] According to a British reporter, "Russian gangsters who smuggle drugs into Britain are buying cheap heroin from Afghanistan and paying for it with guns." The exchange "occurs at a bazaar near the old Afghan-Soviet border, deep in Tajikistan's desert where drug traffickers meet their Taliban suppliers."[38] One kilogram of heroin selling for $1,000 to $1,200 in Afghanistan will double in price at the border trading posts where an AK-47 assault rifle costs approximately $100. According to the same report, "smugglers claimed they are 'untouchable' because their bosses include cabinet-level officials in the government."[38] In effect, the post-Taliban drug trade has become a highly organized and hierarchical business with different layers of players linking the "lower world," which produces, refines, trades, and smuggles opium, to the "upper world" of warlords-turned-politicians and commanders that protect and control the process and extract the lion's share of the profits. As a result, "criminal activities such as trafficking are less overtly the business of political leaders and more the province of an emerging criminal underworld with strong political connections."[39] However, persisting rumors over the years have implicated Ahmed Wali Karzai, the younger bother of Hamid Karzai, as a major player in the drug trade despite being on CIA payroll. According to the *New York Times*, "Ahmed Wali Karzai is a suspected player in the country's booming illegal opium trade . . . Mr. Karzai gets regular payments from the CIA, and has for much of the past eight years . . . for a variety of services, including helping to recruit an Afghan paramilitary force that operates at the CIA's direction in and around Kandahar."[40]

Therefore, the claim that the Taliban now control the bulk of the drug trade business is an oversimplification at best or a convenient fabrication at worst. Like Colombia's guerilla and counter-guerilla groups, the Taliban exploit their country's most lucrative export crop as a source of revenue to fund their enterprise. Yet, they are but one set, albeit growing, within a widespread and diverse group of players. The efficiency of the system relies on a sophisticated pyramidal scheme of protection payments that generally flow from the bottom to the top of participants in the drug trade and on checks and balances that ensure compliance at each level. Farmers pay the local police chief or commander, in currency or as a fraction of their poppy harvest, for the *right* to cultivate and to avoid crop eradication. Traffickers pay the district official, who bribes the provincial administrator, who, in turn, makes payments to one of the 20 to 30 individuals with high-level political connections that keep the system working smoothly, undisturbed by the relevant authorities, and relatively free of competition. Not surprisingly, players' wealth is directly proportional to their place in the pyramid. Hence, while top echelon participants are extremely wealthy, farmers at the bottom of the pyramid rely on poppy cultivation simply to survive at a subsistence level. Under these conditions, most Afghanis view eradication and other counter-narcotics measures as foreign policies directed against the poor of the country who benefit the least from the drug trade and, as a result, have lost any hope that foreign intervention will brighten their future. General discontent provoked by crop eradication, insecurity, and frustration for not sharing in the promised economic and social benefits of peacetime paved the way for the Taliban's return to the poppy-rich south of the country. In fact, it is not ideology that moves Afghanis but a combination of an unstable environment, where bribes to government officials and their cronies are a prerequisite for solving problems, and a dysfunctional administration unwilling or unable to bring fairness and justice to ordinary people.

While the central government's track record on administering justice is scant or nonexistent, the Taliban imposed their brand of justice uniformly in areas under their control. In the words of a lowly villager, "even if it's a minor thing, the Taliban will sort it out. Before [under President Karzai's control], it was not like that. They did not pay attention to us and the poor people were ignored."[41] In addition to having lost confidence in their own government, Afghanis increasingly distrust Western intentions and resent their actions. Indeed, Operation Enduring Freedom (code name of the U.S.-led invasion of Afghanistan that launched the War on Terror) and ISAF focus and spend far more on military missions than on rebuilding the country's physical and social infrastructures. In fact, Army Colonel Hy Rothstein, a 20-year veteran of the Army Special Forces who was commissioned in

2002 by the Pentagon to examine the war in Afghanistan and its outcome, concluded the conflict created conditions that have given "warlordism, banditry, and opium production a new lease on life."[42] Hence, having lost Afghanis' *hearts and minds*, the West has contributed to the return of the Taliban, which now controls nearly half of Afghanistan. Seven years have passed since President Bush declared, only days after 9/11, "We will find those who did it, we will smoke them out of their holes, we will get them running, and we'll bring them to justice." Yet, despite U.S. and ISAF military might and reconstruction aid, Afghanistan is quickly becoming a failed state and a breeding ground for terrorism, Osama bin Laden is alive and hiding in the Afghanistan–Pakistan border region, we are told, al-Qaeda remains a global threat, and the Taliban continue a relentless advance that will likely spill into Pakistan.

In conclusion, the very fact that certain mind-altering drugs were outlawed and their use criminalized has spawned an extremely lucrative international illicit drug market dominated by criminal elements on both sides of the drug trade divide that has profound economic and social consequences for both producer and consumer countries. To combat drug production, trade, and use, the United States, squanders billions of dollars, bullies producer countries into reducing drug production, and coerces the international community into pursuing an unwinnable War on Drugs. Enforcement of antidrug laws and of international conventions in consumer countries varies somewhat according to each country's legal traditions and social sensitivities. The United States, with the most repressive drug laws in the Western world, imposes harsh minimum prison terms on convicts of drug offenses, including marijuana possession, that can be as lengthy as those imposed on rapists and murderers. Additionally, the drug enforcement establishment targets pain-treating physicians as easy and high-profile scapegoats with plenty of forfeitable assets to camouflage its failure to curb drug availability on American streets and to generate additional income. As a result, hundreds of thousands of mostly nonviolent drug users and hundreds of pain-managing physicians are arrested and prosecuted, and many are incarcerated each year. In contrast, in certain European countries where drug use is considered a health, not a criminal, matter, possession has been depenalized or is handled as an administrative offense without increasing overall drug use, which is actually lower than in the United States. The economic and social impact of drugs on consumer countries is the consequence of their societies' insatiable demand for prohibited drugs that created and sustains a highly profitable black market, which in turn fosters crime at home and abroad. Yet, while most drug-related crime is committed by traffickers, drug users must be considered accomplices, albeit unwittingly, for they create demand.

The economic and social impact of drugs on producer countries is far greater than in consumer countries for it involves local military, political, and judicial elites who collude with drug traffickers in the pursuit of riches while trampling on the property, human rights, and lives of the poor and disenfranchised. Such devastating outcomes, and their eventual correction, are directly linked to the economic, social, and political conditions in producer countries; to the inefficiency of their democratic institutions; and to the functional inadequacy of their civil societies. For instance, over the last 20 years Colombia's drug trade has been the main contributor to the crime and corruption that permeates all levels of society, resulting in tens of thousands of human rights violations, kidnappings, assassinations, and massive population displacements reaching into the millions. Yet, Colombia's institutional and social infrastructure and its democratic traditions, albeit imperfect, paved the way for its current president to successfully begin the process of reclaiming control of the country from guerrilla and counterguerrilla groups by combining U.S.-backed military pressure with extending an olive branch to combatants willing to demobilize and reintegrate civil society. During his tenure, several thousand paramilitary combatants have demobilized, and the FARC have being weakened and relegated to scarcely populated jungle areas, considerably reducing crimes committed by these groups (Table 8). However, despite these successes, much remains to be done because, according to the law of supply and demand, producers will continue to supply consumer demand as long as War on Drugs policies remain in place, ensuring an unmatched economic bonanza from the illicit drug trade.

Hence, as long as demand for illicit drugs in consumer countries sustains a lucrative illegal trade, production will follow suit. For instance, should Colombia succeed in reestablishing law and order and drastically reduce cocaine production, both unlikely events in the foreseeable future, cocaine production would simply shift to a different country with its own set of traffickers assisted by the same or different overseas accomplices and supplied by poor farmers eager to grow a profitable and easy to market crop. In contrast, Afghanistan is a country without democratic traditions, institutional infrastructures, or a well-functioning civil society that is controlled by CIA-trained Mujahideen and nominally governed by a central government that is viewed as a powerless and corrupt poppet of *infidel* foreign invaders, only interested in remaining in power even through rigged presidential elections.

Table 8
Violence Indicators in Colombia: 2002–2007[43]

Year	2002	2003	2004	2005	2006	2007
Homicides	28.837	23.523	20.208	18.111	17.479	13.020 (Sept.)
Kidnappings	2.882	2.121	1.440	800	687	393 (Sept.)
Displaced	422.394	217.138	202.919	229.655	242.860	150.940 (Oct·)

The Afghani government has proved unable or unwilling to enforce law and order or to hold back the advance of the socially regressive Taliban despite enormous U.S. and ISAF military and economic assistance. These are propitious grounds and ideal conditions for warlords, common criminals, and Islamic extremists to fill the vacuum, and so they have. Hence, Afghanistan is unlikely to follow Colombia's footsteps, and the country's future looks bleak, as does the goal of instituting a modern, self-sustaining and just democracy in that part of the world as contemplated by the United States and ISAF. Unlike Colombia, Afghanistan is not likely to gain control over its territory in the foreseeable future and risks becoming a failed state, the breeding ground for terrorism, and center stage of an unending and unwinnable War on Terror.

PART IV

Reforming Drug Policy

CHAPTER 9

Reform Proposals

The only purpose for which power can be rightfully exercised over any member of a civilized community, against his will, is to prevent harm to others. His own good, either physical or moral, is not a sufficient warrant.
                                                                —John Stuart Mill

FRAMING THE DISCUSSION

Policy changes are usually incremental rather than sweeping. This is because the latter requires both seldom-achieved consensus on whether goals are being attained or undesirable outcomes outweigh benefits, and political courage to take a stand. This is especially true with regards to drug policy, where prohibitionists have succeeded in dominating the flow of information and public support and where being *tough on drugs* is risk-free because no politician will lose many votes for holding that stance. Additionally, policy discourse is framed by participants' sets of assumptions and biases, which by remaining concealed from the debate preclude openly considering the motivations of discussants when assessing the evidence cited in support of their point of view.[1] This is particularly notorious within drug policy discourse, where sets of beliefs based on ethical, moral, political, and other considerations emphasize and assign relevance to a certain body of knowledge but not to others. Hence, widely divergent positions exist on drug policy,[1] though the literature on the subject suggests polarization of the debate between two opposing viewpoints: prohibitionists versus reformers.

Prohibitionists adopt a *paternalistic* approach based on the premise that the state can and should implement policies that protect individuals from their own actions or behavior, or a *preventive* approach, which emphasizes the principle that justice demands punishing those who engage in activities that risk harm to others. To paternalists, illicit drugs are illicit because they cause harm: end of discussion. Some extreme prohibitionist positions often circulate in the halls of Congress as exemplified by views expressed by members of the Subcommittee on Criminal Justice at its 1999 hearings on "The Pros and Cons of Drug Legalization, Decriminalization and Harm Reduction."[2] For instance, Benjamin A. Gilman (R-NY), expressed the views of most subcommittee members stating, "legalization is a surrender to despair; It cannot and ought not be any topic of serious discussion in our nation's debate of the challenges of illicit drugs." Likewise, Mark Souder (R-IN), expressed his dismay at the very idea of holding hearings on drug legalization arguing, "We do not have hearings called 'the pros and cons of rape." Bob Barr, (R-GA) inquired "whether anti-racketeering laws could be used to prosecute people conspiring to legalize drugs." To preventive justice advocates, drug use exposes others to potential harm and, like drunk driving, is punishable even if no harm results from it.

Alternatively, reformers can be clustered as supporters of the *Public Health, Harm Reduction, Utilitarian,* and *Libertarian* stance on drug use.[1] Public health and harm reduction differ mainly in that while the former advocates policies that generally promote public health, the latter includes collateral harm in the equation. Hence, according to the former, drug use should be reduced without adding public health consequences to the user (e.g., risk of sexual abuse to imprisoned drug offenders); the latter advocates minimizing the overall harm to society of both drug use and of drug policy (e.g., the harm of imprisonment to users and cost to society). Utilitarians take into account the social utility of drugs (e.g., the benefits as well as the harm drugs cause). Libertarians espouse the most radical drug reform ethic, which emphasizes maximum individual liberties as long as they do not expose or cause harm to others or violate their civil liberties.

While this classification stratifies and compartmentalizes, perhaps arbitrarily, the attitudes and mindsets of drug policy debate participants, it nevertheless provides a framework for understanding hidden issues when discussing drug policy, at least in the abstract. I say *at least in the abstract* because a 35-year historical perspective on the meager achievements but devastating consequences of the War on Drugs, described in the preceding chapters, provides solid bases for assessing the economic, social, and political outcomes of drug policy at home and abroad, at least to unbiased observers. From that perspective it seems clear that, having failed on all counts, the War on Drugs should be abandoned and its legal and administrative infrastructures dismantled. Nevertheless, the next section outlines the pros and cons of three drug policy reform proposals that span the spectrum of approaches as a prelude to describing my own. The first proposal tows the official line; the second attempts, unsuccessfully, to solve several opium-related issues at once; and the third follows a libertarian approach.

ILLUSTRATIVE REFORM PROPOSALS
AND POSITIONS

The RAND Corporation Proposal

In their 2005 drug policy analysis paper from the prestigious RAND Corporation's Drug Policy Research Center, the authors state "From 1985 until 2001, 'drugs' was consistently 1 of the top 10 answers when Americans were asked what they thought was the most important problem facing the nation. In response to such concerns, federal and state legislators and executive-branch officials have enacted and implemented policies that, while diverse in approach, are oriented toward enforcement."[3] To pretend that drug policy was enacted in response to public concern is clearly disingenuous and ignores historical facts. As documented in chapter 3, politicians and prominent public figures deliberately and methodically shaped public opinion over many years, portraying drugs as *evil*, *sinful*, and a *plague* that *infected* American streets, the workplace, and schools and would destroy entire generations of *innocent children*. For instance, Harry J. Anslinger, a former Commissioner of the U.S. Bureau of Narcotics during Prohibition, became a tireless and influential if deceitful antidrug crusader. In the 1970s, Nelson Rockefeller was elected Governor of New York on an equally deceitful antidrug campaign against a presumed *epidemic of addiction* in New York State that he claimed had reached plague proportions and threatened the lives of innocent children. Emulating Rockefeller, Richard Nixon promoted the fear of drugs as a political strategy to win popular support for his presidential aspirations. Once elected, he made drug policy the centerpiece of his administration and launched the War on Drugs by implementing the CSA and by creating the DEA. Since then, legions of Anslinger, Rockefeller, and Nixon emulators continue the antidrug disinformation rhetoric at local and national levels, all cheer led by the DEA.

The RAND Corporation report correctly points out, however, that measures adopted "have not led to substantial decreases in the severity of America's drug-related problems, prompting strident denunciations of current policy. Many critics argue that the increased toughness of that policy has done more harm than good. Some go so far as to suggest that drugs should simply be legalized."[3] It also concedes that "programs outside U.S. borders . . . crop eradication and substitution, in particular, show minimal promise" and that "it is not credible to justify an intervention [by the United States] principally on the grounds that it will reduce U.S. drug consumption."[3] The authors tackle issues such as *What the goals have been* (of the War on Drugs) and whether they were achieved (on which they equivocate), "Why hasn't the Drug War been a greater success?" "What about bonuses and collateral damage?" "Why not course corrections?" and "How might US drug problems and policies evolve?" Then, they propose their vision of "How **should** [original emphasis] US drug policy evolve." They point out that because "America is not going to be the world's first drug-free society," the drug problem "must be **managed** [original empha-sis] so as to limit the number of people who use, the frequency or duration of their use, and the damage they do to themselves and others, together with the damage resulting from policy choices."[3] This is to be achieved by tailoring current policy levers (enforcement, treatment, and prevention) according to circumstances. That is, emphasizing enforcement during the beginning of an "epidemic cycle" when there is a "contagious spread" to new users, followed by treatment later in the cycle when there are "more heavy users who are generating substantial social costs"; keeping preven-tion as a measure applicable at all times. Their second recommendation is to "draw strength from cross-State variations in drug policy" under the assumption that "evaluation of open questions and issues regarding varia-tions within the prohibitionist regime might illuminate profitable direc-tions for national and state policy." Finally, the authors make a plea for a "more dispassionate debate" over drug policy.[3]

This drug policy quasi-reform proposal is shaped more by its authors' perceptions and mindsets rather than by facts, some of which they misrep-resent, especially the roots of current drug policy. The authors assert to be "interested primarily in choices at the strategic level-choices, for example, among strict prohibition, moderate prohibition, or decriminalization; choices among goals, for example, those focusing on use reduction or those focusing on harm reduction; decisions as to the appropriate roles of supply and de-mand control."[3] Yet, while acknowledging that U.S.-sponsored foreign pro-grams and interventions to curtail drug production and importation have not and will not reduce U.S. drug consumption, they hold fast to the notion that "measured against its goals, early and more recent, the drug war has had a mixed record, at least superficially."[3] This is a classic prohibitionist stance that points to the negligible benefits of the War on Drugs to justify its contin-uation, albeit with minor adjustments. Such a stance inevitably led to a des-ultory proposal that would harvest tepid results if implemented.

The Senlis Council Proposal

The Senlis Council, an international policy think tank, has achieved noto-riety through its "Afghan village-based Poppy for Medicine" proposal.[4] In it, it presents a carefully researched, though unworkable, counter-narcotics plan with counter-insurgency implications for Afghanistan that, in addition, would address the "global unmet need for morphine." In essence, it consists of setting up pilot projects to assess the feasibility of an opium licensing sys-tem in Afghanistan for the production of opium-derived painkillers such as morphine and codeine. Under the plan, poppy would be turned into valuable medicinal opiates, produced in situ, rather than being diverted to narcotics production destined to supply the illegal drug market. As contemplated, the scheme would give Afghan poppy farmers, and all others involved in the production of medicinal opiates, the opportunity to profit in a legal poppy economy. Presumably, this would encourage all involved to cut ties with drug traffickers while addressing what the authors view as "an extensive morphine shortage for pain associated with cancer and HIV/AIDS."[4]

This proposal draws on licensed poppy cultivation programs established in India in 1947[5] and in Turkey in 1971[6] that were designed to break poppy farmers' reliance on the international illegal heroin market without having to resort to forced crop eradication. With the support of the international community and sustained funding of alternative development programs and effective law enforcement, Turkey switched from production of opium to concentrate of poppy straw to meet legitimate worldwide medical demand. This strategy, which is credited to have brought Turkey's illegal poppy cultivation and illicit trade under satisfactory control within a few short years, remains in place to this day. The underlying rationale of the Senlis council proposal is that abject poverty in Afghanistan and forced crop eradication without a compensatory source of income leaves poor farmers with no alternatives but to rely on drug traffickers and to support the Taliban as survival and self-preservation strategies, respectively. As emphasized in the Senlis report, "the key feature of the Afghan Poppy for Medicine project model is that village-cultivated poppy would be transformed into morphine tablets in the Afghan villages. The entire production process, from seed to medicine tablet, can thus be controlled by the village in collaboration with government and international actors, and all economic profits from medicine sales would remain in the village, triggering economic diversification"[4] free from drug trafficking links.

The report optimistically points out "by triggering economic development in rural communities and integrating these communities within the Afghan legal economy and government system, the Poppy for Medicine projects would decrease insurgents' recruitment bases."[4] It also foresees that taxing a legal opiate industry would create a source of revenue to fund a law enforcement apparatus needed to combat opium diversion into the black market. In turn, this would increase popular support for the central government once it is perceived to look after farmers' livelihood and economic prosperity. If that came to pass, the implications for government stability and for reconstructing and pacifying the country would be considerable. The report also predicts that the Poppy for Medicine plan would "provide emerging and transitional countries with access to affordable essential painkilling medicines . . . **at a price at least 55 percent lower than the market average**" (original emphasis).[4] This aspect of the proposal is significant for, as pointed out by the Senlis council, "in 2005, to meet the pain needs of the end-stage HIV/AIDS and cancer patients in Latin America, 7.1 metric tons of morphine would have been needed, but just 600 kg of morphine was actually used, leaving 91% of these patients' pain needs un-met . . . [and] even in the world's richest six countries, which include the United States and the Western Europe, only 24% of patients' pain needs are being met.[7]

While cogent, innovative, and "a winning solution," according to some of the world press, this proposal remains controversial and is being criticized on several counts. For instance, in a somewhat wordy, inaccurate, and at times contradictory rebuttal, the U.S. State Department drew on four counter arguments.[8] First, the licit opium market is not lucrative enough to entice Afghan farmers. Second, no unmet worldwide need for opiates exists that could be met by Afghanistan. Third, effectively controlling a legal market in Afghanistan is unrealistic. Fourth, legalizing opium would be detrimental to Afghanistan's security and economic development. Of these, the second argument is misleading, the fourth is farfetched and unfounded, and only the first and third are objective and cogent. Indeed, even if the Poppy for Medicine initiative could be made economically competitive and an unmet need for opiates resulted from insufficient supply, the lack of effective legal, economic, and political infrastructures; a weak and corrupt central government distrusted by the population; and growing insecurity would make Afghanistan the least suitable country to implement such a drug control program.

An independent analysis of the Poppy for Medicine initiative provides an unbiased and authoritative critique of the project, which it calls "a rather new, but unrealistic, proposal." It criticizes the proposal as "based on false or inexact premises, on at least two levels: regarding the world market for licit opiates on the one hand, and national and local [Afghan] opium farming communities on the other hand."[9] First, it correctly points out that according to the INCB, "the supply of such opiates has, for years, been 'at levels well in excess of global demand'." This assertion and the Senlis council claim that "un-met worldwide pain needs" exist seem irreconcilable views but in fact are two sides of the same issue. The INCB addresses *supply* in response to *demand* for opiates estimated by each country, whereas the Senlis council refers to a global *unmet need* for opium-derived painkillers due to the fact that "official measurements of 'demand' do not reflect actual morphine 'needs'." Indeed, there is a worldwide pain crisis that is caused by impediments to pain management rather than by an insufficient supply of painkillers. In the United States and other rich countries it is caused mainly by the impact of drug policy on medical practice and by an unfounded fear of addiction nurtured by prohibitionists of various persuasions and affiliations and trumpeted by an uncritical media. In underdeveloped countries it stems primarily from poverty and inefficient, unstructured, and underfunded health care systems unable to provide access to painkillers or even expertise to assess needs. In fact, as acknowledged by the INCB, "most developing countries lack the resources and expertise required for determining medical needs and adjusting drug supply to meet those needs. Medical practice shows undesirably large variations attributable to chronic shortage of staff and inadequate training and information."[9] Given these circumstances, increasing opium supply would have little if any effect on the global pain management crisis in either rich or poor countries. Likewise, out of nearly two dozen countries that cultivate poppy, only four (China, India, Japan, and South Korea) produce opium, and only India exports it. The price paid to Indian farmers in 2004–2005 averaged US$26 per kilogram of opium. Such a low price encourages diversion to the illegal market. In fact, India's production and exportation of licit opium has been plagued by diversion and by increasing unlicensed opium cultivation (7,753 Ha) that exceeded licensed cultivation (6,300 Ha) in 2007 despite the country's Central Bureau of Narcotics' tight regulations. Hence, it is difficult to foresee how such low prices could succeed in weaning Afghan farmers from the illicit drug trade that fetches four to five times higher prices than they could possibly expect under the Poppy for Medicine project, even without taking into account possible additional restrictions and bottlenecks in any government program. Given Afghanistan's economic, social, and political conditions, a rudimentary and corrupt law enforcement establishment and government officials often in collusion with drug traffickers, much of the licensed opium production would undoubtedly find its way to the illicit drug market without significantly impacting the very problems the Poppy for Medicine project seeks to solve.

The Cato Institute's Stance

Soon after its founding in 1977, the Cato Institute, a nonprofit, nonpartisan public policy research foundation, began calling attention to the unintended domestic and international impact of U.S. Drug War policies in books and book chapters, articles and newsletters, opinion and commentaries, Cato studies, legal briefs, and events.[10-14] In an early *Policy Analysis*, dated December 9, 1985,[12] its author noted several major negative outcomes of President Regan's 1981 energetic antiwar "foreign policy that vigorously seeks to interdict and eradicate illicit drugs, wherever cultivated, processed, or transported . . . Despite much rhetorical bravado and a few highly publicized successes," he explained, "the U.S. effort [coordinated by the State Department, the DEA, and the CIA] has been a bitter disappointment. There has been virtually no reduction in the aggregate amount of cocaine, heroin, and marijuana coming into the United States."[12] Looking for an explanation, the author observed, "Congressional conservatives and their ideological brethren in the administration also increasingly identify the narcotics issue with the larger cold war." Such a link is now established with the War on Terror. He also noted, "they assert that Cuba, Bulgaria, Nicaragua, and other Marxist states are trafficking in drugs as part of a conspiracy to 'destabilize' American society."[12] Such a ludicrous, politically motivated claim was no more credible than the temperance movement's assertion that Germany was attempting to addict the entire American population to heroin during World War I, or Harry Anslinger's that Japan had unleashed an opium offensive to do likewise during World War II. In a subsequent drug policy analysis the author observed, "in spite of the greatest anti-drug enforcement effort in U.S. history, the drug problem is worse than ever."[13] Drawing on the Prohibition experience, he proposed drug legalization "as a solution to . . . end crime, corruption, and AIDS caused not by the biochemical effects of illegal drugs but by the attempt to fight drug use with the criminal justice system."[13]

Over the ensuing years, Cato experts and staff have also addressed negative global outcomes of the drug war in publications with titles ranging from *Bad neighbor policy: Washington's futile War on Drugs in Latin America*,[13] to *A society of suspects: The War on Drugs and Civil Liberties*,[14] to *The Drug War and the homicide rate: A direct correlation?*[15] Yet, one of their main rationale for opposing this expensive, ineffective, overreaching, and disastrous U.S. government program of global reach rests on its unconstitutionality, as eloquently stated in a book titled *After Prohibition: An Adult Approach to Drug Policies in the 21st Century*.[16] In it, the author points out that contrary to Prohibition, today's War on Drugs violates the U.S. Constitution. He noted, "It is more than noteworthy, however, that, when the [Temperance] movement reached fruition in the form of national Prohibition, respect for constitutional limits on federal power was still such that it took an amendment to the Constitution to bring federal Prohibition about. No one thought, that is, that the Constitution authorized Congress, by mere statute, to prohibit the manufacture, sale, or transportation of alcoholic beverages. An amendment to the Constitution was required to give Congress that authority. Today, by contrast, we fight the drug war by statute alone."[16] Based on a broad-based series of arguments, the Cato Institute's drug policy stance was articulated in a recent *Handbook for Congress* series titled *The War on Drugs*, where domestic and global policy reform recommendations are made.[17] In the domestic front, Congress is urged to: (1) "Repeal the CSA of 1970"; (2) "Repeal the federal mandatory minimum sentences and the mandatory sentencing guidelines"; (3) "Direct the administration not to interfere with the implementation of state initiatives that allow for the medical use of marijuana"; and (4) "Shut down the Drug Enforcement Administration." At the international level, policy makers are advised to: (1) "Terminate Plan Colombia and other expensive, counterproductive anti-drug programs in the Andean region of South America"; (2) "Not allow anti-drug efforts in Afghanistan to interfere with the far more important effort to destroy the Taliban and Al Qaeda"; (3) "Recognize that prohibition creates a huge black-market premium and potential profit from drug trafficking that terrorist groups will exploit"; (4) "Remove U.S. trade barriers to the products of developing countries"; and (5) "Declare an end to the international war on drugs and assure foreign governments that the United States will no longer pressure them to wage war on their own populations."[17]

The Cato Institute's stance on drug policy is fundamentally libertarian, and its reform proposals reflect it. Not surprisingly, while acknowledging the multifaceted failure of drug policy at home and abroad, despite enormous expenditures and unacceptable human costs, Cato Institute authors emphasize its unconstitutionality and its assault on civil liberties. However, their arguments overlook prohibitionists' false claims that led to drug prohibition in the first place and the pain management crisis caused by current drug policy impact on narcotics prescriptions.

CHAPTER 10

A Rational, Evidence-Driven Drug Policy

Trying to stem the tide of fatuous law that emanates from our incontinent legislatures, at least in the US and the UK, is a luckless and thankless task.
—J. Gardner

Annual drug deaths: tobacco: 395,000, alcohol: 125,000, "legal" drugs: 38,000, illegal drug overdoses: 5,200, marijuana: 0. Considering government subsidies of tobacco, just what is our government protecting us from in the drug war?
—Ralph Nader

Medical and other scientific evidence reviewed in this book support the view that drug use and abuse, whether of licit or illicit drugs, is a personal choice rather than the result of these agents' alleged addictive properties. Moreover, the much-vilified narcotics, far from being dangerous or addictive, are in fact the most potent and safest painkillers on the market today, especially for the treatment of moderate to severe chronic pain. Evidence also confirms that drug-related crime and violence are the result of drug criminalization that created and sustain the highly profitable illegal trade, and of prior antisocial tendencies of some individuals attracted to drugs, rather than of any inherent drug properties compelling to violence by otherwise nonviolent and composed users. Hence, having dispelled the false claims that led to drug prohibition, the question is, what arguments do prohibitionists advance to defend and preserve current drug policy? Overwhelmed by experimental and experiential evidence that drug prohibition has been an extremely costly failure that causes more harm than good, prohibitionists cling to claims of *partial* success in *some* areas and to assert that were it not for current drug policy illicit drug use and addiction would be much worse than it is today. Armed with these assertions rooted in their sets of assumptions and value systems rather than on facts, prohibitionists are unwilling to consider any relaxation of drug laws, much less their depenalization, decriminalization or relegalization. That being the case, two pivotal questions come to mind: Is there any evidence to support protectionists' view that current drug policy acts as a deterrent? If depenalization, decriminalization, or relegalization are to be discarded outright, what new drug policy could succeed and do so without the devastating consequences caused by the current one?

To answer the first question with any degree of certainty would require a head-to-head comparison of drug use prevalence within two comparable populations in the same time frame; one free to use drugs at will, the other not. While such a controlled study has never been done, reasonable guidance can be derived and lessons drawn from marijuana prevalence use in places where it is legal and from comparing the prevalence of alcohol use before and after Prohibition and of legal versus illegal drugs today. As mentioned in chapter 3, the Netherlands considers drug use as a health issue, not a criminal matter, and personal use of cannabis is allowed when purchased by an adult from the country's licensed cannabis cafés (805 in 2002) in amounts up to 5 grams per person per transaction. Yet, despite having being depenalized, cannabis use is not higher in the Netherlands than in most other Western European countries, as revealed by the European Monitoring Center for Drugs and Drug Addiction. According to that report, 3.3% of Netherlanders aged 15 to 64 consumed cannabis *in the last 30 days* in 2005, which ranks it 9th among 27 EU countries behind Spain (8.7%), the United Kingdom (6.2%), Italy (5.8%), the Czech Republic (4.8%), France (4.8%), Luxembourg (4.0%), Austria (3.8%), and Germany (3.4%);[1] all with more severe antidrug laws. Moreover, the prevalence use of cocaine, heroin, and other *hard drugs* is not higher in the Netherlands than in other European countries, dispelling once again the myth that cannabis, marijuana, and other so-called soft drugs are gateways to hard drugs. Additionally, inferences can be drawn from Prohibition with regards to alcohol consumption before and after its repeal. They are applicable to today's drug problem, despite being distanced in time and an American society that has evolved since, because drug use is a universal phenomenon that transcends ethnic, cultural, and time barriers, as outlined in chapter 2. As described in chapter 1, alcohol consumption, especially of the more profitable hard liquors, rose during Prohibition as did the health consequences of adulterated liquors distilled in bootlegged operations. Also, crime and corruption swept the country, and tens of thousands of nonviolent citizens were incarcerated for activities that were legal before and after Prohibition. Furthermore, multiple user surveys conducted in today's drug policy environment confirm undiminished drug availability despite the vigilance of the drug enforcement establishment and harsh penalties for offenders. These surveys and two historical experiments decades apart, one banning alcohol the other allowing cannabis, show that contrary to prohibitionists' assertions, prohibition does not reduce availability and is not a deterrent, nor does free access to drugs increase use or abuse. In fact, just as alcohol consumption decreased markedly after Prohibition, as did overall crime and corruption, repeal of current drug policy would likely be followed by reduced drug use. Moreover, the illicit drug trade fostered and sustained by drug criminalization would come to a standstill, ending drug-related crime and violence in producer and consumer countries alike. Additionally, repealing current drug policy would also contribute to restoring America's former standing in the world; a standing compromised in the last 30 years by foreign adventurism at times funded through covert operations conducted in collusion with drug traffickers.

The answer to the second question is straightforward if one is to adhere to evidence rather than to self-serving preconceptions. Indeed, evidence presented in this book shows that drug policy has failed to achieve the ultimate goal of reducing drug use and addiction rates in America despite an enormous and growing economic cost and human suffering that it causes at home and abroad. In short, current drug policy and drug laws do more harm than good. In fact, they cause indescribable harm wherever they are enforced but little if any good; a situation that is as unacceptable as it is intolerable. Hence, protectionists are left with one of two possible options: (1) better application of current laws and statutes, or "tailoring current policy levers" in hopes of achieving the unachievable; or (2) further tightening drug laws and harsher repression of transgressors. It should be clear to anyone that the first option is a dead-end measure doomed to fail for it doesn't address the underlying culprit of all economic and social ills caused by drug policy: drug criminalization that in turn created a black market, which, given the enormous profits involved, sparks uncontrollable crime and corruption. The alternate option is a classic war posture where more soldiers, more ammunitions, and more financial resources are thrown in hopes to vanquish the *enemy*. Yet, that too is doomed to failure if drug policy experience over three decades is to teach us anything. Indeed, the *drug problem* has actually gotten progressively worse despite efforts by seven U.S. administrations since the creation of the DEA, including Presidents Nixon's and Reagan's major drug war escalations, as described in chapter 3. There are several reasons why further escalation would not significantly impact drug use and addiction trends. First, the lure of mind-altering drugs has been with us for millennia and will likely remain so forever. In fact, in recent times abuse behavior has transcended drugs to involve certain activities (e.g., gambling, sex) and even common foodstuff (e.g., coffee, chocolate). Second, a small segment of the population with impaired self-control is unable to manage use of drugs, food, or activities, increasing their susceptibility to addiction even after becoming aware of the potential health or legal consequences of such a behavior. Third, because the drug trade is driven by demand, any escalation of the War on Drugs that succeeds in reducing the supply to consumers would raise unit price, further enticing

producers and traffickers. Fourth, human behavior is not responsive to legislation even under the threat of harsh penalties, as shown by decades of increasingly repressive U.S. drug laws. Fifth, criminalizing some mind-altering
drugs and demonizing users as enemies of society is the wrong approach.
Indeed, "the martial rhetoric of a 'Drug War' creates a sense of crisis and
urgency that is inimical to rational policy debate . . . martial metaphors not
only stifle dissent, polarize opinion and limit the policy options that can be
discussed."[2] Finally, drugs and drug users are not enemies to be vanquished,
as in a war, but manageable societal problems to be quantified, ranked, and
compared to other social liabilities as a basis for developing appropriate public prevention and nonpunitive interventional policies and for allocating
resources to finance such policies. Yet, while nonpunitive interventional policies would handle drug users and addicts outside the penal code, crimes they
commit would remain punishable. However, punishment must be equitable,
proportionate to the crime and the circumstances, and based on its nature,
type, and gravity and not on prejudice, as is too often the case today for drug
offenders and as was in former times for minority transgressors. Let us not
forget that not long ago young white rapists were often rationalized as *boys
will be boys,* especially if the victim was said to dress or act *provocatively,*
whereas young blacks accused of raping white women were likened to
predators, hunted down, and lynched by mobs seeking revenge rather than
justice.[3]

Clearly, solving the drug problem and alleviating crime, corruption, and
human rights violations linked to the illegal drug trade, itself caused by
current drug policy, requires ending drug prohibition. That is, the depenalization, decriminalization, or relegalization of all illicit drugs; the dismantlement of drug enforcement agencies along with their infrastructures; and the
repeal of all drug laws. Only such a radical change in direction is capable of
ending the economic and social ills caused by current drug policy. Under this
scenario, all drugs would be legal, regulated, and taxed on par with alcohol,
drug use would become a health concern, and users would be eligible for
prevention and educational programs rather than being hunted as criminals.
The following are some of the major benefits that would follow from the repeal of current drug policy.

1. Removing local and foreign traffickers' main source of revenue. In the United
    States and other consumer countries, all drug-related street crime would end,
    restoring peace to neighborhoods taken over by drug pushers and dignity to
    its inhabitants. In producer countries, crime, corruption, and human rights
    violations linked to the drug industry would decline sharply. However, one
    should be under no illusion that social ills ingrained in the societies of cer-
    tain producer countries would be solved by any drug reform. In Colombia, for
    instance, the loss of drug revenues by traffickers linked to guerrilla and counter-
    guerilla groups and to common criminals would likely be substituted, at least
    in part, by a recrudescence in kidnappings for ransom, extortion, and other
    crimes. Colombia's and Afghanistan's dysfunctional societies preceded the

drug trade and require adapted local solutions independently of and in addition to drug policy reform. However, the former is virtually impossible to achieve without the latter.

2. Enabling governments of producer and consumer countries to regulate and tax the production and sale of all drugs, providing a new source of revenue that could be earmarked for drug prevention and education, and to fund socially responsible, nonpunitive interventional policies.

3. Enabling reallocation of billions of dollars wasted each year on the War on Drugs toward social programs designed to assist needy Americans and to aid producer countries in educating and retooling their illegal crop-producing farmers toward profitable alternate crops along with the means to market such crops.

4. Ending the harassment and yearly arrest and prosecution of hundreds of American physicians for issuing prescriptions capriciously deemed "outside the scope of legitimate practice" by untrained drug enforcement agents. In turn, this would empower physicians to prescribe narcotics according to medical criteria rather than as dictated by the DEA, thus ending the pain management crisis in the United States that penalizes tens of millions of chronic pain sufferers and terminally ill patients.

5. Ending the yearly arrest of hundreds of thousands of petty drug offenders and the incarceration of many thousands, enabling law enforcement and the courts to focus on real criminals, and restoring the proper role of prisons as institutions of confinement for criminals and perpetrators of violent crimes.

6. Eliminating drug policy's indirect harm to users such as the health consequences of adulterated drugs and of contaminated needles.

7. Eliminating the forbidden fruit factor that entices many adolescents to experiment with illicit drugs, hence reducing use.

Conclusions

The War on Drugs is a replay of Prohibition at a global scale. While they differ in some important respects, similarities outweigh differences, including their origins, which can be traced back to human nature in terms of both the attraction and opposition to drugs, whether yesterday's prohibited alcohol or today's forbidden drugs. Indeed, the lure of mind-altering drugs has been with us since antiquity and represents a human behavior that cannot be legislated or repressed successfully. Indeed, no amount of intimidation, coercion, or punishment has deterred experimentation with drugs. This is especially the case for adolescents and young adults, most of whom indulge sporadically rather than regularly, few become addicted, and most who do and choose to quit can do so more often than not unassisted. These facts alone render current repressive drug policy entirely unjustifiable. Another similarity is the cynicism and intellectual dishonesty of many promoters of the War on Drugs who impose on others their value system, as did prohibitionists. Both adroitly have used manipulation, disinformation, and outright falsehoods to hold the public hostage to the myths of the dangers of targeted drugs. The modus operandi includes appealing to prejudice, latent racism, and xenophobia to promote a sentiment of *them* vs. *us* in the population. This was the case of the temperance movement, known for its prejudice against immigrants of the early 1900s, especially Catholics, and of Harry J. Anslinger, Commissioner of the U.S. Bureau of Narcotics (1930–1962), who waged an unabashed press campaign during

World War II claiming that Japan had embarked on an Opium Offensive to addict the entire nation.

Today, advocates of the War on Drugs demonize drugs and drug users, instigate in the population a fear of the alleged perils of drugs to self and society, and promote a sense of self-righteousness among drug policy supporters. The strategy includes well-orchestrated and widely publicized arrests of drug traffickers, drug intercepts and seizures, and DEA campaigns against the *drug du jour*, as exemplified by its "OxyContin Action Plan" launched in 2001, which targeted physicians. Such operations are dramatized by an unquestioning and acquiescing media and applauded by a duped public—two essential conditions that ensure the DEA's longevity despite its inability to reduce the amount of drugs on U.S. streets. Another glaring similarity between the two prohibitionist policies is false claims that targeted drugs, whether alcohol of yesteryear or today's mind-altering agents, are inherently addictive and that addiction is caused by a genetic disease. According to this claim, drugs of addiction act on neurocircuitry reward pathways as pleasure reinforcers and, as if to strengthen the notion of their wickedness, incite users to a criminal behavior. Yet scientific and clinical evidence show that drugs are not addictive and that abuse is a choice, as is smoking, unrestrained gambling, or overeating.

Addiction, whether to drugs or to usually normal activities, typifies compulsive or impaired self-control over use linked to the user's personality traits, molded by education and life experiences, the environment, and nonspecific genetic factors, rather than a disease. Intent is a hallmark of addiction (e.g., taking narcotics or food for pleasure rather than for pain relief or nourishment, respectively). For confirmation of this viewpoint, look no further than the extreme rarity of addiction among the millions of pain sufferers, whether from cancer or noncancer illnesses, who take narcotics daily for months to years, not for pleasure but to attain relief from intractable pain and a return to a more functional lifestyle. Likewise, numerous studies over several decades have shown that drugs do not incite violence or criminal behavior in otherwise law-abiding persons. Examples include crime statistics before, during, and after Prohibition and empirical evidence showing that most crimes attributed to drugs are committed by traffickers and by dealers protecting their lucrative turfs. Some drug addicts also engage in mostly nonviolent criminal activities, behaviors that are linked to preexisting delinquent tendencies, as revealed by carefully conducted longitudinal studies of drug-addicted U.S. servicemen during and after the Vietnam War.

Despite these similarities, Prohibition and the War on Drugs differ significantly. The former was promoted mainly by self-righteous rural middle-class activists encouraged by conservative religious leaders, was limited to alcoholic beverages, and was waged within our borders where most of these products were manufactured, sold, and consumed. In contrast, the War on Drugs was created and launched by President Richard Nixon in his quest for power, covers a wide range of psychotropic drugs, and is fought at home and in foreign lands where most of these agents originate. To justify expanding his antidrug crusade beyond our borders, Nixon stated, "Our uncontrollable heroin epidemic . . . is, in other words, a foreign import." More importantly, the War on Drugs and Prohibition are poles apart from a civil liberties standpoint. Indeed, U.S. policy makers of the 1920s and 1930s felt compelled to seek constitutional amendments to both implement Prohibition as the law of the land and to repeal it when confronted with having "prohibition in law but not in fact" and with the social decay it caused. In contrast, President Nixon dispensed of such a formality and created the DEA by executive order, which was followed by an ever-expanding legal and brick-and-mortar infrastructure with funding to match, reaching $13 billion distributed among 11 government departments and agencies involved in the drug enforcement ban in 2008.

More importantly, drug policy has had devastating if unintended consequences far exceeding Prohibition's. During Prohibition, much of the illegal alcohol industry was taken over by home-grown organized criminal groups, often combined with gambling and prostitution, which led to street gangs and to a wave of crime and corruption. Criminalization of today's mind-altering drugs dictates the arrest, prosecution, and incarceration of mostly nonviolent drug offenders each year that divert resources, clutter courts, overcrowd prisons, and cause crime and corruption that far exceeds Prohibition's. More ominously, the DEA's unrestrained enforcement tactics have had a chilling effect on legitimate narcotics prescriptions that interferes with optimal pain management, causing a national pain management crisis where tens of millions of Americans with chronic and terminal illnesses "receive inadequate care because of barriers to pain treatment." In contrast to alcohol Prohibition, which affected the United States, the War on Drugs fostered the emergence of a highly profitable international black market to supply an insatiable global demand for illicit drugs that is exploited by narco-guerillas and narco-terrorists. Involvement of these players and the sheer size of the illicit drug market have enormous geopolitical repercussions not seen during Prohibition. Whereas 1920s America had already developed a well-functioning society governed by the rule of law and capable of confronting Prohibition's challenges, most producer countries, wanting in both, are overwhelmed by their illegal drug industry and its consequences. The consequences are high levels of crime and corruption at all levels of society and massive human rights violations against the poor and disenfranchised perpetrated mainly by narco-guerillas (Colombia) and by drug-funded warlords (Afghanistan). Finally, whereas Prohibition was seen abroad as the product of a puritanical society, the United States is now blamed for the worldwide ravages of drug policy because of its position as a high demand consumer country, the driver of the global War on Drugs, and its counterproductive foreign adventurism.

Given the preceding evidence, the question is: what gives the War on Drugs staying power? The answer is three-fold: the mindset and value systems of promoters; the built-in interests, moral, financial, and otherwise, of supporters; and the acquiescence of a duped public. Hard-core prohibitionists reject the undisputable evidence presented in this book and elsewhere on ideological grounds as illustrated in President Reagan's dismissal of the National Academy of Sciences' "An Analysis of Marijuana Policy 1982" report, stating "Drugs are bad and we are going after them." Drug policy reformers of most persuasions reluctantly accept the notion of relaxing some of its provisions but exclude depenalization, decriminalization, or relegalization of drugs, pointing to dubious partial successes and asserting that were it not for drug policy illicit drug use and addiction would be much worse than it is today. The latter claim also ignores the facts. Indeed, alcohol consumption rose steadily during Prohibition only to fall back to pre-Prohibition levels after its repeal. More germane to drug policy and to our time, legalization of *medical marijuana* in fourteen U.S. states and depenalization of cannabis in the Netherlands since 2000 has not increased use in any of those places. In fact, in 2005 the Netherlands ranked 9th among 27 European countries in cannabis consumption, well behind some with strict penal laws and without increasing hard drugs use.

Any reflective drug policy reform proposal must be anchored on the following incontrovertible facts that redefine the landscape: (1) Drugs of addiction are not intrinsically addictive; (2) black market players cause most crime and corruption attributed to drugs; (3) addiction is not a *disease* over which the *victim* has no control but is rather a compulsion or an impaired control behavior; and (4) human behavior cannot be successfully legislated or repressed regardless of the penalties involved. Acknowledging these facts ineluctably leads to repealing drug policy. As a result, the huge profits commanded by illegal drugs would be eliminated, ending the black market within and between producer and consumer countries, and would do so overnight. Having been rendered obsolete, the drug enforcement apparatus would be dismantled, along with its supporting infrastructures, and all drug laws would be repealed. Profound benefits would ensue at the home front, including (1) ending the DEA's interference with medical practice, placing pain management decisions in the hands of physicians rather than drug policy enforcers, (2) ending drug-related street crime, restoring peace to drug-ridden neighborhoods and dignity to its inhabitants, (3) eliminating the forbidden fruit aspect that entices many youth to experiment with illicit drugs, (4) ending the yearly arrest, prosecution, and incarceration of petty offenders that divert policing resources, clutter courts, and overcrowd prisons at a high cost to society, (5) ending the health consequences of adulterated drugs and of contaminated needles, (6) empowering world governments to control and tax the production and sale of relegalized drugs, creating a new source of revenue that could be earmarked for drug education, prevention, and treatment, and (7) reallocating the billions of dollars wasted on the War on Drugs toward social programs designed to relieve needy Americans and protect the country from real threats, and to help retool illegal crop-producing farmers toward marketable alternate crops. Major benefits for producer countries include removing narco-guerillas' and drug-funded warlords' main source of revenue, hence reducing crime, corruption, and human rights violations perpetrated by these groups. While such groups preceded the War on Drugs and will probably survive the end of the illegal drug trade, their defeat is improbable without it.

Implementation of the radical nonpunitive, socially responsible, and enlightened drug policy reform proposed here entails a monumental undertaking. Indeed, the lack of political will to alter drug policy among today's policy makers, the entrenched public misconceptions about drugs continuously reinforced by detractors' unending disinformation campaigns, and the fierce resistance from those who one way or another benefit from the status quo are formidable barriers. Hence, a momentous struggle looms ahead that ideally should be spearheaded by a new breed of well-informed legislators acting according to society's best interests and with the wisdom and political courage exhibited by policy makers of the 1930s to repeal the far more egregious and socially harmful War on Drugs. However, because such a scenario is improbable, the task will likely require broad-based grassroots initiatives, already underway, or the bold leadership of an enlightened US President. Only then will drug policy "promote the general welfare" mandated by the U.S. Constitution, without penalizing the sick and suffering or confronting a segment of the citizenry as the enemy. Only then will the social mayhem caused by drug policy and the drug trade, at home and abroad, come to an end.

References

PREFACE

1. National Cancer Institute. Risk of abuse and addiction in populations without prior drug abuse histories. In: Substance Abuse Issues in Cancer. 2008. http://www.cancer.gov/cancertopics/pdq/supportivecare/substanceabuse/healthprofessional/allpages#. Accessed December 20, 2007.

2. Porter J, Jick H. Addiction rare in patients treated with narcotics. *N Engl J Med.* 1980;302:123.

3. Perry S, Heidrich G. Management of pain during debridement: A survey of U.S. burn units. *Pain.* 1982;13:267–280.

4. Medina JL, Diamond S. Drug dependency in patients with chronic headaches. *Headache.* 1977;17:12–14.

5. Heather N, Tebbutt JS, Mattick RP, et al. Development of a scale for measuring impaired control over alcohol consumption: A preliminary report. *J Stud Alcohol.* 1993;54:700–709.

6. Chomsky N. *Hegemony or Survival: America's quest for global dominance.* New York, NY: Henry Holt and Company, LLC; 2003.

7. Walsh J. Washington office on Latin America. Reality Check: The U.S. latest coca cultivation estimates make one thing clear: There is *plenty* of coca. http://www.mamacoca.org/docs_de_base/Fumigas/Reality_Check_June_WOLA_2007.pdf. Accessed January 7, 2007.

8. United Nations Office on Drugs and Crime: 2005 World Drug Report, Vol. 1: Analysis. http://www.unodc.org/pdf/WDR_2005/volume_1_web.pdf. Accessed January 7, 2010.

9. Crime in America: FBI Uniform Crime Reports 2005. U.S. Dept. of Justice, Federal Bureau of Investigation Web site. Table 29. http://www.fbi.gov/ucr/05cius/data/table_29.html. Accessed January 15, 2007.

10. Shaffer Library of Drug Policy. The Financial Costs of the War on Drugs Dwarfs the Federal Budget Deficit. http://www.druglibrary.org/schaffer/library/graphs/17.htm. Accessed January 16, 2007.

11. A Survey of Illegal Drugs: First, Inhale deeply. *The Economist.* August 31, 2000. http://www.economist.com/background/displaystory.cfm?story_id=354058. Accessed June 27, 2007.

12. Hall C. Living in pain. *San Francisco Chronicle.* April 5, 1999.

13. American Medical Association. Patients face numerous barriers to receiving appropriate pain treatment. News Release. July 1997.

14. National Association of Attorneys General. Letter to DEA administrator Karen P. Tandy, January 19, 2005. http://www.csdp.org/naagletter.pdf. Accessed January 26, 2010.

15. Wilkinson RA. (Director, Ohio Department of Rehabilitation and Correction). Substance abuse in America's prisons: A case for detection, interdiction, and intervention. The United Nations Office for Drug Control and Crime Prevention and the NGO Alliance for Crime Prevention and Criminal Justice. October 27, 1997.

16. Frontline. *Drug Wars Reports (2000).* http://www.pbs.org/wgbh/pages/frontline/shows/drugs/. Accessed February 23, 2007.

17. Partnership for Responsible Drug Information. *What is the drug problem?* http://www.prdi.org/mission.html. Accessed April 26, 2007.

18. Gardner J. Review of Overcriminalization: The limits of the criminal law, by Huzak, D. Oxford Univ Press, 2008. *Notre Dame Philosophical Reviews*, March 8, 2008. http://ndpr.nd.edu/review.cfm?id=13805. Accessed November 2, 2009.

CHAPTER 1

1. Lee H. *How Dry We Were: Prohibition Revisited.* Englewood Cliffs, NJ: Prentice Hall Inc; 1963.

2. Cherrington EH. *The Evolution of Prohibition in the United States of America.,* Westerville, Ohio: American Issue Press; 1920.

3. Krout JA. *The Origins of Prohibition.* New York, NY: Russell & Russell; 1967:29–30.

4. Dobyns F. *The Amazing Story of Repeal.* Chicago, IL: Willett, Clark & Co.; 1940.

5. Rush B. Inquiry into the effects of ardent spirits upon the human body and mind. *Q J Stud Alcohol.* 1943;4:325–326.

6. Martin J-P. *La vertu par la loi, la prohibition aux États-Unis: 1920–1933.* Dijon: Editions Universitaires de Dijon; 1993.

7. Peterson VW. Vitalizing liquor control. *J Crim Law Criminol* (1931). 1949 Jul–Aug;40(2):119–134.

8. Gerritsen J-W. *The Control of Fuddle and Flash: A Sociological History of the Regulation of Alcohol and Opiates.* Leiden, the Netherlands: Brill; 2000.

9. Odegard PH. *Pressure Politics: The Story of The Anti-Saloon League.* New York, NY: Columbia University Press; 1928.

10. Fournier F. *From alcohol prohibition to regulation*, University of Paris-7, France, July 2002.

11. McGrew JL. *History of Alcohol Prohibition*. Washington DC: National Commission on Marihuana and Drug Abuse; 1972. www.druglibrary.org/schaffer/LIBRARY/studies/nc/nc2a.htm. Accessed August 29, 2007.

12. Epstein JE. *Agency of Fear: Opiates and Political Power in America*. New York, NY: G. P. Putnam and Sons; 1977:14–15.

13. Bureau of the Census. Fifteenth Census of the United States: 1930; Population. In: *Volume II: General Report/Statistical Subjects*. Washington DC: US GPO; 1933:25.

14. Warburton C. *The Economic Results of Prohibition*. New York, NY: Columbia University Press; 1932.

15. Asbury H. *The Great Illusion: An Informal History of Prohibition*. Garden City, NY: Doubleday & Co.; 1950.

16. National Commission on Law Observance and Enforcement. *Report on the Enforcement of the Prohibition Laws of the United States*. Washington, DC: Government Printing Office; 1931. http://www.drugtext.org/library/reports/wick/Default.htm. Accessed October 10, 2007.

17. McWilliams P. *Prohibition: Ain't Nobody's Business If You Do: The Absurdity of Consensual Crimes in Our Free Country*. Los Angeles, CA: Prelude Press; 1996. http://www.mcwilliams.com/books/aint/402.htm. Accessed August 27, 2007.

18. Jurkiewicz C, Painter MJ, eds. *Social and Economic Control of Alcohol: The 21st Amendment in the 21st Century*. Boca Raton, FL: CRC Press; 2007.

19. Tillitt MH. *The Price of Prohibition*. Boston, MA: Harcourt, Brace & Co.; 1932.

20. Rosenbloom MV. *The Liquor Industry: A Survey of Its History, Manufacture, Problems of Control and Importance*. Braddock, PA: Ruffsdale Distilling Co.; 1936.

21. Fisher I. *Prohibition at Its Worst*. New York, NY: Macmillan; 1927.

22. Cowan R. How the narcs created crack; a war against ourselves. *New York National Review*. December 5, 1986:30–31.

23. Licensed Beverage Industry. *Facts about the Licensed Beverage Industry*. New York, NY: Author; 1961:54–55.

24. Woody CH. *The Growth of the Federal Government, 1915–1932*. New York, NY: McGraw-Hill; 1934.

25. Pollock HM. *Mental Disease and Social Welfare*. Utica, NY: State Hospital Press; 1942.

26. Brown FW. Prohibition and mental hygiene: Effects on mental hygiene-specific disorders. *Ann Am Acad Polit Soc Sci*, 1932;163:61–88.

27. Malzburg B. A study of first admissions with alcohol psychoses in New York State 1943–44. *Q J Stud Alcohol*. December 1949;10:294.

28. Feldman H. *Prohibition: Its Economic and Industrial Aspects*. New York, NY: Appleton & Co.; 1927.

29. U.S. Department of Commerce. *U.S. Census Mortality Statistics*. Washington DC: Author; 1924:55.

30. Thornton M. *Alcohol Prohibition was a Failure*. Cato Policy Analysis, No. 157. Washington DC: Cato Institute; 1991.

31. Pandiani JA. The Crime Control Corps: An invisible New Deal program. *Br J Sociol*. 1982:33.

32. Rice SA, ed. *Statistics in Social Studies*. Philadelphia, PA: University of Pennsylvania Press; 1930.

33. Towne CH. *The Rise and Fall of Prohibition: The Human Side of What the Eighteenth Amendment Has Done to the United States.* New York, NY: Macmillan; 1923.

34. Einstein A. My first impression of the USA. An interview for Nieuwe Rotterdamsche Courant. *Berliner Tageblatt,* July 7, 1921.

CHAPTER 2

1. Hamarneh SK. Pharmacy in Medieval Islam and the history of drug addiction. *Med Hist.* 1972;16:226–237.

2. Kritikos PG, Papadaki SN. The history of the poppy and of opium and their expansion in antiquity in the eastern Mediterranean area. *Bull Narc.* 1967;19:17–38.

3. Thompson RC. *The Assyrian Herbal.* London: Luzac and Co.; 1924.

4. Zehnder J. *Le Pavot et son usage chez les Assyriens.* Genève, Switzerland: Bull Soc Bot; 1928.

5. Saber G. *Papaver species and opium through the ages.* Cairo: Bull Inst Égypte; 1956:37,39–54.

6. Howard J. The flowers of ancient Egypt and today. http://www.touregypt.net/featurestories/flowers.htm. Accessed October 31, 2006.

7. Sigerist HE. *A History of Medicine, Vol I: Primitive and Archaic Medicine.* New York, NY: Oxford University Press; 1951.

8. Tschirch A. *Handbuch der Pharmakognosie.* Leipzig: C.H. Tauchnitz; 1933:1208.

9. Hesiod. *Theogony of Hesiod* (II:507–543). Translated by. Evelyn-White HG. 1914. http://www.sacred-texts.com/cla/hesiod/theogony.htm. Accessed November 2, 2006.

10. Jones WHS. *I consulted Hippocrates.* Vol. 4. Cambridge, MA: Harvard University Press; 1953:317.

11. Fragmenta Historica Gr. II. 215, Fragment IX 3.

12. Scott, J.M. *The White Poppy.* New York: Funk & Wagnells, 1969; 5, 46–82, 109–125.

13. Ali ibn Sahl Rabban al-Tabari, *Firdaws al-Hikmah,* edited by MZ Siddiqi. Berlin: Gibb Mem Trust; 1928:154, 157, 232, 234, 406, 444, 447–453, and 464–466.

14. Jabir ibn. Hayyan, *Kitab al-Sumum,* Cairo ms. Tibb Taymur, 393, fols. 47 and 131–132. (cited in reference 1.)

15. Abû'Ali al-Husayn Ibn Sînā. *al-Qānûn fi al-Tibb.* Vol. 1. Cairo: Great Imperial Printing Office (Bülaq); 1877:256–257, 451–453.

16. Hamarneh S. Sources and development of Arabic medical therapy and pharmacology. *Sudhoffs Archiv.* 1970;54:33–35.

17. Lewis B. *The Assassins: A Radical Sect in Islam.* London: Weidenfeld & Nicolson; 1967.

18. Hanes TW, Sanello F. *Opium Wars: The Addiction of One Empire and the Corruption of Another.* Napervile, IL: Sourcebooks; 1954.

19. Lo-shu Fu. *A Documentary Chronicle of Sino-Western Relations, 1644–1820.* Vol. 1. Tucson, AZ: Univ Arizona Press; 1966:380.

20. Wood D. Treaty of Nanjing: Form and the Foreign Office. *J Imp & Commonwealth Hist.* 1996;24:181–196.

21. Cutler JS. *The old clipper days.* In: Lindsey BJ, ed. *Old Marblehead Sea Captains and the Ships in Which They Sailed.* Whitefish, MT: Kessinger Publishing; 2007:P4.

22. Beard M. *Lord Elgin: Saviour or Vandal?* BBC, Ancient History: Greeks. http://www.bbc.co.uk/history/ancient/greeks/parthenon_debate_01.shtml. Accessed February 17, 2007.

23. United Nations Office on Drugs and Crime. World Drug Report 2006. http://www.unodc.org/unodc/fr/world_drug_report.html. Accessed February 17, 2007.

24. Faguet GB. *The War on Cancer: An Anatomy of Failure; A Blueprint for the Future.* Dordrecht, The Netherlands: Springer; 2005.

25. World Health Organization. Global Status Report on alcohol 2004. Geneva: Author; 2004. http://whqlibdoc.who.int/publications/2004/9241562722_(425KB).pdf. Accessed January 17, 2007.

26. Johnston LD, O'Malley PM, Bachman JG, et al. Monitoring the Future: National Survey Results on Drug Use, 1975–2007: Volume II, College Students and Adults Ages 19–45 (NIH Publication No. 08-6418B). Bethesda, MD: National Institute on Drug Abuse; 2008. http://www.monitoringthefuture.org/pubs/monographs/vol2_2007.pdf. Accessed October 1, 2009.

27. Johnston LD, O'Malley PM, Bachman JG, Schulenberg JE. Monitoring the Future: National Survey Results on Drug Use, 1975–2006: Volume I, Secondary School Students. NIH Publication No. 07-6205. Bethesda, MD: National Institute on Drug Abuse; 2007.

28. Midanik LT, Chaloupka FJ, Saitz R, et al. Alcohol attributable deaths and years of potential life lost—United States, 2001. *Morb Mortal Wkly Rep.* 2004;53:866–870. http://www.niaaa.nih.gov/NR/rdonlyres/802A4ECB-D680-4E8B-BF36-319D06412167/0/BriefingBook2.pdf. Accessed October 2, 2009.

29. Centers for Disease Control and Prevention. Annual smoking-attributable morbidity, mortality, years of potential life lost, and economic costs—US 1195–1999. *Morb Mortal Wkly Rep.* 2002;51:300–303. http://www.cdc.gov/mmwr/preview/mmwrhtml/mm5114a2.htm#tab2. Accessed May 14, 2007.

30. National Institute on Drug Abuse. The Economic cost of alcohol and drug abuse in the United States—1992. http://www.nida.nih.gov/economiccosts/Chapter1.html#1.1. Accessed October 2, 2009.

31. Office of National Drug Control Policy. The Economic Costs of Drug Abuse in the United States, 1992–1998. Washington, DC: Executive Office of the President; 2001. Publication No. NCJ-190636.

CHAPTER 3

1. Musto DF. The History of Legislative Controls Over Opium, Cocaine, and Their Derivatives. http://www.druglibrary.org/schaffer/history/ophs.htm. Accessed June 1,2008.

2. The 1912 Hague International Opium Convention. http://www.unodc.org/unodc/en/frontpage/the-1912-hague-international-opium-convention.html. Accessed June 11, 2008.

3. *US 189 Jin Fuey Moy v. United States* (decided Dec 1920). http://openjurist.org/254/us/189/jin-fuey-moy-v-united-states. Accessed June 12, 2008.

4. International Narcotic Education Association. Marijuana or Indian Hemp and its Preparations [pamphlet]. Los Angeles, CA: Author; 1936:3.

5. Gerber RJ. *Legalizing Marijuana: Drug Policy Reform and Prohibition Politics.* Westport CT: Praeger Publishers; 2004:8.

6. The La Guardia Committee Report. The Marihuana Problem in the City of New York. 1944. http://www.druglibrary.org/schaffer/library/studies/lag/lagmenu.htm. Accessed July 20, 2007.

7. Anslinger H. The psychiatric effects of marijuana intoxication. *JAMA.* 1943;101:212–213.

8. Epstein EJ. *Agency of Fear: Opiates and Political Power in America*. Brooklyn, NY: Verso; 1990.

9. Drug Abuse Council, Inc. *The Nation's Toughest Drug Law: Evaluating the New York Experience*. Washington, DC: Author; 1977.

10. The American Presidency Project. Richard Nixon: Special Message to the Congress on Drug Abuse Prevention and Control, June 17, 1971. http://www.presidency.ucsb.edu/ws/index.php?pid=3048&st=narcotic+addict+rehabilitation+act&st1=. Accessed July 18, 2007.

11. Narcotics: The global connection. *Time*. August 28, 1972. http://www.time.com/time/magazine/article/0,9171,906267-1,00.html. Accessed June 19, 2007.

12. Astucia S. *Opium Lords: Israel, the Golden Triangle, and the Assassination of President Kennedy*. Gaithersburg, MD: Ravening Wolf Publishing Co; 2003.

13. Clark E, Horrock N. *Contrabandista! The busting of a heroin Empire*. London: Paul Elek Publishing; 1973.

14. The Federal Reserve Bank of Minneapolis. What Is a Dollar Worth? http://unoccupiedcycle.com/ Accessed June 14, 2007.

15. McCoy AW. *The Politics of Heroin in Southeast Asia*. New York, NY: Harper & Row; 1972. http://www.drugtext.org/library/books/McCoy/book/02.htm. Accessed June 14, 2007.

16. Dixon P. *The truth about drugs*. London: Hodder and Stoughton; 1998. http://www.globalchange.com/drugs/TAD-Intro.htm. Accessed August 7, 2007.

17. Robins LN. The sixth Thomas James Okey Memorial Lecture. Vietnam veterans' rapid recovery from heroin addiction: A fluke or normal expectation? *Addiction*. 1993;88:1041–1054.

18. Biernacki P. Recovery from opiate addiction without treatment: A summary. In: Lambert EY, ed. *The Collection and Interpretation of Data from Hidden Populations*. NIDA Research Monograph 98. 1990. http://www.nida.nih.gov/pdf/monographs/98.pdf. Accessed July 28, 2007.

19. CSDP Research Report, March 2002. Nixon Tapes Show Roots of Marijuana Prohibition: Misinformation, Culture Wars, and Prejudice. http://www.csdp.org/research/shafernixon.pdf. Accessed July 19, 2007.

20. National Commission on Marihuana and Drug Abuse. *Marihuana: A Signal of Misunderstanding*. First Report of the National Commission on Marihuana and Drug Abuse. Washington, DC: U.S. Government Printing Office; 1972.

21. Nixon Tape transcripts: Oval Office Conversation 498–5 with Haldeman and Ehrlichman, May 13, 1971. http://www.csdp.org/research/nixonpot.txt. Accessed July 20, 2007.

22. About ONDCP. Office of National Drug Control Policy Web site. http://www.whitehousedrugpolicy.gov/about/legislation.html. Accessed July 14, 2007.

23. Commission on Behavioral and Social Sciences and Education. *An Analysis of Marijuana Policy*. Washington DC: The National Academies Press; 1982. http://books.nap.edu/openbook.php?record_id=662&page=1. Accessed July 15, 2007.

24. Reagan Aid: Pot can make you gay. *Newsweek*. October 27, 1986:95.

25. Green J. The Bookie of Virtue: William J. Bennett has made millions lecturing people on morality—and blown it on gambling. *Washington Monthly*, June 2003. http://www.washingtonmonthly.com/features/2003/0306.green.html. Accessed July 22, 2007.

26. U.S. Department of Justice—Bureau of Justice Statistics. Drug and Crime Facts, Number of arrests, by drug type, 1982–2005. http://www.ojp.usdoj.gov/bjs/dcf/tables/drugtype.htm. Accessed July 17, 2007.

27. King RS, Mauer M. The war on marijuana: The transformation of the war on drugs in the 1990s. *Harm Reduct J.* 2006;3:6–23. http://www.harmreductionjournal.com/content/3/1/6. Accessed July 20, 2007.

28. Burns S. An open letter to America's prosecutors. Washington, DC: ONDCP; November 1, 2002. http://www.ndaa.org/pdf/alsobrooks_letter_nov_1_2002.pdf. Accessed July 20, 2007.

29. Office of National Drug Control Policy. Policy. http://www.whitehouse drugpolicy.gov/policy/index.html. Accessed July 14, 2007.

30. Office of National Drug Control Policy. Table 2: Drug control funding by agency: FY 2008. http://www.whitehousedrugpolicy.gov/publications/policy/09budget/tbl_2.pdf. Accessed October 6, 2009.

31. The President's National Drug Control Strategy, February 2007. http://www.stayontrack-online.com/images/stories/SOT_ToolKit/ONDCP's%20Presidents%20National%20Strategy%20on%20Drug%20Control%20Policy%2007.pdf. Accessed December 31, 2009.

32. United Nations Office of Drugs and Crime. Drug Control Treaties and Related Resolutions. http://www.unodc.org/unodc/en/treaties/. Accessed January 1, 2007.

33. United Nations Office of Drugs and Crime. Resolutions and Decisions. http://www.unodc.org/unodc/en/commissions/CND/09-resolutions.html. Accessed January 1, 2007.

34. Joranson DE, Gilson AM. Controlled substances, medical practice, and the law. In: Schwartz HI, ed. *Psychiatric Practice Under Fire: The Influence of Government, the Media and Special Interests on Somatic Therapies.* Washington, DC: America Psychiatric Press, Inc.; 1994:173–194.

35. Demand and Supply: Current Poppy-Based Medicines Production System. http://www.poppyformedicine.net/modules/need_morphine Accessed August 22, 2008.

36. United Nations Office of Drugs and Crime. UN International Drug Control Conventions. http://www.unodc.un.or.th/convention/. Accessed July 2, 2007.

37. Report of the International Narcotics Control Board for 1999. New York: United Nations Publication;2000. http://www.incb.org/incb/annual_report_1999.html. Accessed July 29, 2007.

38. Maynard A. Sense and nonsense in British drug policy. *Eurohealth: Tripping on drug policy? Approaches to illicit drugs.* Spring 2001.

39. Brown DK. Tales of Democracy's Dysfunction are Greatly Exaggerated: The Surprisingly Ordinary Politics of Criminal Law. In: Bepress Legal Series, 2006. http://law.bepress.com/expresso/eps/1523/. Accessed July 30, 2007.

40. European Monitoring Center for Drugs and Drug Addiction Thematic Papers—Illicit drug use in the EU: legislative approaches, 2005. http://www.emcdda.europa.eu/attachements.cfm/att_34042_EN_TP_IllicitEN.pdf. Accessed January 7, 2010.

41. The Sentencing Project Web site. Sentencing Policy. http://www.sentencingproject.org/IssueAreaHome.aspx?IssueID=1. Accessed October 6, 2009.

42. U.S. Department of Justice, Office of Justice Programs. Bureau of Justice Statistics: Compendium of Federal Crime Justice Statistics. 2003. http://www.ojp.usdoj.gov/bjs/pub/pdf/cfjs03.pdf. Accessed October 7, 2009.

43. Ibid., Table 5.1.

44. Ibid., Table 5.3.

45. Ibid., Table 7.1.

46. Ibid., Table 4.5.

47. U.S. Census Bureau. US Census Bureau News, June 24, 2004. http://www.census.gov/Press-Release/www/releases/archives/education/001863.html. Accessed July 5, 2007.

48. U.S. Department of Justice—Office of Justice Programs, Bureau of Justice Statistics: Advance for release, November 30, 2006. http://www.ojp.usdoj.gov/bjs/pub/press/pripropr.htm. Accessed July 6, 2007.

49. Human Rights Watch. United States. Punishment and Prejudice: Racial disparities in the War on Drugs. May 2000;12(2). http://www.hrw.org/reports/2000/usa/. Accessed June 15, 2008.

50. National Highway Traffic Safety Administration: Traffic Safety Facts, 2005. http://www.dtadadap.com/PDF/STATS/2005/2005-TSF-Overview.pdf. Accessed June 6, 2007.

51. Traffic Safety Facts: 2006 Traffic Safety Annual Assessment—a Preview. http://www-nrd.nhtsa.dot.gov/Pubs/810791.PDF. Accessed June 6, 2007.

52. Center for Disease Control and Prevention. Impaired driving. http://www.cdc.gov/ncipc/factsheets/drving.htm. Accessed July 9, 2007.

53. Drunk-driving penalties by state. http://info.insure.com/auto/injury/iihsalcohol982.html. Accessed July 10, 2007.

54. Kreca ME. How the US Government Created the "Drug Problem" in the USA. LewRockwell.com. April 2001. http://www.lewrockwell.com/orig/kreca1.html. Accessed August 20, 2008.

55. Carpenter TG. Unsavory Bedfellows: Washington's International Partners in the War on Drugs. Foreign Policy Briefing. Washington DC: The Cato Institute; August 1, 2002.

56. McCoy AW. *The Politics of Heroin in Southeast Asia.* New York, NY: Harper & Row, 1972.

57. The Contras, Cocaine, and Covert Operations: National Security Electronic Briefing Book No. 2. http://www.gwu.edu/~nsarchiv/NSAEBB/NSAEBB2/nsaebb2.htm. Accessed January 7, 2010.

58. Nutt D. Government *vs* science over drug and alcohol policy. *The Lancet.* 2009;374:1731–1733.

CHAPTER 4

1. Merriam-Webster Online Dictionary. http://www.merriam-webster.com/dictionary/addiction. Accessed July 30, 2007.

2. Hyperdictionary. http://www.hyperdictionary.com/search.aspx?define=addiction. Accessed July 30, 2007.

3. Nestler EJ. From Neurobiology to treatment: Progress against addiction. *Nat Neurosci.* 2002;5:1076–1079. http://www.nature.com/neuro/journal/v5/n11s/full/nn945.html. Accessed July 28, 2007.

4. Addiction. Medicalpages.com.au. http://www.medicalpages.com.au/health/1/Addiction/home.aspx. Accessed October 8, 2009.

5. Addiction. Wikipedia: The Free Encyclopedia. http://en.wikipedia.org/wiki/Addiction. Accessed July 30, 2007.

6. Grant JE. Potenza MN. Impulse control disorders: Clinical characteristics and pharmacological management. *Ann Clin Psychiatry.* 2004;16:27–34.

7. Goodman A. Addiction: Definition and implications. *Br J Addict.* 1990; 85:1403–1408.

8. World Health Organization. *International Classification of Diseases* (ICD-10). 2007, Chapter V: Mental and behavioural disorders: Habit and Impulse disorders. http://apps.who.int/classifications/apps/icd/icd10online/index.htm?gf60.htm. Accessed October 8, 2009.

9. Rush B. *An Inquiry Into the Effect of Ardent Spirits Upon the Human Body and Mind, With an Account of the Means of Preventing and of the Remedies for Curing Them.* 8th rev. ed. Boston, MA: J. Loring; 1823.

10. Beecher L. *Six sermons on the Nature, Occasions, Signs, Evils and Remedy of Intemperance.* 3rd ed. New York, NY: American Tract Society; 1828.

11. Woodward S. *Essays on Asylums for Inebriates.* Worcester, MA: Boston Mercantile Journal; 1835.

12. Surry R. Memo to R. Brinkley Smithers. *Christopher D. Smithers Foundation Files.* Mill Neck, NY: 1838.

13. Goodwin DW, Schulsinger E, Hermansen L, et al. Alcohol problems in adoptees raised apart from biological parents. *Arch Gen Psychiatry.* 1973; 28:238–243.

14. Vaillant GE, Milofsky ES. The etiology of alcoholism: A prospective viewpoint. *Am Psychol.* 1982;37:494–503.

15. Schuckit MA. Prospective markers for alcoholism. In: Goodwin DW, van Dusen KT, Mednick SA, eds. *Longitudinal research in alcoholism.* Boston, MA: Kluwer-Nijhoff; 1984.

16. Porjesz B, Begleiter H. Evoked brain potential deficits in alcoholism and aging. *Alcohol Clin Exp Res.* 1982;6:53–63.

17. Peele S, Alexander B. Theories of addiction. In: Peele S, ed. *The Meaning of Addiction: An Unconventional View.* San Francisco: Jossey-Bass; 1998. http://www. peele.net/lib/moa3.html. Accessed August 9, 2007.

18. Lombroso C. *L'Uomo Delinquente.* Milan, Italy: Hoepli; 1876.

19. Nestler EJ. Is there a common molecular pathway for addiction? *Nat Neurosci.* 2005;8:1445–1449.

20. Porter J, Jick H. Addiction rare in patients treated with narcotics. *N Engl J Med.* 1980;302:123.

21. Perry S, Heidrich G. Management of pain during debridement: A survey of US burn units. *Pain.* 1982;13:267–280.

22. Medina JL, Diamond S. Drug dependency in patients with chronic headaches. *Headache.* 1977;17:12–4.

23. Chen K, Kandel DB. The natural history of drug use from adolescence to the mid-thirties in a general population sample. *Am J Public Health.* 1995;85:41–7.

24. Pert CB, Snyder SH. Opiate receptor: Its demonstration in nervous tissue. *Science* (Wash DC). 1973;179:1011–1014. http://www.sciencemag.org/cgi/content/abstract/179/4077/1011. Accessed September 5, 2007.

25. Li X, Keith DE Jr, Evans CJ. Mu opioid receptor-like sequences are present throughout vertebrate evolution. *J Mol Evol.* 1996;43:179–184.

26. Zhang Y, Wang D, Johnson AD, et al. Allelic expression imbalance of human mu opioid receptor (OPRM1) caused by variant A118G. *Biol Chem.* 2005; 280:32618–32624.

27. Uhl GR, Liu QR, Drgon T, et al. Molecular genetics of nicotine dependence and abstinence: Whole genome association using 520,000 SNPs BMC. *Genetics.* 2007;8:10. http://www.pubmedcentral.nih.gov/articlerender.fcgi?artid=1853105. Accessed September 10, 2007.

28. Hamer DH, Hu S, Magnuson V, et al. A linkage between DNA markers on the X chromosome and male sexual orientation. *Science.* 1993;261:321–327.

29. Rice G, Anderson C, Risch N, et al. Male homosexuality: absence of linkage to microsatellite markers Xq 28. *Science.* 1999;284:665–766.

30. Faguet, GB. *The War on Cancer: An Anatomy of failure; a Blueprint for the Future.* Dordrecht, The Netherlands: Springer; 2005.

31. Winger G, Woods JH, Galuska CM, et al. Behavioral perspective on the neuroscience of drug addiction. *J Exp Anal Behav.* 2005;84:667–681.

32. National Institute of alcohol abuse and alcoholism. Twelve-month prevalence and population estimates of DSM-IV alcohol abuse by age, sex, and race-ethnicity: United States, 2001–2002 (NESARC). http://www.niaaa.nih.gov/Re sources/DatabaseResources/QuickFacts/AlcoholDependence/abusdep1.htm. Accessed November 10, 2007.

33. Johnston LD, O'Malley PM, Bachman JG et al. *Monitoring the Future National Survey Results on Drug Use, 1975–2007: Volume II, College Students and Adults Ages 19–45* (NIH Publication No. 08-6418B). Bethesda, MD: National Institute on Drug Abuse; 2008.

34. Robins LN. The sixth Thomas James Okey Memorial Lecture. Vietnam veterans' rapid recovery from heroin addiction: A fluke or normal expectation? *Addiction.* 1993;88:1041–1054.

35. Klingemann H, Sobell L, Barker J, et al. *Promoting Self-Change From Problem Substance Use: Practical Implication for Policy, Prevention, and Treatment.* Dordrecht, The Netherlands: Springer; 2001.

36. Lubman DI, Yucel M, Pantelis C. Addiction, a condition of compulsive behavior? Neuroimaging and neuropsychological evidence of inhibitory dysregulation. *Addiction.* 2004;99:1491–1502.

37. Shoda Y, Mischel W, Peake PK. Predicting adolescent cognitive and self-regulatory competencies from preschool delay of gratification: Identifying diagnostic conditions. *Dev Psychol.* 1960;26:978–986.

38. Mischel W, Shoda Y, Rodriguez ML. Delay of gratification in children. *Science.* 1989;244:933–938.

39. Heather N, Tebbutt JS, Mattick RP, et al. Development of a scale for measuring impaired control over alcohol consumption: A preliminary report. *J Stud Alcohol.* 1993;54:700–709.

40. Hoaken PN, Assaad JM, Pihl RO. Cognitive functioning, and the inhibition of alcohol-induced aggression. *J Stud Alcohol.* 1998;59:599–607.

41. Edwards G, Taylor C. A test of the matching hypothesis: Alcohol dependence, intensity of treatment, and 12-month outcome. *J Stud Alcohol.* 1977;38:1004–1031.

42. Robins LN, Helzer JE, Hesselbrocl M, Wish E. Vietnam veterans three years after Vietnam: how our study changed our view of heroin. In: Brill L, Winick C, eds. *The Yearbook of Substance Use and Abuse.* 2nd ed. New York, Human Sciences Press, 1980; vol 2.

43. Lettieri DJ, ed. Theories on drug abuse, selected contemporary perspectives. National Institute on Drug Abuse 1980. Research Monograph 30.

44. Biernacki P. *Pathways From Heroin Addiction: Recovery Without Treatment*. Philadelphia, PA: Temple University Press; 1986.

45. Hennrikus DJ, Jeffery RW, Lando HA. Occasional smoking in a Minnesota working population. *Am J Public Health*. 1996;86:1260–1266.

46. Erickson PG, Alexander BK. Cocaine and addictive liability. In: Schaler JA, ed. *Drugs: Should We Legalize, Decriminalize or Deregulate?* Amherst, NY: Prometheus Books; 1989:271–287.

47. Miller WR, Heather N, eds. *Treating Addictive Behaviors*. 2nd ed. Dordrecht: Springer; 1998.

48. McLellan AT, Arndt IO, Metzger DS, Woody GE, O'Brien CP. The effects of psychosocial services in substance abuse treatment. *JAMA*. 1993;269:1953–1959.

49. Schaler J. *Addiction is a Choice*. Chicago, IL: Open Court; 2000.

50. Davies JB. *The Myth of Addiction*. Newark, NJ: Harwood Academic Publishers; 1997.

CHAPTER 5

1. Libby RT. *Treating Doctors as Drug Dealers: The DEA's War on Prescription Pain killers*. Cato Policy Analysis, No. 545. Washington DC: Cato Institute; 2005.

2. Hall CT. Living in Pain Addiction. *San Francisco Chronicle*. April 5, 1999.

3. American Medical Association. Patients face numerous barriers to receiving appropriate pain treatment [news release]. July 1997.

4. World Health Organization. Access to controlled medications programme: Briefing note. Geneva, Switzerland: Author; March 2007. http://www.who.int/med icines/areas/quality_safety/AccessControlledMedicationsBrNote.pdf. Accessed June 11, 2008.

5. American Pain Foundation. Talking points on pain. *AM News*. September 23–30, 2002.

6. Stewart WF, Ricci JA, Chee E, et al. Lost productive time and cost due to common pain conditions in the US workforce. *JAMA*. 2003;290:2443–5414.

7. The Harrison Narcotics Act. PL 223, 63rd Congress, December 17, 1914.

8. Schaffer Library of Drug Policy. Cannabis medicines from pharmaceutical history. http://www.druglibrary.org/mags/medical_marijuana_throughout_his. htm. Accessed June 11, 2008.

9. Epstein JE. *Agency of Fear: Opiates and Political Power in America*. New York, NY: G. P. Putnam and Sons; 1977.

10. Drug Enforcement Administration. Authority to control; Standards and schedules. Sec. 812. Schedules of controlled substances. http://www.usdoj.gov/ dea/pubs/csa/812.htm#c. Accessed October 9, 2009.

11. Drug Enforcement Administration. Mission statement. http://www.dea. gov/agency/mission.htm. Accessed June 11, 2008.

12. U.S. Department of Justice, Drug Enforcement Administration. Action Plan to Prevent the Diversion and Abuse of OxyContin, 2001. http://www.deadiver sion.usdoj.gov/drugs_concern/oxycodone/abuse_oxy.htm. Accessed January 7, 2010.

13. Roche T. The potent perils of a new drug. *Time*. January 8, 2001:47.

14. Cohen G. The poor man's heroin. *US News and World Report*. February 12, 2001:27.

15. Clines F, Meier B. Cancer painkillers pose new abuse threat. *New York Times.* February 9, 2001:A21.

16. Dad arrested in son's OxyContin death. WDSU.com. http://www.wdsu.com/news/896462/detail.html. Accessed June 12, 2008.

17. CBS News' "48 HOURS" and MTV News and Docs' "TRUE LIFE," as Part of a Continuing Cooperative Project, "Prescription Pain-Killing Drug OxyContin," Dec. 12 and 13. http://www.prnewswire.com/cgibin/stories.pl?ACCT=104&STORY=/www/story/12-06-2001/0001629104&EDATE. Accessed April 21, 2007.

18. Bloodsworth D. OxyContin under Fire (five-part series). *Orlando Sentinel.* October 19–23, 2003.

19. Sentinel overstated deaths caused solely by Oxycodone. *Orlando Sentinel.* August 1, 2004.

20. Bazilchuk N. The OxyContin dilemma: A drug's dangers justify unusual controls [Editorial]. *The Burlington Free Press.* August 10, 2001.

21. PurduePharma.com. OxyContin dismissals and withdrawals exceed 400. January 5, 2006. http://www.purduepharma.com/pressroom/news/20060105.pdf. Accessed January 7, 2010.

22. Laidler J. Grants to help combat drug use. *Boston Globe.* August 8, 2004.

23. Mandal V, Antle R. "Hillbilly Heroin" Target of Alert: Oxycontin Blamed for 250 Deaths in Ontario. *Ottawa Citizen.* August 4, 2004.

24. Pinsky D, Seppala M, Meyers R, et al. *When Painkillers Become Dangerous: What Everyone Needs to Know About OxyContin and Other Prescription Drugs.* Center City, MN: Hazelden Foundation and Educational Services; 2004.

25. The U.S. Attorney's Office, Western District of Virginia. The Purdue Frederick Company, Inc. and top executives plead guilty to misbranding OxyContin; will pay over $600 million. May 10, 2007. http://www.vawd.uscourts.gov/OPINIONS/JONES/107CR00029.PDF. Accessed January 7, 2010.

26. Van Zee A. Purdue Pharma, profits, and the public domain. *Tricities.com.* June 18, 2007.

27. Testifying before the United States Senate Caucus on International Narcotics Control, Executive Summary, April 11, 2002. http://www.dea.gov/pubs/cngrtest/ct041102p.html. Accessed January 26, 2007.

28. Balko R. Fisking the DEA. May 15, 2005. http://www.theagitator.com/archives/021071.php#021071. Accessed January 26, 2007.

29. U.S. Department of Justice. A guide to equitable sharing of federally forfeited property for state and local law enforcement agencies. March 1994. http://www.usdoj.gov/jmd/afp/07federalforfeiture/index.htm. Accessed January 26, 2007.

30. U.S. Department of Justice, Drug Enforcement Administration. Title 21 USC Controlled Substances Act. Section 802. *Definitions.* http://www.deadiversion.usdoj.gov/21cfr/21usc/802.htm. Accessed December 23, 2009.

31. National Cancer Institute. Risk of abuse and addiction in populations without drug abuse histories. In: *Substance Abuse Issues in Cancer.* http://www.cancer.gov/cancertopics/pdq/supportivecare/substanceabuse/healthprofessional/allpages#Section_42. Accessed January 27, 2007.

32. Cone EJ, Fant RV, Rohay JM, et al. Oxycodone involvement in drug abuse deaths: A DAWN-based classification scheme applied to an Oxycodone postmortem database containing over 1000 cases. *J Anal Toxicol.* March 2003;27:57–67.

33. Balko R. Drug war police tactics endanger innocent citizens. *Foxnews.com.* June 21, 2006.

34. From painkillers to prison [Editorial]. *St. Petersburg Times.* April 5, 2004.

35. Markon J. Pain doctor convicted of drug charges, *Washington Post.* December 16, 2004:A1.

36. White J. McLean doctor facing drug trafficking charges. *Washington Post.* September 25, 2003:B3.

37. Portenoy RK, Campbell JN, Foley K, et al. Letter from Past Presidents of American Pain Society denouncing testimony against Dr. Hurwitz—12/29/2004. http://www.aapsonline.org/painman/hurwitzletter.htm. Accessed May 27, 2007.

38. U.S. Drug Enforcement Administration. Virginia Pain Doctor Sentenced to 25 Years [news release]. April 14, 2005. http://www.dea.gov/pubs/pressrel/pr041405.html. Accessed December 23, 2009.

39. Markon J. Pain doctor 'cavalier,' jury foreman says. *Washington Post.* December 21, 2004:B3.

40. O'Dell L. Appeals court orders new trial for pain specialist. *The Associated Press.* August 22, 2006.

41. Drug Enforcement Administration. Prescription Pain Medications: Frequently Asked Questions and Answers for Health Care Professionals and Law Enforcement Personnel. http://aapsonline.org/painman/deafaq.pdf. Accessed December 30, 2007.

42. Thierny J. Trafficker or dealer? And who is the victim? *The New York Times* March 27, 2007.

43. Hall CT. Jury acquits doctor in pain-control test case. *San Francisco Chronicle.* May 20, 2004:A1.

44. Fisher FB. Pain killer. *Harvard Medical Alumni Bulletin.* June 22, 2006.

45. Drug Enforcement Administration. The Myth of the Chilling Effect; Doctors Operating Within Bounds of Accepted Medical Practice Have Nothing to Fear from DEA [news release]. October 30, 2003. http://www.usdoj.gov/dea/pubs/pressrel/pr103003p.html. Accessed January 1, 2007.

46. Libby RT. *The DEA's "One-tenth of One Percent" myth of doctors who are sanctioned in drug cops and doctors: Is the DEA hampering the treatment of chronic pain?* Cato Institute Conference. Washington, D.C. September 9, 2005.

47. U.S. Department of Justice, Drug Enforcement Administration. Cases against doctors: 2005 fact sheet. http://www.deadiversion.usdoj.gov/crim_admin_actions/crim_actions.htm. Accessed January 1, 2007.

48. American Board of Internal Medicine. Number of candidates certified (valid Medical Oncology certificates). http://www.abim.org/pdf/data-candidates-certified/all-candidates.pdf. Accessed January 7, 2009.

49. National Institutes of Health. *State-of-the-Science Conference on Symptom Management in Cancer: Pain, Depression, and Fatigue.* Bethesda, Maryland. July 15–17, 2002.

50. Joranson DE, Gilson AM. Drug crime is a source of abused pain medications in the United States. *J Pain Symptom Manage.* 2005;30:299–301.

51. Office of National Drug Control Policy. *The Economic Costs of Drug Abuse in the United States, 1992–2002.* Washington, DC: Executive Office of the President; 2004. Publication No. 207303. http://www.ncjrs.gov/ondcppubs/publications/pdf/economic_costs.pdf. Accessed January 7, 2010.

52. The Drug War in the Andes. http://www.einaudi.cornell.edu/LatinAmer ica/outreach/pdf/DrugWarintheAndes.pdf. Accessed January 11, 2010.

53. Brennan F, Cousins MJ. Pain relief as a human right. *Pain*. 2004;12(5).

54. Faguet GB. *The War on Cancer: An Anatomy of Failure; A Blueprint for the Future*. Dordrecht, The Netherlands: Springer; 2005.

55. PPSG receives letter from DEA requesting removal of FAQ from our website. http://www.medsch.wisc.edu/painpolicy/DEA/Mr.%20David%20Joranson. PDF. Accessed 7, 2010.

56. Kaufman M. Specialists decry DEA reversal on pain drugs. *Washington Post*. December 21, 2004:A8.151.

57. National Association of Attorneys General. Letter to DEA administrator Karen P. Tandy. January 19, 2005. http://www.csdp.org/naagletter.pdf. Accessed January 26, 2010.

58. Libby RT. *The Criminalization of Medicine: America's War on Doctors*. Westport, CT: Greenwood Publishing Group; 2007.

59. Mechanic D, McAlpine DD, Rosenthal M, et al. Are patients' office visits with physicians getting shorter? *N Engl J Med*. 2001;344:198–204.

60. Dispensing controlled substances for the treatment of pain; Notice. *Federal Register* September 6, 2006;71(172). http://www.csdp.org/research/E6-14517.pdf. Accessed January 26, 2010.

CHAPTER 6

1. International Association for the Study of Pain. What Is Pain? http://www. iasp-pain.org/AM/Template.cfm?Section=Pain_Definitions&Template=/CM/ HTMLDisplay.cfm&ContentID=1728. Accessed January 7, 2010.

2. Harstall C, Ospina M. How prevalent is chronic pain? *Pain*. 2003;11:1–4.

3. Vera RL. Brief reports from the pain management symposium: Opioid therapy in chronic pain management. *Proc (Bayl Univ Med Cent)*. 2000;13:249–250.

4. American Medical Association. Patients Face Numerous Barriers to Receiving Appropriate Pain Treatment [news release]. July 1997.

5. Zech DF, Grond S, Lynch J, et al. Validation of World Health Organization guidelines for cancer pain relief a 10-year prospective study. *Pain*. 1995;63:65–76.

6. World Health Organization. *WHO Guidelines: Cancer pain relief (2nd ed.), with a guide to opioid availability*. Geneva, Switzerland: Author; 1996.

7. World Health Organization. *Cancer pain relief*. Geneva, Switzerland: Author; 1986.

8. The American Occupational Therapy Foundation. The Thesaurus of Occupational Therapy Subject Headings. http://www.taxonomywarehouse.com/ vocabdetails_include.asp?vVocID=479. Accessed January 7, 2010.

9. The Free Dictionary by Farlex. http://www.thefreedictionary.com. Accessed December 23, 2009.

10. Britannica online. Narcotic. http://www.britannica.com/EBchecked/topic/ 403484/narcotic. Accessed April 12, 2007.

11. World Health Organization. *Achieving Balance in National Opioids Control Policy: Guidelines for Assessment*. Geneva, Switzerland: Author; 2000.

12. Morgan G, Ward R, Barton M. The contribution of cytotoxic chemotherapy to 5-year survival in adult malignancies. *J Clin Oncol*. 2004;16:549–560. http://

fiocco59.altervista.org/images/studi_effetti_chemio_5_anni.pdf. Accessed October 25, 2008.

13. Faguet GB. *The War on Cancer: An Anatomy of Failure; A Blueprint for the Future.* Dordrecht, The Netherlands: Springer; 2005.

14. Kruger L. *Methods in Pain Research.* Boca Raton, FL: CRC Press; 2001:50.

15. Collet BJ. Chronic opioid therapy for non-cancer pain. *Br J Anaesth.* 2001;87:133–143. http://bja.oxfordjournals.org/cgi/content/full/87/1/133. Accessed October 25, 2008.

16. National Cancer Institute. Pain (PDQ), Health Professional Version. http://www.nci.nih.gov/cancertopics/pdq/supportivecare/pain/HealthProfessional. Accessed January 26, 2007.

17. Long SP. American Society of Anesthesiologists; Committee on Pain. *ASA Newsletter.* 2005;69:9. http://www.asahq.org/Newsletters/2005/09-05/long09_05.html. Accessed April 5, 2007.

18. Joranson DE, Cleeland CS, Weissman DH, et al. Opioids for chronic cancer and non-cancer pain: A survey of state medical board members. *Fed Bull.* 1992;79:15–49.

19. Joranson D, Ryan E, Gilson KM, et al. Trends in medical use and abuse of opioid analgesics. *JAMA.* 2000;283:1710–1714. http://jama.ama-assn.org/cgi/content/abstract/283/13/1710. Accessed May 10, 2007.

20. Teno JM, Fisher ES, Hamel MB, et al. Medical care inconsistent with patients' treatment goals: Association with 1-year Medicare resource use and survival. *J Am Ger Soc.* 2002;50:496–500.

21. U.S. Department of Justice, Drug Enforcement Administration, Office of Diversion Control. Cumulative Distribution by State in Grams per 100,000 Population; Reporting Period: 01/01/2005 to 12/31/2005. http://www.deadiversion.usdoj.gov/arcos/retail_drug_summary/2005/05_rpt4.pdf. Accessed October 30, 2009.

22. National Cancer Institute. Cancer Topics: Pain PDQ®. http://www.nci.nih.gov/cancertopics/pdq/supportivecare/pain/healthprofessional/allpages#Section_1. Accessed February 12, 2007.

23. Radbruch L, Sabatowski R, Loick G, et al. Constipation and the use of laxatives: a comparison between transdermal fentanyl and oral morphine. *Palliat Med.* 2000;14:111–119.

24. Daeninck PJ, Bruera E. Reduction in constipation and laxative requirements following opioid rotation to methadone: a report of four cases. *J Pain Symptom Manage.* 1999;18:303–309.

25. Aparasu R, McCoy RA, Weber C, et al. Opioid-induced emesis among hospitalized nonsurgical patients: effect on pain and quality of life. *J Pain Symptom Manage.* 1999;18:280–288.

26. Porter J, Jick H. Addiction rare in patients treated with narcotics. *N Engl J Med.* 1980;302:123.

27. Bouckoms AJ, Masand P, Murray BG, et al.: Chronic non-malignant pain treated with long-term oral narcotic analgesics. *Ann Clin Psychiat.* 1992;4: 185–192.

28. National Cancer Institute. Clinical management of patients with substance abuse histories. In: *Substance Abuse Issues in Cancer.* http://www.cancer.gov/cancertopics/pdq/supportivecare/substanceabuse/HealthProfessional/page7. Accessed October 26, 2008.

29. U.S. Department of Justice. Office of Justice Programs. Bureau of Statistics. Drugs and Crime Facts: Drug Use. http://www.ojp.usdoj.gov/bjs/dcf/du.htm. Accessed January 29, 2007.

30. The NORML Almanac of Marijuana Arrests Statistics. US Marijuana Arrests. http://www.norml.org/pdf_files/state_arrests_2004/NORML_US_Marijuana_ Arrests.pdf Accessed November 2, 2007.

31. Johnston, LD. O'Malley PM, Bachman JG, et al. *Monitoring the Future: National Survey Results on Drug Use, 1975–2007: Volume II, College Students and Adults Ages 19–45* (NIH Publication No. 08-6418B). Bethesda, MD: National Institute on Drug Abuse; 2008. http://www.monitoringthefuture.org/pubs/monographs/ vol2_2007.pdf. Accessed October 1, 2009.

32. Wettering T, Backhaus J, Junghanns K. Addiction in the elderly—an underestimated diagnosis in clinical practice? *Nervenarzt*. 2002;73:861–866.

33. Perry S, Heidrich G. Management of pain during debridement: A survey of U.S. burn units. *Pain*. 1982;13:267–80.

34. Medina JL, Diamond S. Drug dependency in patients with chronic headaches. *Headache*. 1977;17:12–14.

35. Trescot AM, Boswell MV, Atluri SL, et al. Opioid guidelines in the management of chronic non-cancer pain. *Pain Phys*. 2006;9:1–39.

36. Gabriel SE, Jaakkimainen RL, Bombardier C. The cost-effectiveness of misoprostol for nonsteroidal anti-inflammatory drug-associated adverse gastrointestinal events. *Arthritis Rheum*. 1993;36:447–459.

37. CSM Update. Non-steroidal anti-inflammatory drugs and serious gastrointestinal adverse reaction. *Br Med J (Clin Res Ed)*. 1986;292:1190–1191.

38. Gabriel SE, Jaakkimainen RL, Bombardier C. *National Totals for Prescriptions of Antiarthritic Drug Therapies in Canada*. Montreal: IMS Canada; 1997.

39. Tamblyn R, Berkson L, Dauphinee D, et al. Unnecessary prescribing of NSAIDs and the management of NSAIDs-related gastropathy in medical practice. *Ann Int Med*. 1997;127:429–438.

40. Miniter R. Business Europe: A German conspiracy theory with no "legs." *The Wall Street Journal Europe*. August 27, 2001.

41. Gotlieb D. Cox 1 and Cox 2: The cyclo-oxygenase systems. http://www. arthritis.co.za/cox.html. Accessed October 26, 2008.

42. The Oxford League Table of analgesics in acute pain. http://www.medi cine.ox.ac.uk/bandolier/booth/painpag/Acutrev/Analgesics/Leagtab.html. Accessed February 4, 2007.

43. Food and Drug Administration. Database. Center for evaluation and research. Maximum Recommended Therapeutic Dose (MRTD). http://www.fda. gov/aboutfda/centersoffices/cder/ucm092199.htm. Accessed February 4, 2008.

44. Bonica JJ. General considerations of chronic pain. In: Bonica JJ, ed. *The Management of Pain*. Philadelphia, PA: Lea & Ferbiger; 1990:186–196.

45. Richy F, Bruyère O, Ethgen O, et al. Time dependent risk of gastrointestinal complications induced by non-steroidal anti-inflammatory drug use: a consensus statement using a meta-analytic approach. *Ann Rheum Dis*. 2004;63:759–766.

46. Wolfe M, Soll AH. The physiology of gastric acid secretion. *N Engl J Med*. 1988;319:1707–1715.

47. Wolfe MM, Lichtenstein DR, Singh G. Gastrointestinal toxicity of nonsteroidal anti-inflammatory drugs. *N Engl J Med*. 1997;340:1888–1899.

48. Gabriel SE, Jaakkimainen L, Bombardier C. Risk for serious gastrointestinal complications related to use of nonsteroidal anti-inflammatory drugs. A meta-analysis. *Ann Intern Med.* 1991;115:787–796.

49. Bateman DN, Kennedy JG. Non-steroidal anti-inflammatory drugs and elderly patients [Editorial]. *BMJ.* 1995;310:817–818.

50. Bandolier. NSAIDS and Adverse Effects. http://www.medicine.ox.ac.uk/bandolier/booth/painpag/nsae/nsae.html. Accessed February 10, 2007.

51. Singh G, Ramey DR, Terry R, et al. NSAID-related effects on the GI tract: an ever widening spectrum. *Arthritis Rheum.* 1997;40(Suppl):S93.

52. Lanas A, Perez-Aisa MA, Feu F, et al. A nationwide study of mortality associated with hospital admission due to severe gastrointestinal events and those associated with nonsteroidal anti-inflammatory drug use. *Am J Gastroenterol.* 2005;100:1685–1693.

53. Laporte J-R, Vidal X, Carne X. Gastrointestinal bleeding is common. *BMJ.* 1995;311:391.

54. McNicol E, Strassels S, Goudas L, et al. Nonsteroidal anti-inflammatory drugs, alone or combined with opioids, for cancer pain: a systematic review. *J Clin Oncol.* 2004;22:1975–1992.

55. Green CR, Pandit SK, Levy L, et al. Intraoperative ketorolac has an opioid-sparing effect in women after diagnostic laparoscopy but not after laparoscopic tubal ligation. *Anesth Analg.* 1996;82:732–737.

56. Tighe KE, Webb AM, Hobbs GJ. Persistently high plasma morphine-6-glucuronide levels despite decreased hourly patient-controlled analgesia morphine use after single-dose diclofenac: Potential for opioid-related toxicity. *Anesth Analg.* 1999;88:1137–1142.

CHAPTERS 7

1. Wren CS. Anti-drug effort criticized as more harm than help. *The New York Times.* June 9, 1008.

2. Ibañez AM, Moya A. La Población desplazada en Colombia: Examen de sus condiciones socioeconómicas y análisis de las políticas actuales. Colombia; Departamento Nacional de Planeación; 2007.

3. Entrevista: Colombia tiene la situación humanitaria más grave de toda América Latina. *Semana,* January 15, 2007.

4. Gutiérrez F. Organized crime and the political system in Colombia (1978–1998). In: Welna C, Gallón G, eds., *Peace, Democracy, and Human Rights in Colombia.* Notre Dame, IN: University of Notre Dame Press; 2007:267–308.

5. Peterson S. People and ecosystems in Colombia: Casualties of the drug war. *The Independent Review.* Winter 2002;6(3).

6. Gómez H, de Roux CV, Franche M-A, et al. *El conflicto, callejón con salida.* Informe Nacional de Desarrollo Humano, 2003. SBN 958-97196-7-8, Bogotá, Colombia, September 2003. http://www.pnud.org.co/indh2003. Accessed March 3, 2007.

7. Tierra, poder político y reformas agraria y rural, Cuadernos Tierra y Justicia, ILSA, Bogotá, 2002 and Colombia Forum. http://www.kus.uu.se. Accessed March 5, 2007.

8. Departamento Nacional de Planeación. Estimación de pobreza en Colombia, 2006. http://www.scribd.com/doc/124049/Pobreza-en-Colombia. Accessed March 5, 2007.

9. Pobre País: Pobres cifras. *Semana*. October 16–23, 2006.

10. Index Mundi. Colombia Population Below Poverty Line. http://www.index mundi.com/colombia/population_below_poverty_line.html. Accessed March 12, 2007.

11. Niños y Jóvenes: Por qué ingresan a grupos armados? *Hechos del Callejón*, August 1, 2008. http://indh.pnud.org.co/files/boletin_hechos/Ninos_y_jovenes. pdf. Accessed March 12, 2007.

12. Human Rights Watch. *You'll Learn Not to Cry: Child Combatants in Colombia, Girls.* September 2003. http://hrw.org/reports/2003/colombia0903/10.htm#_ ftn168. Accessed March 12, 2007.

13. Amnesty International. Colombia: Scarred Bodies, Hidden Crimes: Sexual Violence Against Women in the Armed Conflict—Testimonies [press release]. October 13, 2004. http://news.amnesty.org/index/ENGAMR230492004. Accessed March 15, 2007.

14. BBC News. Colombia's most powerful rebels. September 19, 2003.http:// news.bbc.co.uk/2/hi/americas/1746777.stm. Accessed April 1, 2007.

15. Amnesty International. The AK-47: The World's Favourite Killing Machine. June 26, 2006. http://www.controlarms.org/en/documents%20and%20files/re ports/english-reports/the-ak-47-the-worlds-favourite-weapon. Accessed January 7, 2010.

16. Parte de guerra de las FARC. October 23, 2007. http://www.abpnoticias. com/index.php?option=com_content&task=view&id=2327&Itemid=98. Accessed April 1, 2007.

17. Programa de las Naciones Unidades para el desarrollo: Informe Nacional de Desarrollo Humano. National Human Development Report 2003 for Colombia. http://hdr.undp.org//es/informes/nationalreports/americalatinacaribe/co lombia/name,3213,es.html. Accessed January 1, 2010.

18. Verdad Colombia. Mayors Under Threat: Documentos. http://www.ver dadcolombia.org/archivos/VerDocumento.php?Id=9. Accessed April 1, 2007.

19. Amnesty International. Colombia. Reporting, Campaigning, and Serving without Fear: The Rights of Journalists, Election Candidates and Elected Officials. February 9, 2006. http://www.amnesty.org/en/library/asset/AMR23/001/2006/ en/d9feb583-fa0d-11dd-b1b0-c961f7df9c35/amr230012006en.pdf.   Accessed April 5, 2007.

20. Mackensie E. Las FARC asesinan electos y candidatos en Colombia—(2007-10-23). Articulos, *Verdad Colombia*. http://www.verdadcolombia.org/archivos/ VerArticulo.php?Id=200. Accessed Januuay7, 2010.

21. Verdad Colombia. Guerillas attack Bojayá. June 1, 2002. http://www. verdadcolombia.org/archivos/VerDocumento.php?Id=7. Accessed April 23, 2007.

22. Oficina en Colombia del Alto Atrato Comisionado de la Naciones Unidas para los Derechos Humanos: *Informe de la Oficina en Colombia del Alto Atrato Comisionado de las Naciones Unidas para los Derechos Humanos sobre su Misión de Observación en el Medio Atrato*, 20 Mayo de 2002. http://www.hchr.org.co/ documentoseinformes/informes/tematicos/bojaya.pdf. Accessed January 29, 2010.

23. Mariner J. The EU, the FARC, the PKK, and the PFLP: Distinguishing Politics from Terror. *FindLaw's Legal Commentary*. May 13, 2002. http://writ.news.find law.com/mariner/20020513.html. Accessed June 24, 2007.

24. Un pueblo a la espera. *Semana*. April 30, 2007.

25. Los diputados del Valle fueron asesinados con 95 disparos de fusil AK-47, el arma usada por las Farc. *Semana*. November 28, 2007.

26. Enigma sangriento. *Semana*. September 15, 2007.

27. Halvorssen T. Guerrilla Nation: The arrest of FARC terrorist Ricardo Granda sheds new light on Hugo Chávez's ongoing support of terrorism. *The Weekly Standard*. January 26, 2005.

28. Sumas y Restas. *Semana*. March 12, 2007. http://www.semana.com/wf_In foArticulo.aspx?idArt=106270. Accessed December 23, 2009.

29. Chávez, A. Colombia: Secuestros S.A. http://contacto.canal13.cl/contacto2/html/Reportajes/secuestro_colombia/index.html. Accessed June 25, 2007.

30. Álvaro Uribe convirtió el manejo de las estadísticas en una de sus herramientas de gobierno. *El Tiempo*. February 11, 2006.

31. Informe Nacional de Desarrollo Humano. Las víctimas: Una Guerra injusta. El conflicto, callejón con salida. 2003. http://www.pnud.org.co/2003/full/capitulo_5.pdf. Accessed July 1, 2007.

32. Fundación País Libre. *Estadisticas del secuestro*. September 2007. http://www.paislibre.org/images/PDF/secuestrogenerales%201996%20-%202007%20 septiembre.pdf. Accessed July 5, 2007.

33. Rey P. La Nación y El Mercurio. *Colombia: La Radio de los Secuestrados*. http://www.lanacion.com.ar/nota.asp?nota_id=995780. Accessed January 29, 2010.

34. Granda R. Entrevistas. Guerilla en Colombia: El fin y los medios. http://www.tinku.org/content/view/2315/88/. Accessed August 2, 2008.

35. Posada MS. El Proceso de Paz del Gobierno Pastrana—El Fracaso y sus consecuencias. *Centro de Análisis Sociopolíticos*. March 10, 2002. http://www.cas.org.co/articulos/articulos/VerArticulo.php?Id=9. Accessed August 18, 2007.

36. Society for Irish Latin American Studies. Explosive Journey: Los tres monos. http://www.irlandeses.org/21stC2.htm. Accessed August 20, 2007.

37. Peters N. CIA Cash Funded Drugs Trade. *Scotland on Sunday*. July 8, 2001.

38. Imponen 20 años a Montesinos por venta de armas a las FARC. *Diario El Comercio* (Perú). September 22, 2006.

39. Various sources cited in: Rudqvist A. ELN and the current peace talk scenario in Colombia. *The Collegium for Development Studies of Uppsala University*. February 2006.

40. Relevo Presidencial en Colombia: Trece muertos y una treintena de heridos ensombrecen la investidura. *El País*. August 8, 2002. http://www.cesarsalgado.net/200208/020808.htm. Accessed August 20, 2007.

41. Youtube.com. Video Ingrid Betancourt Alive December 2007. http://www.youtube.com/watch?v=a2hRQdU98Uk. Accessed January 5, 2008.

42. Isacson A, trans. Excerpts: Letter by Ingrid Betancourt. *Washingtonpost.com*. December 17, 2007. http://www.washingtonpost.com/wp-dyn/content/article/2007/12/17/AR2007121701220.html. Accessed December 20, 2007.

43. Los narcoguerrilleros de las FARC aceptaron que no tienen a Emanuel. Nueva burla al pueblo. *El Caminante*. January 5, 2008. http://argentina.indyme dia.org/news/2008/01/575899.php. Accessed January 20, 2008.

44. Un noruego y cinco colombianos son los seis turistas secuestrados por las Farc en Nuquí (Chocó). *El Tiempo.* January 14, 2008.

45. La Gran Marcha. *Semana.com.* http://www.semana.com/wf_InfoArticulo. aspx?IdArt=109319. Accessed February 22, 2008.

46. Final feliz? *Semana.* March 10, 2008.

47. El computador de Reyes. *Semana.* March 4, 2008.

48. Colombia: The prospects for peace with the ELN. *International Crisis Group; Latin America Report, no. 2.* October 4, 2002.

49. Revela la Fundación PAÍS LIBRE de Colombia: Las Farc secuestraron a 326 personas entre 2000 y 2008. http://www.cope.es/noticia_pdf.php5?not_codigo= 44702. Accessed January 11, 2010.

50. International Crisis Group. Colombia: The prospects for peace with the ELN, 4 October 2002. http://www.reliefweb.int/library/documents/2002/icg-col-4oct.pdf Accessed January 11, 2010.

51. Moor M, Zumpolle L. *The Kidnap Industry in Colombia: Our Business?* p. 26 *in* Pax Christi, Utrecht, The Netherlands, November 2001. http://74.125.93.132/ search?q=cache:TqJHQlCDo3wJ:www.ikvpaxchristi.nl/catalogus/uploaded_file. aspx%3Fid%3D167+www.ikvpaxchristi.nl/catalogus/uploaded_file.aspx%3Fid %3D167&cd=1&hl=en&ct=clnk&client=safari. Accessed January 29, 2010.

52. Radiografía del ELN. *El País.* July 5, 1998.

53. Colombia captures rebel commander opposed to peace talks, army says. *International Herald Tribune.* January 9, 2008.

54. Un Acuerdo Nacional es la salida a la crisis. *Central Command.* April 27, 2008. http://www.eln-voces.com/index2.php?option=com_content&do_pdf=1&id=223 Accessed March 1, 2008.

55. Weiss A. Colombia's paramilitary: Profile of an entrenched terror network. *Znet.* April 22, 2002. http://www.zmag.org/znet/viewArticle/12172. Accessed January 21, 2010.

56. Leech G. Colombie: Cinquante ans de violence. http://www.legrandsoir. info/Colombie-Cinquante-ans-de-violence.html. Accessed March 2, 2008.

57. Ibáñez AM, Moya A. *La población desplazada en Colombia: Examen de sus condiciones socioeconómicas y análisis de las políticas actuales.* Bogotá, Colombia: Departamento Nacional de Planeación; 2007.

58. Comisión Colombiana de Juristas. *Colombia 2002–2006: Situation regarding human rights and humanitarian law.* http://www.coljuristas.org/documentos/doc umentos_pag/situacioningles.pdf. Accessed March 10, 2008.

59. Memorias de un para. *Semana.* March 19–26, 20007.

60. Rohter L. Colombians tell of massacre, as Army stood by. *New York Times.* July 14, 2000.

61. Centro de Investigación y Educacion: Paramilitarismo de Estado en Colombia. http://www.nocheyniebla.org/files/u1/casotipo/deuda/html/pdf/2000.pdf. Accessed March 5, 2008.

62. Amnesty International. Colombia: Scarred bodies, Hidden crimes: Sexual violence against women in the armed conflict—Testimonials. October 14, 2004. http://www.amnesty.org/en/library/info/AMR23/040/2004. Accessed January 11, 2010.

63. El 8000 de los paras: El ventilador. *Semana.* November 27, 2006.

64. Congreso en la picota. *El Tiempo.* April 13, 2008.

65. El cartel de "40." *Semana.* October 23, 2006.

66. Pacto con el Diablo. *Semana.*, January 22, 2007.

67. Amnesty International. 2007 Annual report for Colombia. http://www. amnestyusa.org/annualreport.php?id=ar&yr=2007&c=COL. Accessed March 5, 2008.

68. Laplante L, Theidon K. Transitional justice in times of conflict: Colombia's Ley de Justicia y Paz. *Michigan J Intl Law.* 2004;28:49–107. http://students.law. umich.edu/mjil/article-pdfs/v28n1-laplante-theidon.pdf. Accessed March 5, 2008.

69. Amnesty International. Justice & Peace Law and decree 128. http://www. amnestyusa.org/all-countries/colombia/justice-and-peace-law-and-decree-128/ page.do?id=1101862. Accessed January 11, 2010.

70. Logan S, Shoemaker M. Colombia's AUC: From irregular army to mafia. ISN Security Watch, Bogotá. April 9, 2005. http://www.isn.ethz.ch/isn/Current-Affairs/Security-Watch/Detail/?id=107221&lng=en. Accessed March 5, 2008.

CHAPTERS 8

1. Faguet JP. *Building democracy on quicksand: Altruism, Empire, and the United States. Challenge.* May/June 2004;47(3):73–93.

2. Central Intelligence Agency. The CIA World Factbook: Afghanistan. May 15, 2008. https://www.cia.gov/library/publications/the-world-factbook/geos/af. html. Accessed March 6, 2008.

3. Rainwater J. Afghanistan: Terrorism and Blowback: A Chronology. http:// www.janrainwater.com/htdocs/afghan2p1.htm. Accessed March 3, 2008).

4. Nyrop RF, Seekins DM, eds. *Afghanistan: A Country Study. Foreign Area Studies.* Washington DC: The American University; 1986.

5. Cooley JK. *Unholy Wars: Afghanistan, America, and International Terrorism.* London: Pluto Press; 2002.

6. Fry MJ. *The Afghan Economy.* Leiden, Netherlands: E.J. Brill; 1974:4.

7. Galster S. Afghanistan: The Making of U.S. Policy, 1973–1990. October 9, 2001 http://www.gwu.edu/~nsarchiv/NSAEBB/NSAEBB57/essay.html. Accessed January 11, 2010

8. Savranskaya S. 1. The Soviet Experience in Afghanistan: Russian Documents and Memoirs. In John Prados and Svetlana Savranskaya (eds), Vol II: *Afghanistan: Lessons from the Last War*, October 9, 2001. http://www.gwu.edu/~nsarchiv/ NSAEBB/NSAEBB57/index.html. Accessed January 29, 2010.

9. Lyakhovsky A. *The Tragedy and Valor of Afghan.* Moscow: Iskon; 1995. http:// www.gwu.edu/~nsarchiv/NSAEBB/NSAEBB57/soviet.html (document 8). Accessed March 8, 2008.

10. Gates R. *From the Shadows: The Ultimate Insider's Story of Five Presidents and How They Won the Cold War.* New York: Simon & Schuster; 1997.

11. Interview with Vincent Javert. *Le Nouvel Observateur* (Paris). January 15–21, 1998:76 (translated from the French by William Blum).

12. The American Presidency Project. Reagan R. Proclamation 5033—Afghanistan Day, 1983, March 21, 1983. http://www.presidency.ucsb.edu/ws/index. php?pid=41077. Accessed March 10, 2008.

13. The American Presidency Project. Message on the Observance of Afghanistan Day, March 21, 1983. http://www.presidency.ucsb.edu/ws/index.php?pid=41078. Accessed March 10, 2008.

14. Moran M. Bin Laden comes home to roost. *MSNBC*. August 24, 1998.

15. US next superpower foe for Terrorist Leader. *Associated Press*. August 23, 1998.

16. Chernyaev A. *My Six Years with Gorbachev*. English R, Tucker E, trans. University Park, PA: Penn State University Press; 42. http://www.gwu.edu/%7Ensarchiv/NSAEBB/NSAEBB57/soviet.html. Accessed March 10, 2008.

17. Bradsher H. *Afghan Communism and Soviet Interventions*. Oxford: Oxford University Press; 1999:185.

18. Leupp G. *Meet Mr. Blowback: Gulbuddin Hekmatyar, CIA Op and Homicidal Thug*. *CounterPunch*. February 2003. http://www.counterpunch.org/leupp02142003.html. Accessed December 23, 2009.

19. Seumas Milne. They can't see why they are hated: Americans cannot ignore what their government does abroad. *The Guardian*. September 13, 2001. http://www.guardian.co.uk/politics/2001/sep/13/september11.britainand911. Accessed March 12, 2008.

20. Rawa. Treatment of women in Taliban [film]. http://en.wikipedia.org/wiki/Taliban. Accessed March 12, 2008.

21. Masjid Al-Muslimiin. *The Islamic Dress Code*. Islamic Center of Columbia, SC. http://www.iopal.net/forum/archive/index.php/t-2060.html. Accessed March 12, 2008.

22. Harrison F. Crackdown in Iran over dress code, 27 April, 2007. http://news.bbc.co.uk/2/hi/6596933.stm. Accessed March 14, 2008.

23. Human Rights Watch Report: *Afghanistan, the massacre in Mazar-e-Sharif*. November 1, 1998. Incitement of violence against Hazaras by Governor Niazi. http://www.hrw.org/en/reports/1998/11/01/afghanistan-massacre-mazar-i-sharif. Accessed March 15, 2008.

24. How the Taliban slaughtered thousands of people. *The Sunday Times*. November 1, 1998.

25. UN report details Taliban "killing frenzy." *The News International*. November 6, 1998.

26. Amnesty International. Afghanistan: Thousands of civilians killed following Taleban takeover of Maxar-e Sharif. September 3, 1998.

27. Human Rights Watch Report. *Massacres of Hazaras in Afghanistan*. February 2001;13(1(C)). http://www.hrw.org/reports/2001/afghanistan/. Accessed March 17, 2008.

28. CNN.com. Transcript of President Bush's address. September 21, 2001. http://archives.cnn.com/2001/US/09/20/gen.bush.transcript/. Accessed March 20, 2008.

29. Bin-Laden video. *Falschuberstzung als Beweismittel?* WDR, Das Erste, Monitor Nr. 485 am December 20, 2001.

30. Federal Bureau of Investigation. The FBI's Ten Most Wanted Fugitives. http://www.fbi.gov/wanted/topten/fugitives/fugitives.htm. Accessed March 20, 2008.

31. Federal Bureau of Investigation. Bin Laden not wanted for 9/11? *MG The Milli Gazette*. June 11, 2006. http://www.milligazette.com/dailyupdate/2006/20060612_bin_laden_911_fbi.htm. Accessed March 21, 2008.

32. Rashid A. *Taliban: Militant Islam, Oil and Fundamentalism in Central Asia*. New Haven, CT: Yale University Press; 2000.

33. The five dancing Israelis arrested on 9/11. http://www.whatreallyhap pened.com/fiveisraelis.html. Accessed March 21, 2008.

34. Goodhand J. Frontiers and wars: The opium economy in Afghanistan. *J Agrarian Change.* 2005;5(2):191–216. http://www.gtz.de/de/dokumente/en-opi um-economy-2005-afg.pdf. Accessed October 25, 2009.

35. United Nations Office on Drugs and Crime. Afghanistan: Opium Survey 2007. October 2007.

36. Kamminga J, van Ham P. How to beat the opium economy. *International Herald Tribune.* November 30, 2006.

37. Mili H, Townsend J. Afghanistan's drug trade and how it funds Taliban operations. *Terrorism Monitor, The Jamestown Foundation.* May 10, 2007;5(9).

38. Starkey J. Drugs for guns: How the Afghan heroin trade is fuelling the Taliban insurgency. *The Independent.* April 29, 2008. http://www.independent.co.uk/ news/world/asia/drugs-for-guns-how-the-afghan-heroin-trade-is-fuelling-the-taliban-insurgency-817230.html. Accessed March 22, 2008.

39. Shaw M. Drug trafficking and development of organized crime in post-Taliban Afghanistan *in* Afghanistan: Drug Industry and Counter-Narcotics policy. *World Bank Afghanistan Opium Report.* November 28, 2006.

40. Ahmed Wali Karzai. *The New York Times.* October 29, 2009. http://topics.ny times.com/topics/reference/timestopics/people/k/ahmed_wali_karzai/index. html. Accessed October 30, 2009.

41. Loyn D. Why the Afghan Taleban feel confident. *BBC News.* February 1, 2008. http://news.bbc.co.uk/2/hi/south_asia/7222194.stm. Accessed March 23, 2008.

42. Pentagon Report on Afghanistan Criticizes War Strategy: Report. *Agence France Presse.* April 5, 2004.

43. Observatorio de Minas Antipersonal, Observatorio de Derechos Humanos. http://indh.pnud.org.co/files/boletin_hechos/fin_opt.pdf. Accessed October 25, 2009.

CHAPTER 9

1. Chacksfield AJ. Ethical Frames for Drug Policy and the Salience of Competing Bodies of Knowledge. *Paper presented at the annual meeting of The Midwest Political Science Association,* Chicago, IL, April 2004. http://www.allacademic.com/ meta/p83837_index.html. Accessed April 15, 2008.

2. Supporters of Drug Policy Reform Should Be Considered for RICO Prosecutions; Compared to Pedophiles and Rapists at House Hearing. http://www.ndsn. org/summer99/capitol1.html. Accessed January 11, 2010.

3. Caulkins JP, Reuter P, Iguhi MY, et al. *How Goes the "War on Drugs"? An Assessment of U.S. Drug Problems and Policy.* Los Angeles: The RAND Corporation; 2005.

4. *Poppy for Medicine. Licensing poppy for the production of essential medicines: an integrated counter-narcotics, development, and counter-insurgency model for Afghanistan.* London: The Senlis Council; 2007.

5. Bhattacharji R. *India's experiences in licensing poppy cultivation for the production of essential medicines. Lessons for Afghanistan.* London: The Senlis Council;

2007. http://www.poppyformedicine.net/documents/india_case_study. Accessed April 20, 2008.

6. Kamminga J. *The Political History of Turkey's Opium Licensing System for the Production of Medicines: Lessons for Afghanistan.* London: The Senlis Council; 2006. http://www.poppyformedicine.net/documents/Political_History_Poppy_Li censing_Turkey_May_2006. Accessed April 20, 2008.

7. *Poppy for Medicine: Part B: Afghan-made medicines to meet the global need for painkillers.* London: The Senlis Council; 2007. http://www.icosgroup.net/docu ments/poppy_medicine_technical_dossier.pdf. Accessed April 21, 2008.

8. U.S. Opposes Efforts to Legalize Opium in Afghanistan. http://kabul.usem bassy.gov/uploads/images/SyEqN3nIAYh1yFpxMBvfTA/fact_sheet_070307. pdf. Accessed January 29, 2010.

9. Chouvy P-A. Licensing Afghanistan's opium: Solution or fallacy? *Caucasian Review of International Affairs.* Spring 2008;2(2).

10. Cato Institute. Law and Civil Liberties: Drug War. http://www.cato.org/ subtopic_display_new.php?topic_id=10&ra_id=9. Accessed April 25, 2008).

11. Ostrowski J. *Thinking About Drug Legalization.* Cato Policy Analysis, No. 121. Washington DC: The Cato Institute; 1989.

12. Carpenter TG. The US Campaign Against International Narcotics Trafficking: A Cure Worse Than the Disease. Washington DC: The Cato Institute; 1985.

13. Boaz D, Lynch T. Bad neighbor policy: Washington's futile War on Drugs in Latin America. In: *Cato Handbook for Congress.* 6th Edition. Washington DC: The Cato Institute; 2005. http://www.cato.org/subtopic_display_new.php?topic_id=10& ra_id=9. Accessed April 25, 2008.

14. Wisotsky S. A Society of Suspects: The War on Drugs and Civil Liberties. Cato Policy Analysis, No. 180. Washington DC: The Cato Institute; 1992. http:// www.cato.org/subtopic_display_new.php?topic_id=10&ra_id=9. Accessed April 26, 2008.

15. Brumm HJ, Cloninger DO. The Drug War and the homicide rate: A direct correlation? *Cato Journal.* Winter 1995;14(3). http://www.cato.org/pubs/journal/ cj14n3/cj14n3-8.pdf. Accessed April 27, 2008.

16. Pilon R. The illegitimate war on drugs. In: *After Prohibition: An Adult Approach to Drug Policies in the 21st Century.* Washington DC: The Cato Institute; 2000. http://www.cato.org/pubs/books/after-pro-chpt3.pdf. Accessed April 28, 2008.

17. Boaz D, Lynch T. The war on drugs. In: *Cato Handbook for Congress.* 6th ed. Washington DC: The Cato Institute; 2005.

CHAPTER 10

1. 2007 Annual Report: The State of the Drug Problem in Europe. European Monitoring Center for Drugs and Drug Addiction, Lisbon, November 2007. http:// www.emcdda.europa.eu/publications/annual-report/2007. Accessed January 2010.

2. Hall W. Creating space for a more reasoned debate about drug policy. *Policy Options.* October 1998.

3. Davis G. *America Lynchings: A documentary feature.* http://www.american lynching.com/main.html. Accessed April 30, 2008.

Index

Addiction, 7, 17–21, 24, 27, 30, 35, 40–45, 48, 50, 52–55, 66, 69–82, 87, 88, 90, 96, 100–102, 106–9, 111, 112, 114, 117, 118, 124, 125, 189, 192, 196, 197, 202, 204; genetic(s), 72, 73, 75–77, 79–82, 202; marshmallow test, 79; physical dependence, 86, 90, 108, 109, 111, 117; reward circuitry, 73–74; self-control, 78–80, 82, 202; theories, 69–82; tolerance, 56, 57, 62, 70, 71, 74, 90, 109, 114–17, 176

Afghanistan, 26, 49, 127, 128, 165–84, 190–94, 198, 203; Anglo-Afghan wars, 166–67; Durand Line, 167–68; early days, 166–67; Gandamak treaty, 167; Hekmatyar, Gulbuddin, 168, 171, 173–74; human rights violations, 173, 176, 183; Karmal, Babrak, 169–70, 172; bin Laden, Osama, 166, 171–72, 177, 178, 182; massacres, 176; Mujahideen, 64, 165, 168, 170–74, 176, 179, 183; Northern Alliance, 173–74, 177; Omar, Mullah Muhammad, 175–77, 179; Operation Cyclone, 171;

Operation Enduring Freedom, 181; opium under the Taliban, 179–82; Pashtun, 166–68, 174, 176; People's Democratic Party of Afghanistan, 168; rise and fall of, 174–78; Taliban, 26, 165, 166, 171, 173–82, 184, 191, 194. *See also* Brzezinski, Zbigniew; Soviet-Afghan war

Al-Birûnî, 19

Alcohol, 3–12, 23, 25, 27, 30, 35, 37, 38, 40, 46, 53, 55, 56, 63, 64, 66, 71, 72, 77, 78, 80, 81, 84, 90, 123, 194–98, 201–4

Alexander the Great, 20

Al-Tabari, 18

AMA. *See* American Medical Association

American Medical Association (AMA), 40, 42, 44, 84, 85, 101, 106

American Society of Addiction Medicine (ASAM), 110

Amphetamines, 25, 35

Anslinger, Harry J. *See* Prohibition

Arabia/Muslims, 18–20, 169, 171, 173–76, 178; Al-Birûnî, 19; Ali Ibn

About the Author

DR. FAGUET is a retired clinician and researcher who was funded by the National Cancer Institute and the Department of Veterans Affairs. He was a member of numerous professional organizations and a reviewer for federal and private granting agencies and for prestigious medical journals. He published many peer-reviewed articles, several book chapters, and three previous books, including the acclaimed *War on Cancer: An Anatomy of Failure; A Blueprint for the Future*. As a pain expert, he witnessed the enormous contribution of narcotics to pain management despite the general albeit erroneous perception of their lurking dangers and the increasing interference of drug policy on medical practice. His professional experience and his insightful knowledge of the devastating affect of the drug trade on Colombian society, producer of 80% of worldwide cocaine, complemented by an exhaustive literature search, are the bases of his reflections and recommendations.